T0289768

Traditional Chinese Medicine in the Treatment of Post-COVID-19 Syndrome

中医诊治新冠长期病症

Traditional Chinese Medicine in the Treatment of Post-COVID-19 Syndrome

中医诊治新冠长期病症

Dan Jiang
Hallam Institute of TCM, UK

Fanyi Meng
Lincoln College, UK

Kerry Webster
Cinnabar Therapies, UK

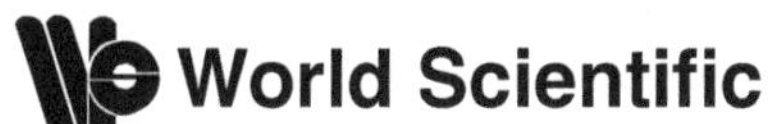

NEW JERSEY • LONDON • SINGAPORE • BEIJING • SHANGHAI • HONG KONG • TAIPEI • CHENNAI • TOKYO

Published by

World Scientific Publishing Europe Ltd.
57 Shelton Street, Covent Garden, London WC2H 9HE
Head office: 5 Toh Tuck Link, Singapore 596224
USA office: 27 Warren Street, Suite 401-402, Hackensack, NJ 07601

Library of Congress Cataloging-in-Publication Data
Names: Jiang, Dan, 1952– author. | Meng, Fanyi (Of University of Lincoln) author. | Webster, Kerry, author.
Title: 880-01 Traditional Chinese medicine in the treatment of post-COVID-19 syndrome = Zhong yi zhen zhi xin guan chang qi bing zheng / Dan Jiang, Fanyi Meng, Kerry Webster.
Other titles: 880-02 Zhong yi zhen zhi xin guan chang qi bing zheng
Description: New Jersey : World Scientific, [2023] | Includes bibliographical references and index.
Identifiers: LCCN 2022041066 | ISBN 9781800613485 (hardcover) | ISBN 9781800613492 (ebook for institutions) | ISBN 9781800613508 (ebook for individuals)
Subjects: MESH: COVID-19--complications | Medicine, Chinese Traditional--methods | Phytotherapy--methods | Drugs, Chinese Herbal--administration & dosage | Acupuncture Therapy | Case Reports
Classification: LCC RA644.C67 | NLM WC 506.5 | DDC 616.2/4144--dc23/eng/20221109
LC record available at https://lccn.loc.gov/2022041066

British Library Cataloguing-in-Publication Data
A catalogue record for this book is available from the British Library.

For any available supplementary material, please visit
https://www.worldscientific.com/worldscibooks/10.1142/Q0398#t=suppl

Desk Editors: Nimal Koliyat/Adam Binnie/Shi Ying Koe

Typeset by Stallion Press
Email: enquiries@stallionpress.com

Preface

In 2019, when one of the authors joined a group meeting of experts in TCM to plan and prioritise the publishing of a series of TCM textbooks, the book on Warm Diseases — the one dealing with pandemics — was put on the back burner and it was decided that it will be the last book published as it had only historic value. The reason was simple — pandemics were no longer a major threat to human health. It was an obvious consensus because after the Second World War, we had successfully tamed most infectious diseases and non-infectious diseases were the most important topics and at the top of the public health and medical practice agenda. This was true in Chinese medicine practice all over the world as well.

It was a big surprise that a new virus can cause a dramatic change to human life and medical focus in such a short time. The emergence of COVID-19 has moved the whole world into a new era and everything changed, including TCM practice. Over time, the catastrophe worldwide has been gradually controlled with great effort in terms of prevention and restriction of contact. The waves of infections have abated. Although the threat of death is not imminent, the damage to our body, our psyche, and our society will linger on for many years and cast a shadow on the rest of the life of many.

Since spring 2020, many COVID-19 survivors have been expressing their agony and struggling to return to normal life due to long-lasting mental and physical weakness. The challenge is great and they did not find pre-made answers and available medications for their suffering. Meanwhile, the medical precession and resources have been drawn into the acute cases and therefore do not have enough resources to spare to tend to the survivors. With such a desperate need for solutions to the post-COVID-19 situation, many of the survivors turned to TCM for help, and the outcomes are considered to be the right ones for most people in search of answers.

The authors have been standing alongside the patients since the pandemic started and have treated many cases within such contexts by applying ancient wisdom recorded during the past pandemic periods, with full knowledge that this situation could become a world-wide problem later and affect a bigger population from ancient observations. The authors' early practice was directed by their experience and knowledge, without guideline from authority. But their efforts seemed to be on the right track and many patients got satisfactory outcomes and could return to their normal life. Eventually, the conditions were recognised by the WHO and many other countries. Many cases treated by the authors turned out to be post-COVID-19 syndrome (PCS) on hindsight. Since the guidelines became available, there have been more patients with PCS in mind, and the authors have made a good effort in dealing with their issues with much attention being paid to such presentation in clinic observations in the hope of formulating some approaches for better understanding and treatment.

The diagnosis methods and treatment ideologies constitute a whole-system approach of TCM, meaning that acupuncture, Chinese herbal medicines, manual therapy, Qigong/Taiji, and lifestyle adjustments are used in combination specific to reach individual to help them make a complete recovery. The use of acupuncture was limited until after the summer of 2020 due to its physical contact nature. Then, it soon became the most demanded treatment for the COVID-19 "hangover" and provided a great level of immediate relief from pain/aches and many other symptoms. Chinese herbal medicine (CHM) was the main treatment from ancient documents and would provide an internal route to boost the Qi and blood production and establish the body's defence function. The therapeutic effects delivered from the meridian/channel (on surface of the body) and from the inner mechanism (herbs and Qigong from inner world of the body) are combined in a synchronised action, which is the whole-system TCM approach. This is the main experience of the authors and has been tested and proved to be the best available in terms of TCM approach.

Jiang, a popular online practitioner, local to Sheffield, has accumulated more than 200 cases at the time of first draft of this book with full records of clinical information and treatment. She has summarised all her experience of the post-COVID-19 syndrome and presented her findings in several academic seminars on individual topics within PCS, which have been condensed into the body of this book.

Meng, practising at Lincoln College teaching clinic and also helping his mentees in various clinical encounters, has accumulated many cases in cardiological impairment, loss of smell, and restricted respiratory conditions, with most cases treated by acupuncture and dozens with CHM, which have been drafted into the introductory parts.

Webster has been continuously practising since the summer of 2020 when a lot of her existing patients complained about long-lasting problems after the initial COVID-19 infection. Her experience is also positive and valuable. She has been the main editor of the drafts.

All the authors believe that the pandemic will move to a stage of regular onset, but its devastating effect will remain for those who are vulnerable. However, evidence revealed by new research suggests that after the infection, even without symptoms in the acute stage, people have continued to suffer from brain damage, lung impairment, and the contrary immune system behaviour. The change did not simply go away as time passed in a large proportion of people. They need decent treatment and care.

The medical field and healthcare practice have been fundamentally changed due to the COVID-19 pandemic. The authors would also like to elaborate on the changes in some practices in a separate publishing. The observed clinical experiences of the authors will be a positive contribution to all practitioners of complementary medicine and also to those who find themselves in poor health due to COVID-19.

Our practice experience and observations are mainly from our own independent small clinical setting (no more than 5 treatment rooms, with fewer than 20 regular treatment sessions per day) which might not suit practice in other circumstances. For example, the legal requirements might be different in other European countries compared to the UK where the authors are practising. We welcome all criticisms and contributions on our limited findings.

About the Authors

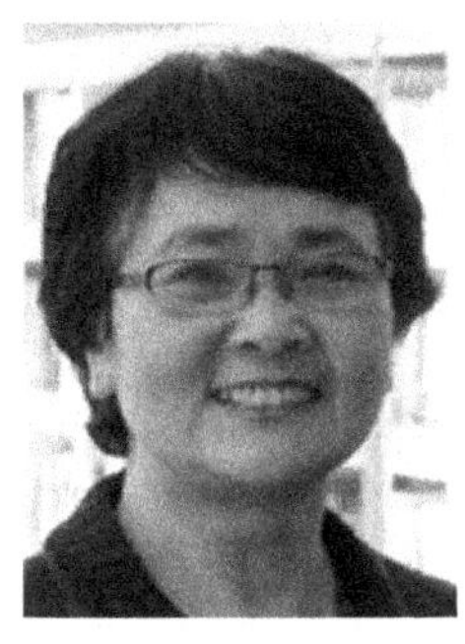

Dan Jiang is a TCM consultant (awarded by WFCMS), Fellow of the British Acupuncture Council, and Fellow and Mentor at Association of Traditional Chinese Medicine (ATCM). She graduated from Beijing University of Chinese Medicine in 1978 and continued her post-graduate studies, receiving her Medical Masters Degree in 1987. She has been practising acupuncture and TCM since 1991 in Sheffield and Harley Street, London, UK. She is a Visiting Professor and Special Appointed TCM Consultant in Beijing University of TCM; Vice-Principal of Pan European Federation of TCM Consultants; Editor-in-Chief for the book of *Principle & Practice TCM in the West*; Co-author of *Neurobiology of Chinese Herbal Medicine*, and Author of more than 50 professional papers published in international journals of medicine and sciences.

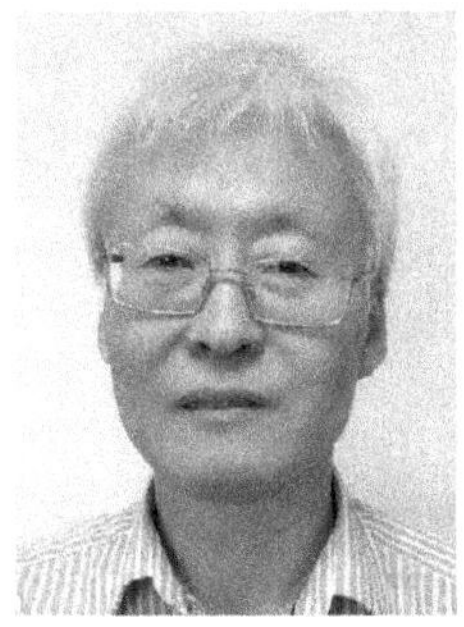

Fanyi Meng graduated from Beijing University of Chinese Medicine in 1983 and became a senior academic in the TCM diagnostic department of the university. He has 40 years of clinical experience and 30 years as a teacher/researcher in China and the UK. He was the programme leader of BSc (Hons) Complementary Medicine at the University of Lincoln. Fanyi's clinical speciality is infertility and cancer support management. His research focused on acupuncture treatment of the above conditions. He has published more than 40 papers in peer-reviewed journals, 8 book chapters, and 4 books on the theory and practice of Chinese medicine. He has treated more than 40 patients affected by COVID-19 with acupuncture and Chinese herbs, now categorised as post-COVID-19 syndrome, and achieved satisfactory results. His approach is whole-system TCM management which is presented in this book.

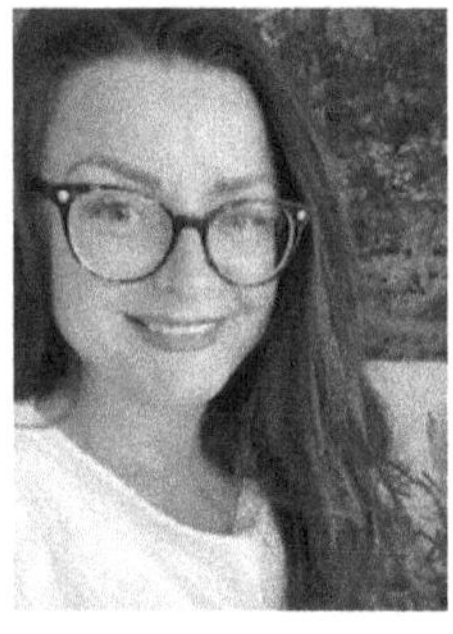

Kerry Webster started her Chinese Medicine education in 2018, at Lincoln College, where she studied BSc (Hons) Acupuncture, completing her degree in 2021 with a First-Class Honours. She continued her education in 2021 with a post-graduate Herbal Medicine Diploma with the Phoenix Academy of Acupuncture & Herbal Medicine. Kerry began her education in health and well-being at the Grimsby Institute of Further and Higher Education in 2000, studying Sports Therapy and Exercise. In 2015, her interest in body work led her to study in Brighton with Jing Advanced Massage Training, completing with a foundation in Advanced Clinical Massage. She also studied Nuad Bo Rarn with the Sussex Thai Massage School. Deepening her knowledge of movement, she completed a 10-month series on Myofascial Anatomy and Movement education in Leeds with Natural Bodies from 2017 to 2018.

Contents

Introduction

In November 2019, a new infectious disease was reported in China which was later identified to be caused by a novel coronavirus, SARS-CoV-2. The clinical condition was formally named by the World Health Organization as COVID-19, an infectious disease that mainly affects the respiratory system. The disease spread across the entire world in 2020 and caused a new global pandemic. As the disease evolved into new varieties, its clinical feature changed from pneumonia and acute respiratory distress syndrome in the early reports to broad damage in the respiratory and other systems. The pandemic developed at an unprecedented scale, infecting 370 million people and causing the death of more than 5 million people as of the drafting of this work. It is the most devastating new global disease in the past 50 years, worse than AIDS, and is the first priority of the public health sector in most countries worldwide, also an important topic in social and political life.

In the middle of 2020, survivors of the acute stage of COVID-19 realised that their nightmare was not over yet as many of them struggled to return to normal life. At that point, the long-term damage of COVID-19 emerged, and it was realised that post-COVID-19 suffering needs to be recognised and managed in an effective way. The survivors found that their temperature was normal, the test of the antigen was negative, and they were no longer labelled as COVID-19 patients, but they struggled to supply air and breathe when they performed physical work. Others were in poor health, suffering from severe fatigue and a lack of mental capacity to carry out daily duties and work. They no longer have the disease, nevertheless they are still ill and, most importantly, the medical community could not accommodate their clinical suffering into a proper diagnosis, not to mention a treatment. Facing such a challenge, clinical interest groups, formed mainly by those medical and healthcare professionals who suffered from COVID-19 (Assaf *et al.*, 2020), started the discussion on the post-infectious suffering and proposed the terms of long COVID and post-COVID-19 syndrome (PCS) in the hope of raising the awareness of public health authorities, for better understanding of the nature through proper research investment and eventually better management of the illness (Calland and Perego, 2021).

The pandemic did not vanish as many wished; it waxes and wanes and cunningly evolves from alpha to omicron, and so on. A considerable proportion of the population has now experienced COVID-19. Taking the UK as an example, in the last week of March 2022, 21 million people had tested positive thus far (*BBC*, 2022) among a national population of 67 million, which is 31% (21/67) of the total number. A continuous increase of COVID-19 cases, and therefore a corresponding mounting numbers of survivors after the acute infection, is expected. The survivors who still suffer from the damage left by COVID-19 are officially counted in the millions. The vast number of sufferers and their healthcare demands could no longer be neglected and many research projects were then commissioned focusing on the scale of the damage left by acute COVID-19, the spectrum of the symptoms, the mechanism of multi-organ/system damage, and a way in which to effectively manage such conditions. As clinical and laboratory research reports accumulated enough data for further analysis, health authorities could now evaluate the evidence and make guidelines and recommendations for the management of post-COVID-19 conditions.

According to research based on the UK Primary Care electronic record covering 95% of England's population (Walker *et al.*, 2021), among all patients who reported illness after COVID-19, 64% of them were eventually diagnosed as PCS and 17% were further referred by their GPs to post-COVID Assessment Clinics, which were set up after the government initiatives to address problems in the secondary care system as the treatments provided by GPs were not satisfactory. Less than 3% were cleared of illness at the end of the research.

Up to the point of drafting the manuscript, there are two guidelines available, one from the UK's health and clinical guidance centre, the NICE, and the other from the World Health Organization (WHO). The two institutions hold a similar opinion on the definition of ill health. However, the UK NICE guideline is more comprehensive and inclusive, and more suitable for clinicians.

From all available evidence, it is obvious that the early and original SARS-CoV-2 was more devastating than the recent Delta and Omicron variations, and the infection was more likely to lead to hospitalisation and severe cases. As a result, more people who survived the early episode of the pandemic would be left with a poorer health profile, with a significant percentage of them dying within one year. The new variations, on the other hand, cause a relatively small percentage of sufferers to suffer from severe conditions, and the aftermath has therefore been more optimistic in the recent months.

The main reason to raise the awareness for utilising Traditional Chinese Medicine (TCM) is that the treatment and care of the post-COVID-19 conditions are not ideal with mainstream medical solutions. As lessons learnt from the management of borderline conditions such as ME and fibromyalgia have shown, the disease-centred model of the medical practice is struggling and the holistic medical/healthcare model is providing an alternative solution. This experience is now easily extended to the new situation. Moreover, the authors' personal clinical observations have added weight supporting the clinical effectiveness of TCM treatment of PCS, in the absence of large-scale RCT.

TCM is a holistic medical system whose clinical judgement is made by looking not only into clinical manifestations presented currently but also the patient's overall health status in the four dimensions of the social and physical environment the person lives in, seasonal change associated to the ill health, the development route and interventions the patient received, and the response to the intervention/treatment. Hence, treatment would not be possible without the information of the development of the post-COVID-19 conditions from the beginning.

Regarding the route of development of the post-COVID-19 conditions, some key concepts are essential for clear understanding and transferable communication in this book. Those key concepts are acute COVID-19, post-COVID-19 syndrome, and long COVID.

Key Clinical Terms

Acute COVID-19

Clinical manifestations are positive test, inflammation in lung as pneumonia, difficulty in breathing, elevated temperature, general aching, loss of smell, etc. However, after two years of evolution, the new variants show a hugely different picture in clinical manifestations. A substantial portion of people who tested positive show no symptoms, known as asymptomatic, although they are infected patients. The displayed symptoms are like those of cold or flu.

Long COVID-19

Clinical manifestations are continuing of acute conditions lasting more than 4 weeks, remaining in the need of medical care, and lower blood oxygen level, with many presenting a negative test. In USA, this term is broadly used to cover any long suffering after acute COVID-19 episode. PCS was not introduced to their medical system yet.

Post-COVID-19 Syndrome (PCS)

Clinical manifestations are varies symptoms focusing on exhaustion and brain fog, after 12 weeks, testing negative, with no severe clinical indication to be hospitalised, no need for constant oxygen inhalation, but in very poor health and unable to return to the previous level of work output. These are the key factors in UK NICE guidelines (2022). Furthermore, the WHO holds a similar opinion, as it defines the time length of 3 months.

The study of the trajectory of the COVID-19 symptom recovery validates the necessity of early assessment and intervention. It has only been two years since the start of the COVID-19 pandemic and the post-COVID-19 conditions are constantly being reviewed and more information has been made available on how the symptoms have recovered. In the last few months, it has become clear that a majority of the COVID-19 sufferers will not continue into a post-infection condition or chronic condition, and only a small proportion of patients have persisting symptoms, leading to the post-COVID-19 stage and necessitating medical treatment and good healthcare.

From experience of other infectious diseases, it is easy to use reasoning methods to conclude that the remaining symptoms will go away as times goes on, and that people do not need treatment. However, in the case of PCS, evidence suggests that the effect of "time" might not be as powerful as many had thought. The statistical figures of how the conditions have improved in the natural recovery course suggest that natural recovery over time is not optimistic. It follows different patterns, and the dropping curve might not happen if there are more than 12 symptoms reported in the early stage. This was not recorded in the case of influenzas or similar infections before. The reality is that more than 20% (Mayer *et al.*, 2020) to 29% (Davis *et al.*, 2021) of all patients will not recover at all, and will develop PCS (although the diagnosis standards are different from the newly established WHO guideline). Three symptoms dominate the list of symptoms, explicitly, fatigue (87%), brain fog (85%), and breathlessness (71%). The three symptoms lead to serious impairment in physical and mental capacity, particularly in the workplace, leading to absence from work. According to official figures reported by the British authority ONS, 1.3 million people reported symptoms 4 weeks after catching COVID-19, while 892,000 (70%) are still suffering problems after 12 weeks, which is PCS. Some of them are presenting worse, with 506,000 (40%) having the condition for more than a year. According to these figures, if the patients experience symptoms for more than 4 weeks, 70% of them will eventually develop PCS. Significantly, the current

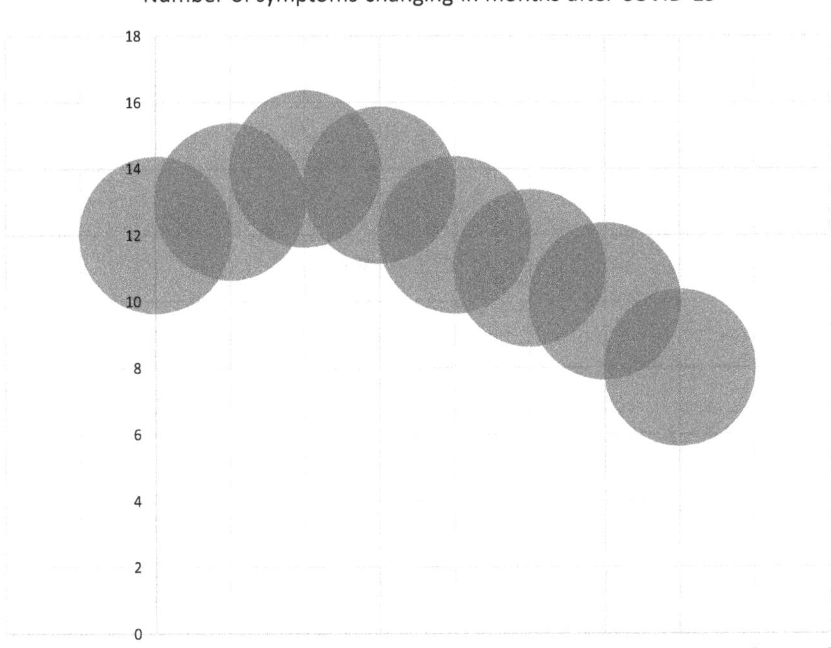

Figure 1. The recovery trend of COVID-19 survivors (Davis *et al.*, 2021).

treatment/care approaches do not appear ideal, coupled with 40% of people not having recovered even after a year (ONS, 2022). The figure might be higher than the worldwide average, because the reality in many other countries could be remarkably similar if free testing is provided to the entire population.

Figure 1 taken from Davis *et al.* (2021) shows the recovery curve in 7 months after the onset and the number of symptoms related to the recovery pattern. When patients reported less than 12 symptoms of PCS, they will be highly likely to make a full recovery in 7 months, while those reporting more than 12 symptoms tend to not recover with symptoms lasting 7 months or more. At the point of 7 months, they will have even more symptoms, with an average reporting of 14 symptoms.

The data were extracted from Davis *et al.* (2021) as percentages of patients experiencing the symptoms at the beginning and at the 79-day point (Table 1).

From the recovery curve, more than half the patients showing symptoms in the 4th week will continue into the 12th week without natural recovery. Furthermore, after 12 weeks, the conditions will remain with no improvement. If the study continued into 18 months, it is predicted that more than half of the sufferers will not recover to the level before the infection.

This is unambiguous evidence that PCS needs to be diagnosed and treated, highlighting that simply resting and maintaining diligent care might never be enough for most patients.

Table 2 shows the broad spectrum of distributions of the symptoms. According to the broad spectrum of damage after acute COVID-19, more

Table 1. Prevalence of symptoms of PCS.

	Beginning of COVID-19	79 days after
Fatigue	95	87
Breathlessness	90	71
Chest tightness	75	44
Cough	68	29
Muscle pain	65	36
Palpitation	55	32
Brain fog	n/a*	85

Note: *Confusion and brain fog are mostly reported in week 3–6, lasting into week 12. Could not trace from the beginning.

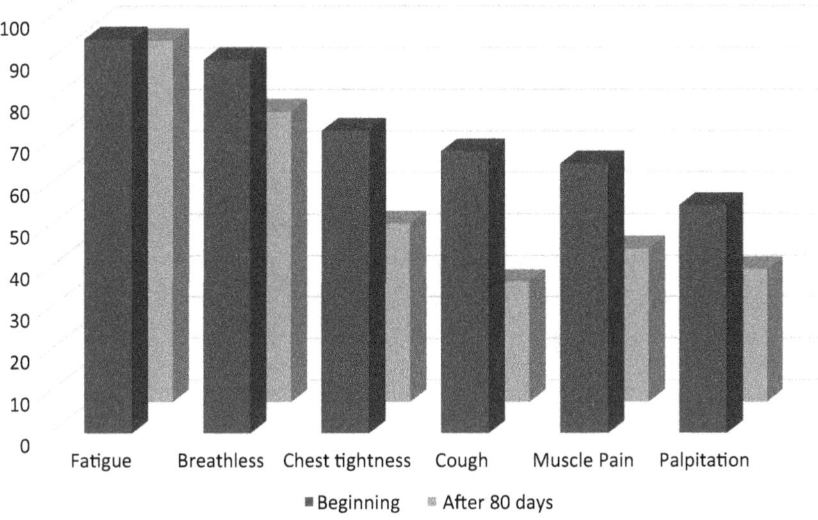

Figure 2. The decline of key symptoms of PCS after 80 days.

than 50 symptoms have been recognised within several systems of the body. Some symptoms are abating with the "time" effect more easily than others, for example, cough and muscular pain can do well with natural recovery. While the two main symptoms, the fatigue and breathless are stubborn as Figure 2 demonstrated. They eventually become the main complaints of COVID survivors.

Clinical Symptoms and Characteristics — Statistic View of PCS

The data in columns 2 and 3 of Table 3 have been extracted from the NICE report (2022, pp. 13–16), and the data in column 4 have been produced from various sources.

From available research reports, it seems that the severity of acute COVID-19 is not linked to PCS occurrence. Many asymptotic patients have also developed PCS. But, some do suggest that hospitalisation and ICU experience are linked to a significantly higher risk of developing new and serious illness and a higher chance of being readmitted to the hospital. The reason might be a fundamental personal condition before the COVID-19 infection.

Table 2. Distribution of PCS symptoms.

General health	Respiratory	Cardiovascular	Neurological	Digestive	Skin	Psychological	Others
Fatigue	Breathlessness	Palpitation	Brain fog*	Nausea	Hair loss	Anxiety	Hearing loss
General aching	Cough	Chest pain	Sleeping problems	Poor appetite	Rashes	PTSD	Tinnitus
Lower fever	Sore throat	Chest tightness	Pins and needles numbness	Diarrhoea		Depression	Vision change
				Indigestion			Allergy
			Tastelessness				Menstruation cycle change** (CDC, 2022)
			Dizziness				

Notes: *Brain fog is a summative term of a range of malfunctions including cognitive impairments, poor concentration, poor memory, poor mathematical ability, lack of spirit, and slow reactions (NICE, 2022). **Menstruation cycle changes are included in the CDC's list (CDC, 2022), not in the NICE report.

Table 3. The frequency of common PCS symptoms.

Symptom	Average prevalence (%)	Range of prevalence in different reports (%)	Prevalence in general population (%)	Increase compared to non-COVID situations (%)
Dyspnoea (breathing difficulty) (4–12 weeks after COVID diagnosis) (Francesca *et al.*, 2021)	38	27–51		
Dyspnoea (12 weeks after diagnosis)	22	12–35	9–13 [11]	8
Cough (Michelen *et al.*, 2020)	28	22–35	10 [12]	18
Sleeping problem (Francesca *et al.*, 2021; Taquet *et al.*, 2021)	36	10–74	6–10 [13]	24
Anxiety/depression (Francesca *et al.*, 2021; Whitaker *et al.*, 2021; Whittaker *et al.*, 2021)	36	10–74	No data for the combined symptoms	
Hair loss (Francesca *et al.*, 2021)	22	20–24	<6 [14]	14
Cognitive impairment (Francesca *et al.*, 2021)	24	18–21	11 [15]	13
Poor concentration (Francesca *et al.*, 2021; Nasserie *et al.*, 2021)	25	22–28	No data available	

Quality of Life (QoL) Is the Centre of the Problem

When research projects report symptoms in PCS patients, most of them focus on how many symptoms are presented and how long they remain. Concerns about the overall quality of life (QoL) and how PCS leads to damaged function in work, social, and family activities, and managing one's own life, come from other authorities rather than the department of health and health services. The QoL overlaps with the symptom list but is more useful to understand how severely the overall functioning of daily life is affected.

Aimed at understanding the general picture of QoL among the PCS population, Malik *et al.* (2021) conducted a systematic review and meta-analysis to reveal the prevalence of those with poor QoL. From 12 studies consisting of 4828 patients, patients with poor QoL measured by (EQ-VAS) amounted to 59%; among them, mobility problems presented in 36% and 8% were unable to manage personal care. Only 28% of them considered that they were in their usual status, which means they managed their life "ok", although they still had symptoms.

Not restricted to PCS, Ziauddeen *et al.* (2021) found in 2550 patients in the long COVID stage that the impairments and severe symptoms caused an inability to carry out domestic duties for 84% of patients, a limitation in social activities for 77%, absence from work for 74%, and 50% were not able to maintain an independent life. They saw improvement at week 6. However, at week 6, 32% were still unable to live independently.

A longer follow-up study by Vaes *et al.* (2021) reported that 62% of PCS patients reported moderate to extreme difficulty in their daily life and required help from family or care from others. Furthermore, there is a sharp contrast to the QoL before they were infected. Overall, there was working impairment (reduced working hours) in 71% at 3 months and 60% after a 6 month follow-up.

In the UK and many European countries, when facing such a problem of QoL in the workforce and the lack of ability of people to go back to work, a phased return-to-work scheme (National Education Union, 2019) or similar policy was introduced in organisations, which allowed people to go back to work with a reduced workload (reduced hours or lighter duties) to suit their damaged capacity of work. This scheme is typically planned in two phases to suit the individuals; phase one is for the first 3 months (initial phase of reduced work commitment, usually a larger proportion of workload), and phase two is 4–6 months, with much closer to normal workload (pre-full duty stage).

Lambert *et al.* (2021) conducted a Patient-Led Research Collaborative survey (n = 3762) looking at the factors that triggered a relapse of PCS symptoms and reported that physical exertion in 70% of the people, stress in 58%, poor mental activity in 46%, and poor menstruation in 34% were the main factors leading to a deterioration of conditions. Davis *et al.* (2021) reported similar findings, suggesting that relapse is 77% related to physical activity, 55% to stress, 42% to poor cognitive activities, and 35% to poor menstruation. This can partially explain why exerting oneself physically and/or mentally becomes a problem to more than half of the sufferers, preventing them from returning to normal work along with managing daily life effectively.

Figure 3 was drawn using data extracted from the report by Alkodaymi *et al.* (2022).

Another point worthy of discussion is the reactions experienced to COVID vaccination, which has been a lingering topic for the last two

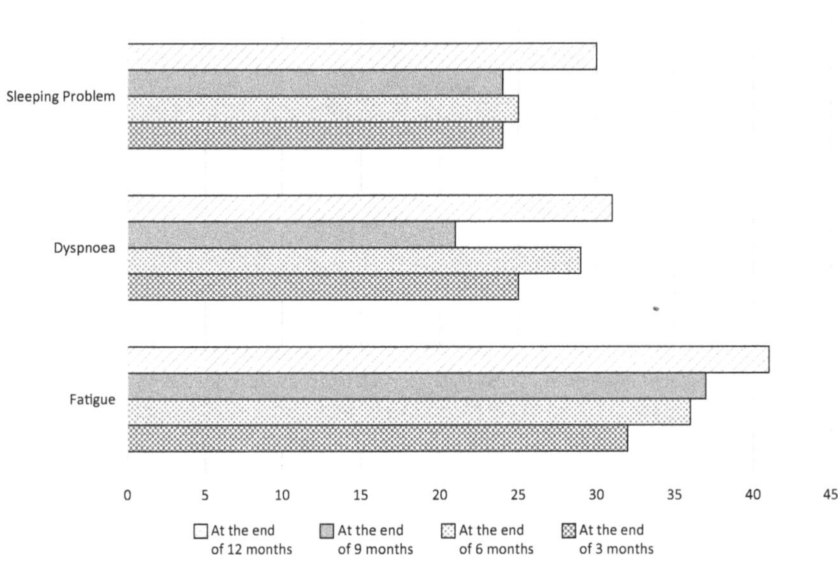

Figure 3. Prevalence of PCS symptoms in follow-up times.

years, with people experiencing various bodily and mentally uncomfortable feelings lasting from a few hours to many days. For some, the long-lasting reaction shows a similarity to the post-COVID-19 syndrome. Although the evidence is not enough to lead to a unanimous judgement, some of the sufferers need good medical treatment and high-quality care to recover. Their main concerns include brain fog, loss of smell and taste, fatigue, and palpitation, after the brief period of flu-like symptoms. According to the authors' clinical observations, these clinical conditions are in line with post-COVID-19 syndrome and should be treated using the same principles proposed in the following chapters.

References

Alkodaymi, M., Omrani, O., and Fawzy, N. (2022). Prevalence of post-acute COVID-19 syndrome symptoms at different follow-up periods: A systematic review and meta-analysis. *Clinical Microbiology and Infection.* https://doi.org/10.1016/j.cmi.2022.01.014.

Assaf, G., Davis, H., McCorkell, L., *et al.* (2020). COVID-19 prolonged symptoms survey — Analysis report (2020 11 May). Patient-Led-Research-Collaborative. Available at: https://patientresearchcovid19.com/research/report-1/.

BBC. (2022). COVID-19 in the UK: How many coronavirus cases are there in my area? *BBC News*. Available at: https://www.bbc.co.uk/news/uk-51768274. (Accessed 30 March 2022).

CDC. (2022). Subjective cognitive decline — A public health issue. Centers for Disease Control and Prevention (USA). Available at: https://www.cdc.gov/aging/data/subjective-cognitive-decline-brief.html#:~:text=The%20prevalence%20of%20subjective%20cognitive,compared%20to%2010.6%25%20among%20women.

Davis, H., Assaf, G., McCorkell, L., *et al.* (2021). Characterizing long COVID in an international cohort: 7 months of symptoms and their impact. *E-Clinical Medicine (Lancet Discovery Science)*, 38, 101019. https://doi.org/10.1016/j.eclinm.2021.101019. https://www.thelancet.com/journals/eclinm/article/PIIS2589-5370(21)00299-6/fulltext.

Francesca, D., Waddell, L. A., Cheung, A. M., *et al.* (2021). Prevalence of long-term effects in individuals diagnosed with COVID-19: A living systematic review. *medRxiv* [Preprint]. https://doi.org/10.1101/2021.06.03.21258317.

Lambert, N., Corps, S., El-Azab, S. N., *et al.* (2021). COVID-19 survivors? Reports of the timing, duration, and health impacts of post-acute sequelae of

SARS-CoV-2 (PASC) infection. *medRxiv*. https://doi.org/10.1101/2021.03.22.21254026.

Malik, P., Patel, K., Pinto, C., *et al.* (2021). Post-acute COVID-19 syndrome (PCS) and health-related quality of life (HRQoL) — A systematic review and meta-analysis. *Journal of Medical Virology*, 94, 253–262. https://doi.org/10.1002/jmv.27309.

Mayer, K. P., Sturgill, J. L., Kalema, A. G., *et al.* (2020). Recovery from COVID-19 and acute respiratory distress syndrome: The potential role of an intensive care unit recovery clinic: A case report. *Journal of Medical Case Reports*, 14, 161. https://doi.org/10.1186/s13256-020-02481-y.

Michelen, M., Manoharan, L., Elkheir, N., *et al.* (2020). Characterising long-term COVID-19: A rapid living systematic review. *medRxiv* [Preprint]. https://doi.org/10.1101/2020.12.08.20246025.

Nasserie, T., Hittle, M., and Goodman, S. N. (2021). Assessment of the frequency and variety of persistent symptoms among patients with COVID-19: A systematic review. *JAMA Network Open*, 4(5), e2111417.

National Education Union. (2019). Phased return to work. National Education Union (UK). Available at: https://neu.org.uk/media/2556/view.

NICE. (2022). Common symptoms in COVID-19 rapid guideline: Managing the long term effects of COVID-19. NICE. Available at: https://app.magicapp.org/#/guideline/EQpzKn/rec/jMpVDq.

ONS. (2022). Prevalence of ongoing symptoms following coronavirus (COVID-19) infection in the UK. (6 January 2022). Office for National Statistics (UK). Available at: https://www.ons.gov.uk/peoplepopulationandcommunity/healthandsocialcare/conditionsanddiseases/bulletins/prevalenceofongoingsymptomsfollowingcoronaviruscovid19infectionintheuk/6january2022.

Taquet, M., Geddes, J. R., Husain, M., *et al.* (2021). 6 month neurological and psychiatric outcomes in 236 379 survivors of COVID-19: A retrospective cohort study using electronic health records. *The Lancet Psychiatry*. https://doi.org/10.1016/S2215-0366(21)00084-5.

Vaes, A., Delbressine, J. M., Houben-Wilke, S., *et al.* (2021). Recovery from COVID-19: A sprint or marathon? 6 month follow-up data from online long COVID-19 support group members. *ERJ Open Research*, 7(2), 00141.

Walker, A. J., MacKenna, B., Inglesby, P., *et al.* (2021). Clinical coding of long COVID in English primary care: A federated analysis of 58 million patient records in situ using OpenSAFELY. *medRxiv* [Preprint].

Whitaker, M., Elliott, J., Chadeau-Hyam, M., *et al.* (2021). *Persistent symptoms following SARS-CoV-2 infection in a random community sample of 508,707 people*. http://hdl.handle.net/10044/1/89844.

Whittaker H. R., Gulea, C., Koteci, A., *et al.* (2021). Post-acute COVID-19 sequelae in cases managed in the community or hospital in the UK: A population based study. *medRxiv* [Preprint]. https://doi.org/10.1101/2021.04.09.21255199.

Ziauddeen, N., Gurdasani, D., O'Hara, M. E., *et al.* (2021). Characteristics of long Covid: Findings from a social media survey. *medRxiv* [Preprint]. https://doi.org/10.1101/2021.03.21.21253968.

Chapter 1

The Diagnosis and Treatment of Post-COVID-19 Syndrome in Biomedical Medicine

The National Guidelines on Post-COVID-19 Syndrome (NICE)

According to NICE (2022), post-COVID-19 syndrome involves multi-systems and some of the impairments are not fully understood yet. The diagnosis of PCS could not be made based on simple blood tests/biomarkers. It needs a diagnosis approach of excluding all other obvious causes which can produce the key symptoms. Therefore, the history and current symptoms provide the essential evidence of the diagnosis.

Although there are no biomarkers agreed upon for diagnosis purposes, some of the key information is nonetheless more valuable than other information. With regard to the diagnosis procedures, a consensus has been reached which suggests a holistic way of processing the individual suffering and prefers face-to-face assessment being essential for both clinicians and patients. The diagnosis criteria and the exclusive assessments give direction to the search for biomarkers, focusing on respiratory functional test, image investigation of lungs by CT, MRI, PET, etc., in both clinical evaluation and further research. Considering the large population of COVID-19 survivors and the demand for diagnosis, it would be impossible to carry out a thorough investigation on each patient concerned due to resource limitation.

The guidance actually suggests that the diagnosis is principally on the shoulder of the clinician who has the direct duty of care for the patient, namely, the general practitioners (GP) in most countries. NICE have set a rough criterion for the diagnosis which was thereafter accepted by the WHO. There is only one difference between the NICE criterion and the WHO recommendation, and that is the length of time from onset of COVID-19, which is stipulated as 12 weeks by the WHO and 3 months by NICE. The two guidelines are interchangeable in clinical practice.

It is worth highlighting that in those patients presenting no symptoms for the first couple of days but testing positive for COVID-19, later onset of symptoms is common and develops into post-COVID-19 syndrome eventually within the 12-week period.

According to the updated research reports on the diagnosis and treatment standards of PCS, there are four key factors that are needed to establish a diagnosis of post-COVID-19 syndrome.

They are as follows:

a. A clear diagnosis of COVID-19 via established testing.
b. Minimum 3 months after COVID-19 (acute stage) diagnosis, with symptoms lasting at least 2 months, and still present.
c. Presenting with the 3 key symptoms: cognitive dysfunction (brain fog), fatigue, and breathlessness.
d. The above-mentioned symptoms are not inherited from previous illnesses such as ME, fibromyalgia, or diabetes, and could not be explained by an alternative diagnosis (WHO, 2021a, 2021b).

There is currently no well-recognised biomarker, or imaging diagnosis for PCS. Therefore, case history and exclusive diagnosis are the accepted method for medical and healthcare professions.

It is interesting that one of the world's most influential health authorities, the Centers for Disease Control and Prevention (CDC, 2021) of the USA, has not formally developed a national guideline or definition to date on this topic. They use a term "Post-COVID Conditions" to describe all poor health conditions remaining after 4 weeks of an acute COVID-19 episode. The CDC have been open to all potential terms from Long COVID to Chronic COVID. Also, interestingly, there has been no revision of their policy since September 2021. As a matter of fact, the CDC have not established the condition as a medical diagnosis and prefer to deal with those symptoms accordingly. Many national authorities are in agreement with the USA, and have not issued any formal recognition of PCS or the post-COVID-19 suffering in different terms.

What Could Be Learnt from Previous Similar Clinical Topics

Post-intensive care syndrome (PICS)

In the early stage of the COVID-19 pandemic (2020), up to 15% patients were hospitalised and nearly half of those in hospital were in the ICU. For those people who recovered from the ICU, the average number of days spent in the ICU was much longer than any other respiratory disorders, approximately 20 days. Due to the critical stage of the respiratory distress and multi-organ damage, the patients suffered various conditions which are generalised as Post-Intensive Care Syndrome (PICS). PICS is not a new phenomenon; however, in the last two years, due to the widespread nature of COVID-19 and the large number of patients admitted to hospital, and eventually the ICU, PICS became a health concern as it needs a better understanding along with multi-disciplinary care and treatment.

The similarity and difference between PICS and PCS are illustrated in Table 1 (Stam *et al.*, 2020; WHO, 2021b). From Table 1, it can be seen that the two actually overlap, except for the lack of definition of two symptoms in the PCS symptom list, impulsivity and muscle waste.

According to Inoue *et al.* (2019), three major impairments last long into the rehabilitation stage, namely, physical capacity impairment, cognitive impairment, and mental impairment. The physical impairment is

Table 1. Comparison of the symptoms between PICS (Stam *et al.*, 2020) and PCS (WHO, 2021b).

Symptoms (Stam *et al.*, 2020)	PICS	PCS
Fatigue	Y	Y
Breathlessness	Y	Y
Cognitive impairment	Y	Y
Impulsivity	Y	n/a
Anxiety/depression	Y	Y
PTSD	Y	Y
Pain	Y	Y
Intolerance in exercise	Y	Y
Muscle waste	Y	n/a

possibly due to the restricted use of skeleton muscle. The pathology of cognitive impairment is unknown, but is linked to the stress experienced, causing hormonal fluctuation, the fluctuation of the blood sugar level, and interruption of blood supply to the brain. Similarly, mental impairment is typically part of the post-trauma stress disorder (PTSD).

Lessons have been learnt and most reports agreed (Van Der Schaaf *et al.*, 2015) that a multi-disciplinary team is the possible solution to provide care and management for the conditions as well as treatment being maintained in the long term.

Post-viral syndrome (PVS)

Viral infections are a relatively new area in biomedicine. Reliable diagnosis methods in clinical practice were only established in the 1980s (Rasmussen, 2015) for clinically diagnosing hepatitis by using antibodies. Since then, numerous diseases have been identified as being caused by viral infections. Retrospectively, many other diseases were reviewed and considered to be caused by viruses as well. Among those mass infections, or global pandemics of viral infections, some of the records in the last century might provide valuable clues for us to deal with COVID-19 and its PCS.

Post-infectious fatigue was widely observed with SARS, a viral infection similar to COVID-19. Tansey *et al.* (2007) found that 64% of survivors of SARS had experienced fatigue at the point of 3 months after the acute illness, and the symptom remained for up to 12 months, with 60% still suffering from fatigue. Furthermore, a study following up on survivors to their 4th year after initial infection in Hong Kong stated that 40% still have fatigue and 27% were eventually diagnosed as having ME or chronic fatigue syndrome (CFS) (Liam *et al.*, 2009).

Another well-researched viral infection and its long-term impairment of health was Epstein–Barr (glandular fever), which is an infectious mononucleosis. At the point of 6–12 months after the onset, between 9% and 12% patients could not fully recover and met the diagnosis criteria of ME/CFS (White *et al.*, 1998; Buchwald *et al.*, 2000).

ME and fibromyalgia

As discussed above, as many as 10% of all patients surviving the initial infection will continue to suffer from various problems and will eventually be diagnosed as having ME or CFS at the point of 12 months after the infection. However, before the diagnosis of ME/CFS, a majority of survivors will be managed under PCS, until a diagnosis of ME can be established. From historical studies of viral infections, it has been suggested that a similar percentage of survivors with symptoms lingering into this stage indicates the illness has remained long enough to qualify such a diagnosis. In other words, those suffering from PCS will have a 50% chance, or one in two chances, of gradually recovering to a status allowing them the capacity to manage their daily life and return to work, and another 50% or half of the survivors will eventually be diagnosed as ME/CFS, or fibromyalgia (FM) if pain is the main symptom. In other words, those do not recover will continue their suffering and live with a poor quality of life, very likely to be a lifelong illness without cure.

One of the commonly circulated mechanisms of ME/CFS is about the abnormal control of the Glymphatic System (a drainage system in the central nervous system). This allows pro-inflammatory cytokines to pass through the blood brain barrier which causes high fever in the acute stage and impairment of cognitive, alertness, (Holmes, 2017) and many other changes featured in the later stage, including ME/CFS (Lam, 2009; Magnus, 2015).

From previous clinical practice and observation, the authors and their colleagues have fine-tuned our understanding of ME and its clinical approaches with a whole-system TCM approach in treating ME/CFS, and achieved a high level of satisfactory outcomes. And the core understanding of the ME/CFS syndrome patterns shows the level of overlap with observed PCS cases; therefore, a similar approach is validated for our clinical treatment whereas no clinical trial results could be made available yet.

Acupuncture, herbs, and manual therapy (Tuina) should all be employed for improved and quicker recovery. It was also noticed from a therapeutic point of view that manual techniques could be used to aid lymphatic drainage, influencing the CNS and stimulating the sympathetic tone to raise functions of the nervous system (Perrin *et al.*, 2020).

References

Buchwald, D. S., Rea, T. D., Katon, W. J., *et al.* (2000). Acute infectious mononucleosis: Characteristics of patients who report failure. *The American Journal of Medicine*, 109(7), 531–537. https://doi.org/10.1016/S0002-9343(00)00560-X.

CDC. (2021). Post COVID conditions. Centers for Disease Control and Prevention, USA. Available at: https://www.cdc.gov/coronavirus/2019-ncov/long-term-effects/index.html.

Cope, H., Mann, A., David, A., *et al.* (1994). Predictors of chronic "postviral" fatigue. *Lancet*, 344(8926), 864–868. https://doi.org/10.1016/S0140-6736(94)92833-9.

Holmes, T. H. and Anderson, J. N. (2017). Cytokine signature associated with disease severity in chronic fatigue syndrome patients. *Proceedings of the National Academy of Sciences*, 114, E7150–E7158.

Inoue, S., Hatakeyama, J., Kondo, Y., Hifumi, T., Sakuramoto, H., *et al.* (2019). Post-intensive care syndrome: Its pathophysiology, prevention, and future directions. *Acute Medicine and Surgery*, 6, 233–246. https://doi.org/10.1002/ams2.415.

Lam, M. H. B., Wing, Y. K., Yu, M. W. M., *et al.* (2009). Mental morbidities and chronic fatigue in severe acute respiratory syndrome survivors: Long-term follow-up. *Archives of Internal Medicine*, 169(22), 2142–2147. https://doi.org/10.1001/archinternmed.2009.384.

Magnus, P., Gunnes, N., Tveito, K., *et al.* (2015). Chronic fatigue syndrome/myalgic encephalomyelitis (CFS/ME) is associated with pandemic influenza infection, but not with an adjuvanted pandemic influenza vaccine. *Vaccine*, 33, 6173–6177. https://doi.org/10.1016/j.vaccine.2015.10.018.

NICE. (2022). Covid-19 rapid guideline: Managing the long term effect of Covid-19/Identification. National Institute of Clinical and Care Excellence. Available at: https://app.magicapp.org/#/guideline/EQpzKn/rec/jMpVDq.

Perrin, R., Riste, L., Hann, M., Walther, A., Mukherjee, A., and Heald, A. (2020). Into the looking glass: Post-viral syndrome post COVID-19. *Medical Hypotheses*, 144, 110055. https://doi.org/10.1016/j.mehy.2020.110055.

Rasmussen, A. L. (2015). Probing the viromic frontiers. *mBio*, 6(6), e01767-15. doi:10.1128/mBio.01767-15.

Stam, H. J., Stucki, G., and Bickenbach, J. (2020 April). Covid-19 and post intensive care syndrome: A call for action. *Journal of Rehabilitation Medicine*, 15;52(4), jrm00044. doi: 10.2340/16501977-2677.

Tansey, C. M., Louie, M., Loeb, M., *et al.* (2007). One-year outcomes and health care utilization in survivors of severe acute respiratory syndrome. *Archives of Internal Medicine*, 167(12), 1312–1320. https://doi.org/10.1001/archinte.167.12.1312.

Van Der Schaaf, M., Bakhshi-Raiez, F., Van Der Steen, M., Dongelmans, D. A., and De Keizer, N. F. (2015). Recommendations for intensive care follow-up clinics: report from a survey and conference of Dutch intensive cares. *Minerva Anestesiologica*, 81, 135–144.

White, P. D., Thomas, J. M., Amess, J., *et al.* (1998). Incidence, risk and prognosis of acute and chronic fatigue syndromes and psychiatric disorders after glandular fever. *British Journal of Psychiatry*, 173(6), 475–481. https://doi.org/10.1192/bjp.173.6.475.

WHO. (2021a). *A Clinical Case Definition of Post COVID-19 Condition by a Delphi Consensus*. Geneva: World Health Organisation, pp. 20–21.

WHO. (2021b). *Clinical Case Definition Working Group on Post COVID-19 Condition. Towards a Universal Understanding of Post COVID-19 Condition*. Geneva: World Health Organisation.

Chapter 2

Other Common Health Concerns After Acute COVID-19 Stage

Increased Risk of Some Chronic Diseases

According to large-scale follow-up studies of patients discharged from hospital after the acute stage of COVID-19, their health was seriously damaged, not limited to the lungs. A large percentage (29.4%) of them were rehospitalised for various serious diseases within a one-year period and as 1 in 8 people died of the illness (Ayoubkhani *et al.*, 2021). The damage was observed in a pattern of multiple-system weakness, from the respiratory system and circulation system to the liver and kidney (Figure 1). Subsequently, the risk of adding a new disease like diabetes, heart attack, stroke, kidney disorder, and liver damage has been significantly increased; in addition, this is not limited to the aged population. The risk of developing a new disease, like diabetes, heart failure or attack, stroke, or kidney and liver diseases, is 2–3-fold higher than the population who did not have COVID-19 (Alkodaymi, 2022).

Although the study subjects were severe cases that required hospital treatment, the study can still reveal the nature of the disease associated with multiple organ/system damage.

Apart from the common symptoms considered in post-COVID-19 syndrome (PCS), various clear clinical diagnoses were established. The PCS diagnosis excluded any other established diseases, which were not in the range of PCS, but can lead to increased significant damage in the patients. Hence, the conditions added after COVID-19, PCS, or non-PCS are long-lasting themes in the management of health among the population that suffered and recovered from COVID-19 infection. The reason is that those after-COVID-19 conditions are all chronic and life-long and out of the purview of cure with current available treatment. The management should always be considered in the context of the post-COVID-19 stage, taking the viral infection, the damage in the cardiovascular tissues, the immune system response, and the mental/psychological aspects into overall consideration.

The disease will subsequently be managed together with PCS in a holistic view. That is the advantage of TCM. Indeed, TCM has demonstrated its clinical effects in treating many conditions listed here, from diabetes and arrhythmia to liver and kidney impairments. The evidence of the clinical effectiveness will be reviewed in the corresponding sections as the volume of evidence is large.

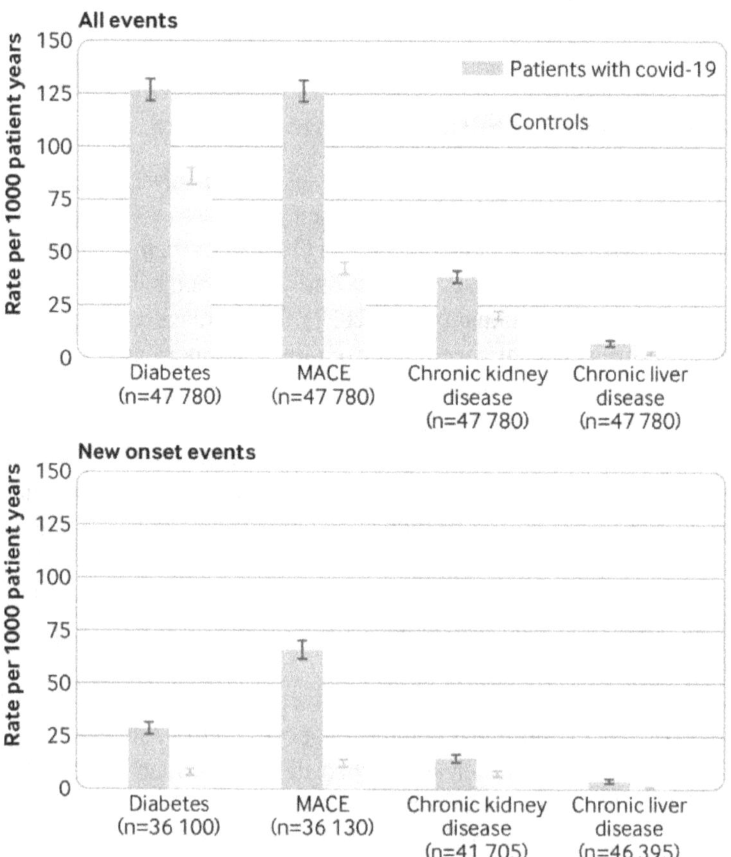

Figure 1. The numbers and rates of the major categories of increased damage due to COVID-19 reported in Ayoubkhani *et al.*'s report (2021).

Note: MACE: Major adverse cardiovascular events.

The Cochrane Review conducted its own study on COVID-19 and its damage to the cardiovascular system led by Pellicori *et al.* (2021), which includes 220 studies from China (47.7%), the USA (20.9%), and Italy (9.5%). A majority (89%) of the studies were clinical observation/retrospective. However, three RCTs were found and 20 were prospective. In this very extensive study, it was found that hypertension at 36%, diabetes at 22%, and ischaemic heart disease at 10% presented in patients hospitalised with COVID-19; furthermore, those conditions increased the risk of death.

Heart impairments

Heart attack, heart failure, and arrhythmia are very commonly reported among the population after COVID-19 infection. Some studies suggest that the likelihood of having a new heart condition like heart failure, arrhythmia, and heart attack, which did not exist before the COVID-19 infection, is much higher in those who suffered from COVID-19 infection.

Pathological studies suggest that the SARS-CoV-2 virus invades into myocardium tissue via the ACE-II receptor, then causes direct damage of heart tissue. There are plenty of ACE-II receptors in both the heart and lungs. This invasion pathway allows the virus to enter the heart tissues from blood. However, with regard to the delayed damage after the acute stage of COVID-19, the mechanism is not clear yet.

Stroke

Developing a stroke is much more common in the post-COVID-19 population than the non-COVID-19 population of same-age individuals. The circumstances are an addition to the impairment of the heart conditions, and is part of the cardio-vascular system impairments. Clinical observation finds more “clotting” (thrombosis/embolism) than “bleeding” (haemorrhage) in the brain after COVID-19.

The major incidents related to COVID-19 also concern the practice of vaccination. Research into the side effects of the COVID-19 Vaccine, particularly in the 49 cases of CVST and VITT after the Oxford CoV-19 vaccine, has been conducted. It tends to affect women, and the onset is within 1 week of the first dose of injection. Symptoms start with headache and progress in severity. Subarachnoid haemorrhage (SAH) and Intracerebral haemorrhage (ICH) were confirmed in half of the patients. The platelet count dropped significantly, and PF4 IgG Assay and d-Dimer, indicators of immune system involvement were positive in a majority of the cases. Around nineteen patients died (39%) of complications relating to CVST and VITT (Sharifian-Dorche *et al.*, 2021). This report led to the hypothesis that immune-reaction-led damage in the blood clotting mechanism might already exist in the COVID-19 pathology, although it has not been revealed yet.

The Circulating System Conditions

Evidence suggests that preexisting circulatory system conditions made the COVID-19 infection more likely to be severe, leading to hospitalisation and a higher death rate.

However, the co-relation is not limited to pre-infection; the chance of developing a new circulatory system condition or developing into a major incident (heart attack or stroke) is much higher among those who recovered from COVID-19.

Runucci *et al.*'s (2020) report finds that the levels of d-dimer, interleukin-6 (IL-6), C-reactive protein (CRP), fibrinogen, and platelet were increased in COVID-19 patients, which are clear indicators of hypercoagulability and linked to thrombosis. This could affect patients during the acute stage of COVID-19, and it could lead to higher risk of blood clot long after the infection. Connor and Levy (2020) echoed their support of the study. In clinical practice, corresponding to the findings of the hypercoagulability, anticoagulant treatment has shown to decrease the mortality of COVID-19 patients (Tang *et al.*, 2020; Helms *et al.*, 2020).

Figueroa *et al.* (2020) examined the national statistics in Scotland and found excess deaths for cardiovascular disease at about 4 weeks after the first wave of the pandemic, and this excess disappeared in week 17. These observations suggest that the short-term increase in excess cardiovascular deaths might be associated with undetected/unconfirmed deaths related to COVID-19. It suggests cardiovascular disease patients are more susceptible to infection and are likely to have severe results. When the same investigation was carried out by Banerjee *et al.* (2021) in England, Italy, and China, the results suggested that the direct increased death numbers could be 31,205 and 62,410 respectively in the year 2020. As of February

2022, no other national-level study on the increased death rate is available. Nevertheless, the studies are convincing that COVID-19 leads to more death directly after infection. There are also non-direct effects causing increased suffering from cardiovascular illness and death.

Among the reported conditions relating to the cardiovascular system due to COVID-19 are heart failure, arrhythmia, atrial fibrillation, myocardial infarction, myocarditis, and thromboembolism. The Cochrane Database's very own review included 220 studies that paid particular attention to the damage caused by COVID-19 and reported details of cardiovascular conditions. Biomarkers of cardiac tissue damage are abnormal in most patients even though they did not show clinical signs. The incidence of cardiovascular complications displayed a wide range, in particular for arrhythmias (9.3%), heart failure (6.8%), and thrombotic complications (7.4%). These spectra of conditions were confirmed by many other research reports (Cenko *et al.*, 2021).

The Mental and Emotional Effect of COVID-19: PTSD and Depression

The mental health situation is a major aspect of post-COVID-19 syndrome (PCS). The negative effects have been widely agreed upon from clinical observations and reports. An acute disease like COVID-19 involves whole-body response, and many of the responses are harmful to the mental status. It was also found that the SARS-II virus could also enter the central nervous system causing potential impairment directly.

Among those hospitalised, PTSD is highly possible for several reasons. The first is that there are many cases of mortality which can inevitably cause mental shock. Second, because of the high infection rate, a non-visiting policy has been applied to all hospitals around the world. This leads to the feeling of fear, helplessness, and despair. The alien feeling of been supplied oxygen in a hospital setting could be linked to near-death scenarios due to the media (Malik *et al.*, 2021). Patients who survive acute COVID-19 and are discharged from hospital tend to have PTSD with a high level of prevalence between 15% and 20% (Bellen *et al.*, 2021; Chang & Park, 2020). However, detailed analysis is lacking from specialists. All available evidence suggests that PTSD is a bad form of anxiety and can be the causation of many additional developments, including depression and bodily complaints.

Anxiety, sleeping problems, and depression are complicated, interconnected, and entangled aspects of mental and emotional changes.

Immune System Abnormality

Cytokine Storm is a frequently mentioned term when discussing COVID-19 and is considered to be the key development of the worse outcomes in acute COVID-19. It was defined as an overreaction of the immune system in fighting against the pathogens, mostly viruses. But in the context of COVID-19, a Cytokine Storm (CS) is the commonly used term. Cytokine refers to a range of small proteins released by cells in different part of the body tissues, particularly the immune cells. Their main purpose is to coordinate the body's defence response against infection and trigger inflammation (George, 2022). When the defence response is appropriate, it effectively clears the virus or bacteria that could potentially cause the illness. However, when the reaction is well over what is needed, namely, excessive, or uncontrolled levels of cytokines are released, resulting in hyperinflammation, it causes great difficulty to the individual, causing more damage to the involved tissues/organs, with the potential for death. In the instance of COVID-19, it not only creates severe damage in the lungs, immediately causing lungs to be congested with blood, but can also leave long-lasting damage of fibrosis in the lungs, both of which reduce the efficiency of oxygen/carbon dioxide exchange and prompt a reduction of oxygen levels in the blood, in the short and long term.

When the storm is over, the overexcited immune system will experience an exhaustion period, not reacting to pathogens as quickly as previously, increasing the risk of catching cold or flu, or another variant of SARS-II easily. This is a stage of immune deficiency. The deficiency is a major contributor to the fatigue of PCS (Mohammed *et al.*, 2020).

Mehta *et al.* (2020) reported elevated levels of IL-2, IL-7, interferon, macrophage inflammatory protein-α, granulocyte-colony stimulating, factor, and tumour necrosis factor-α. Together, those biomarkers indicate a hyperinflammation correlated to lung and heart failure.

Reviewing the research in ME/CFS patients, it has become clear that the damage to immune function is a major contributor to the long-lasting fatigue and lower resistance to cold/flu. Problem is shown in the form of polymorphisms in IFN-γ+874T/A and the IL-10−592C/A was corresponding to the energy problem (Vollmer-Conna *et al.*, 2008). In another analysis, a portfolio of immune measurements, including genes and proteins (IL-6, IL-10, etc.) to cells, revealed the link between fatigue and the immune dysfunction after infection (Piriano *et al.*, 2012).

Immune dysfunctions have been a clinical theme in health promotion and disease prevention in TCM for a couple of millennia. Therapeutic methods were broadly tried, and many effective protocols are used in current practice, including herbs, therapeutic food, external/skin stimulation with moxibustion, acupuncture, Dao yin (self-message according to channel theory), and Qigong exercise. Treatment and lifestyle management together will be most beneficial.

Diabetes

To date, nearly all surveys from various countries have revealed that among the post-COVID-19 population, the newly added diagnosis of diabetes (type-II, mainly) is noticeable. The patients did not have concerns of diabetes before they were infected with COVID-19. They also may not show typical post-COVID-19 syndrome (PCS), as their symptoms are mainly about fatigue. Some studies (Ayoubkhani, 2021; Pellicori, 2021) revealed that among the patients with post-COVID-19 Syndrome who had been discharged from the hospital, around 20% of them could be diabetic, which is much higher than the population level of their age. This leads to a suggestion that in individuals newly diagnosed with diabetes, the causation is being infected with COVID-19. However, the long-term link between non-hospitalised patients and diabetes is not clear at this stage.

According to the WHO and UK guidelines, when diabetes is diagnosed, many of the symptoms the patients suffer from will be explained, such as fatigue, intolerance to exercise, and lack of capacity to work and participate in social activities. The patients might be diagnosed with diabetes alone, or are more likely to be diagnosed with PCS and diabetes together. In clinical management with TCM, the co-existing of the two might be a bit broad to treat, but it is not a problem of the holistic approach.

The mechanism of developing diabetes has been explored by scholars and Sathish *et al.* (2021) have summarised the understanding and findings to help understand the pathology of such development. The SARS-II virus could enter the pancreatic β cells directly via ACE-II receptors and laboratory research has confirmed the distribution of ACE-II on pancreatic cells (Tikellis *et al.*, 2004) and this is proven in real cases (Yao *et al.*, 2020). Another route of impairment is by triggering an excess inflammatory reaction feature by cytokines (eInterleukin-6) and C-reactive protein, leading to auto-immuno-attack. The third possibility is about the restriction measures' negative impacts. Due to the illness and stay home policy, the patients reduced their physical activity, are unable to maintain a healthy diet, and gain weight. These negative lifestyle changes can cause some known pathophysiological effects, including insulin resistance and triggering inflammatory pathways, which have been proven to be linked to type-II diabetes.

Secondary Problems: Skin Response, Hair Loss, Loss of Smell, etc.

Skin rashes

Skin rashes are one of the commonly reported symptoms/conditions among PCS. It might be triggered by the stress response (fight/flight, adrenaline response) or an abnormal untuned immune system, which allows autoimmune problems to take place. Immune storm is another main mechanism of auto-immune problem. The skin conditions mostly start in the acute COVID-19 stages and some start later.

According to a dermatologist's studies, the skin conditions that occur during COVID-19 are broad, from exanthema (48%), vascular (33%), to urticaria (12%) (Gisondi *et al.*, 2021). 92% of the conditions start within 4 weeks of COVID-19 onset. The review suggests that the diversity of skin conditions and their different patterns of onset could only be explained by multi-pathway pathology.

Doykov *et al.* (2020) have observed long-lasting above-normal inflammation biomarkers in patients months after COVID-19. This persistent inflammatory over-reaction could provide a clue in explaining why skin conditions are common, as those biomarkers are also presented in all autoimmune/allergy skin conditions, although they might not be the cause. Contrarily, the prolonged virus presence redirects the immune system resource, and the immune system will act eccentrically, failing to maintain the normal protection of the skin (Oronsky *et al.*, 2021).

TCM has demonstrated efficacious results in treating many autoimmune-caused skin conditions from skin allergy, urticaria, to eczema. Internal/oral herbs, external/atopic herbal creams, and acupuncture are used in the therapeutic portfolio, according to individual constitutions (lifelong body characters) and syndrome patterns (reaction status reflecting the current situations). The authors have seen numerous cases in their practice and are confident to offer TCM treatment and management to help PCS patients. According to historical TCM records, it was mostly caused by the residual, although not powerful, of the pathogens, which may be akin to or altered from its initial form, in combination with latent/long hiding pathogens that cause the problems. Damp-heat, heat in blood, and wind-heat are common types of patterns in TCM because they all cause red colour skin changes, as heat attempts to exit from the skin.

Loss of hair — Telogen effluvium (TE)/alopecia

Searching research reports, it is that clear hair loss is not mentioned in the acute stage of COVID-19, but is a common concern in long COVID-19 and post-COVID-19 syndrome. According to Abrantes *et al.* (2021), most cases were patchy alopecia, and 70% of the sufferers were women of about 40 years of age. Only 26.7% of them had a previous history of androgenetic alopecia. Trichologist reports showed empty hair follicles confirming the diagnosis. The onset of the TE occurred between 32 and 58 days (average 45 days) after a positive RTC test. With dermatological treatment and care, most of them have been recovered between 12 and 100 days (average 47.5 days). Pressure alopecia was also considered in some cases. Moreno-Arrones *et al.* (2021) reported similar results from a multicentre clinical study. Among 214 patients, the average age was 47.4 years, and 78% were women. There is a clear link between TE and fever reported in the acute stage (86%). The onset or clearly evident hair loss is after 57 days. On average, it took 4 weeks to stabilise.

To investigate if COVID-19 increased the risk of hair loss, Trüeb *et al.* (2020) carried out a big clinical survey on hair loss and grey hair comparing COVID-19 patients and a non-COVID-19 population; the outcomes confirmed that the risk of suffering from hair loss is significantly higher than the non-COVID-19 population, while greying hair is not significantly higher. However, the study did not reveal the status of how long after COVID-19 the samples reported their experience, which could be explained as a post-COVID-19 phenomenon.

However, the above-mentioned studies were limited to people reporting their condition to dermatologists, not including the post-COVID-19 periods. According to NICE, hair loss is among the common symptoms in PCS, and most of the patients were not referred to specialist. Their treatment/management should be considered in a holistic way, considering the whole PCS rather than simple methods of healing the condition of skin and hair root (follicles).

The mechanisms were studied as well. Several studies pointed to the androgen receptor which regulates the transmembrane protease, serine 2 (TMPRSS2), the pigment-producing mechanism. Androgen receptor is required for SARS-CoV-2 infectivity (Baratchian *et al*., 2021). This pathway was considered for developing drugs to combat COVID-19. Thus, hyperactivation of androgen receptors, AGA, could lead to a significantly high risk of severe outcomes in COVID-19, in addition to developing hair loss. Others are pointing out the imbalance of autonomic nerve functions, as it was commonly observed in the population after childbirth, or experience traumatic events. Hormonal fluctuation was also considered, as a majority of the sufferers are women.

For a long history, hair loss was observed and treated with TCM. It was linked to childbearing, ageing, and emotional upheaval, which led to syndrome patterns of blood deficiency, kidney essence deficiency, and heat in blood. Many TCM herbal formulas were introduced for the recovery of hair. Skin acupuncture, seven stars needling, was also applied and better than natural recovery was observed. The TCM diagnosis and treatment are illustrated in a later chapter.

Loss of smell (anosmia) and taste

Anosmia is a symptom coming in the early stage of COVID-19 in more than half of all cases, and most of them could spontaneously recover without treatment within 2 weeks (8 days on average). However, when the symptom is not cleared with other symptoms and getting into the long COVID-19 stage, the symptom seems a lasting one, with very slow recovery. In the authors' observations, many patients have experienced good recovery 6 months after COVID-19, even though the sense of smell is still not fully recovered.

It is also important that in many cases the patients have both smell and taste problems, while some of them report a metallic taste. And some of them only have taste problems. This is partially due to the requirement of TCM practice to collect a feeling of taste in the case history for diagnosis purposes.

Long ago before COVID-19, research endeavouring to find the pathway of a virus getting into the brain and causing brain damage, after the SARS pandemic, found that a possible route to reach the brain was through the olfactory nerve (Desforges *et al.*, 2014). Since the SARS-II virus is extremely similar to the SARS-CoV-2 virus, the same pathway could be through the brain. Meanwhile, the olfactory (responsible for function of smelling) nerve could be damaged when the virus diffuses in it.

Another possible explanation of loss of smell is the finding related to the ME/CFS in COVID-19, the lymphatic drainage in the brain via the perivascular space, which is next to the olfactory nerve into the nasal mucosa. When the drainage is in trouble, a physical pressure could depress the olfactory nerve and cause the smell dysfunction (Valiee, 2021).

Persistent anosmia observed among long COVID-19 patients may be involved via a cascade of effects generated by dysautonomia leading to ACE2 antibodies enhancing a persistent immune activation.

References

Abrantes, T. F., Artounian, K. A., Falsey, R., *et al.* (2021). Time of onset and duration of post-COVID-19 acute telogen effluvium. *Journal of the America Academy of Dermatology*, 85(4), 975–976. https://doi.org/10.1016/j.jaad.2021.07.02.

Alkodaymi, M. S., Omrani, O. A., Fawzy, N., *et al.* (2022). Prevalence of post-acute COVID-19 syndrome symptoms at different follow-up periods: A systematic review and meta-analysis. *Clinical Microbiology and Infection*, 28(5), 657–666. https://doi.org/10.1016/j.cmi.2022.01.014. https://www.sciencedirect.com/science/article/pii/S1198743X22000386.

Ayoubkhani, D., Khunti, K., Nafilyan, V., *et al.* (2021). Post-covid syndrome in individuals admitted to hospital with covid-19: Retrospective cohort study. *BMJ*, 372, n693. doi:10.1136/bmj.n693. PMID: 33789877; PMCID: PMC8010267.

Banerjee, A., Chen, S., Pasea, L., *et al.* (2021). Excess deaths in people with cardiovascular diseases during the COVID-19 pandemic. *European Journal of Preventive Cardiology*, 28(14), 1599–1609. https://doi.org/10.1093/eurjpc/zwaa155.

Baratchian, M., McManus, J. M., Berk, M. P., *et al.* (2021). Androgen regulation of pulmonary AR, TMPRSS2 and ACE2 with implications for sex-discordant COVID-19 outcomes. *Scientific Reports*, 11, 11130. https://doi.org/10.1038/s41598-021-90491-1.

Cenko, E., Badimon, L., Bugiardini, R., *et al.* (2021). Cardiovascular disease and COVID-19: A consensus paper from the ESC Working Group on Coronary Pathophysiology & Microcirculation, ESC Working Group on Thrombosis and the Association for Acute CardioVascular Care (ACVC), in collaboration with the European Heart Rhythm Association (EHRA). *Cardiovascular Research*, 117(14), 2705–2729. https://doi.org/10.1093/cvr/cvab298.

Chang, M. C. and Park, D. (2020). Incidence of post-traumatic stress disorder after coronavirus disease. *Healthcare*, 8(4), 373.

Desforges, M., Le Coupanec, A., Stodola, J. K., *et al.* (2014). Human coronaviruses: Viral and cellular factors involved in neuroinvasiveness and neuropathogenesis. *Virus Research*, 194, 145–158.

Doykov, I., Hällqvist, J., Gilmour, K. C., *et al.* (2020). "The long tail of COVID-19" — The detection of a prolonged inflammatory response after a SARS-CoV-2 infection in asymptomatic and mildly affected patients. *F1000Research*, 9, 1349. doi:10.12688/f1000research.27287.2.

Figueroa, J. D., Brennan, P. M., Theodoratou, E., *et al.* (2020). Distinguishing between direct and indirect consequences of COVID-19. *BMJ*, 369, m2377. doi:10.1136/bmj.m2377.

George, A. (2022). Cytokine storm. *NewScientist*. Available at: https://www.newscientist.com/definition/cytokine-storm/. (Accessed 18 February 2022).

Gisondi, P., Di Leo, S., Bellinato, F., *et al.* (2021). Time of onset of selected skin lesions associated with COVID-19: A systematic review. *Dermatology and Therapy (Heidelberg)*, 11, 695–705. https://doi.org/10.1007/s13555-021-00526-8.

Helms, J., Tacquard, C., Severac, F., *et al.* (2020). High risk of thrombosis in patients with severe SARS-CoV-2 infection: A multicenter prospective cohort study. *Intensive Care Medicine*, 46(6), 1089–1098.

Malik, P., Patel, K., Pinto, C., *et al.* (2021). Post-acute COVID-19 syndrome (PCS) and health-related quality of life (HRQoL) — A systematic review and meta-analysis. *Journal of Medical Virology*, 94, 253–262. https://doi.org/10.1002/jmv.27309.

Mehta, P., McAuley, D. F., Brown, M., *et al.* (2020). COVID-19: Consider cytokine storm syndromes and immunosuppression. *International Health Regulations*, 395, 1033–1034.

Moreno-Arrones, O. M., Lobato-Berezo, A., Gomez-Zubiaur, A., *et al.* (2021). SARS-CoV-2-induced telogen effluvium: A multicentric study. *Journal of the European Academy of Dermatology and Venereology*, 2021, 35, e181–e183. https://doi.org/10.1111/jdv.17045.

Oronsky, B., Larson, C., Hammond, T. C., *et al.* (2021). A review of persistent post-COVID syndrome (PPCS). *Clinical Reviews in Allergy & Immunology*, 1–9. doi:10.1007/s12016-021-08848-3.

Pellicori, P., Doolub, G., Wong, C. M., *et al.* (2021). COVID-19 and its cardiovascular effects: A systematic review of prevalence studies. *Cochrane Database of Systematic Reviews*, 3(3), CD013879. doi:10.1002/14651858.CD013879.

Sathish, T., Tapp, R. J., Cooper, M. E., and Zimmet, P. (2021). Potential metabolic and inflammatory pathways between COVID-19 and new-onset diabetes. *Diabetes & Metabolism*, 47(2), 101204. https://doi.org/10.1016/j.diabet.2020.10.002.

Sharifian-Dorche, M., Bahmanyar, M., Sharifian-Dorche, A., *et al.* (2021). Vaccine-induced immune thrombotic thrombocytopenia and cerebral venous sinus thrombosis post COVID-19 vaccination; a systematic review. *Journal of the Neurological Sciences*, 428, 117607. https://doi.org/10.1016/j.jns.2021.117607.

Tang, N., Bai, H., Chen, X., *et al.* (2020). Anticoagulant treatment is associated with decreased mortality in severe coronavirus disease 2019 patients with coagulopathy. *Journal of Thrombosis and Haemostasis*, 18(5), 1094–1099.

Tikellis, C., Wookey, P.J., Candido, R., *et al.* (2004). Improved islet morphology after blockade of the renin- angiotensin system in the ZDF rat. *Diabetes*, 53, 989–997.

Trüeb, R. M., Rezende, H. D., and Dias, M. F. (2020). Comment on alopecia and grey hair associated with COVID-19 Severity. *Experimental Dermatology*, 29, 1250–1252. https://doi.org/10.1111/exd.14220.

Vallée, A. (2021). Dysautonomia and implications for anosmia in long COVID-19 disease. *Journal of Clinical Medicine*, 10(23), 5514. doi:10.3390/jcm10235514. PMID: 34884216; PMCID: PMC8658706.

Vollmer-Conna, U., Piraino, B. F., Cameron, B., *et al.* (2008). Cytokine polymorphisms have a synergistic effect on severity of the acute sickness response to infection. *Clinical Infectious Diseases*, 47(11), 1418–1425. https://doi.org/10.1086/592967.

Yao, X. H., Li, T. Y., He, Z. C., *et al.* (2020). A pathological report of three COVID-19 cases by minimal invasive autopsies. *Zhonghua Bing Li Xue Za Zhi*, 49, 411–417.

Zou, L., Ruan, F., Huang, M., *et al.* (2020). SARS-CoV-2 viral load in upper respiratory specimens of infected patients. *New England Journal of Medicine*, 382, 1177–1179. https://doi.org/10.1056/NEJMc2001737.

Chapter 3

General TCM View on Post-COVID-19 Syndrome (PCS)

Post-COVID-19 Syndrome from the TCM Point of View and the Evolving Understanding of COVID-19 in TCM

In the history of TCM, many pandemics have been recorded, and TCM was the only medical system existing in practice to help the people fight against the various conditions, thus a rich experience has been accumulated. In the first book to systematically discuss an infectious disease of "Cold Attack Disease", the acute stage was classified into the three yang pattern systems of *Taiyang*, *Yangming*, and *Shaoyang* with the corresponding treatment plans. The remaining unfavourable conditions are either the chronic continued sufferings due to the nature of the infections, or the poorly cared/treated cases prolonging into long struggles. These conditions are classified into the three *Yin* pattern systems of *Taiyin*, *Shaoyin*, and *Jueyin*. The conditions of the three *Yin* system are the post-acute stage of most infectious diseases which are later confirmed by the experience/observation of TCM in many pandemics. Hence, this three *Yin* pattern system is the timely tested precious experience that can be lent to TCM practice regarding PCS. Detailed subtypes/syndrome patterns and corresponding treatments using herbal formulas were listed. Those principles and treatment methods have been continuously used till now.

Similar to the "Cold Attack Disease", "Warm/Heat Diseases" were also systematically reviewed and summarised using a Four-Phase Syndrome Pattern system (*Wei-Qi-Ying-Xue* system) and the reaction was discussed as well.

According to those sources, the post-acute illness was mainly caused in three ways: the residual pathogen continuing its damage but at a very minimum level; the overconsumption of our defensive system and the weakness of the defensive *Qi* as a result of the reaction to the invasion; and the depletion of nutrition/materials for balancing the whole body's system, which is the *Yin Deficiency.*

Learning from the ancient theory and experience, it is easy to find the similarity between the numerous pandemics caused by invasion of external factors. The SARS-II virus spread through air and through contact to enter the human body, which is exactly what is described as an external pathogenic factor, although the nature of the SARS-II virus could be explained by many scholars in their own understanding. The three key characteristics of "external", "pathogenic", and "infectious" were all agreed upon. Popular ideas of defining the virus as per TCM concepts include *Cold-Damp*, *Wind-Cold*, *plague Qi*, *damp-plague*, and *damp-heat-toxic* hypotheses. The *cold-dampness* hypothesis is mainly based on its character of being worse in the winter season, and it is true that the worldwide epidemic peaks were worst in the winter season. The *plague-toxic* hypothesis gives a good rationalisation of its direct damage to the internal organ of the lung (pneumonia) which is different compared to most other infections starting from the upper respiratory tracts. The *heat-damp* hypothesis focuses more on its course which is longer than the usual flu, and this characteristic is considered to be the stubborn feature of the illness.

From ancient experience, whenever an infectious disease lasts longer than usual, it increases the consumption of *Qi* in general, which supports the *defensive Qi (Wei-Qi)* hypothesis, the over consumption then will lead to fatigue and exhaustion. Information indicates that COVID-19 is showing this correlation between the long course of the disease and fatigue afterwards.

Experience also suggests that if the pathogen in the lung is cleared but breathlessness and cough remain, it is most likely due to the pathological response or the disrupted function of the lung, which is the main site of infection and defence response. Along with the weakened lung, allowing the waste to stay in the body will eventually lead to *phlegm* accumulation. If the cough is not accompanied by phlegm or sputum, the damage is of the opposite nature in which the lung failed to retain body fluid to keep it moistened. This in TCM is the *Yin Deficiency* of the *Lung*.

Loss of smell or taste is commonly explained to be the result of the channel in the head and the brain being smudged by dampness. This is another reason why dampness appears in several hypotheses.

The mental and emotional impairments in PCS were much deeper changes caused by the severe interruption to the functioning of the internal organs, which leads to the abnormal flow of *Qi*. Furthermore, the liver function is exhausted due to the high demand for exertion required to keep *Qi* flow in order.

Common Syndrome Patterns of TCM Relevant to Post-COVID-19 Syndrome

Lung Qi/Yin Deficiency

The damage of the lung system in TCM is a straightforward consideration because the acute stage of COVID-19 illness mainly takes place in the respiratory system, which is the domain of the *Lung* system in TCM. The prolonged battling consumes/exhausts the whole system eventually, and this exhaustion in TCM is understood to be the lack of essential *Qi* to maintain its functions of breath and defence of the airway, which is manifested as shallow breathing or breathlessness when carrying out daily routines. While the longer than normal duration of the normal immune response indicates a lack of regulation and resting/repairing mechanism, a typical imbalance in TCM, where the *Yin* is failing to restrain the *Yang* representing the fighting force. The *Yin* Deficiency results in the aftermath of all febrile diseases, which are characterised by high temperature, or the later stage of hyper functional diseases, such as hyperthyroidism.

The key characteristic of *Lung Qi Deficiency* is the shortness of breath, increased sweating (spontaneous sweating), frequent relapse of common-cold-like symptoms like sneezing and sore throat, and easily becoming exhausted.

The characteristic of *Lung Yin Deficiency* is dry cough, itchy/ticklish throat, night sweating, hot sensation during night/hot flushes, a red tongue with little coating/peeled coating, and a rapid thin pulse.

The general treatment plan is straightforward, tonifying the *Qi* and *Yin* in the *Lung*.

Acupuncture points: LU2, LU9, RN6, ST36, BL13.

Tonifying methods in needling: Acupressure could be taught to patients to enable them to apply the same at home.

The LU2 and LU9 are the two acupuncture points listed in ancient classics for making the *Lung* channel and *Lung* organ stronger; therefore, they should be used for all weakness in the *Lung* System, from *Qi Deficiency* to *Yin Deficiency*. BL13 is the back-shu point of the Lung with direct effect over the lung system. However, this point could not be used in acupressure by the patients at home. RN6 and ST36 are the common supporting acupuncture points for all weakness, particular *Qi*, and *blood Deficiency*. RN6 is the "sea of *Qi*" which indicates that the ancient TCM practitioners approached this point for mobilising the *Qi* from storage. ST36 is the point with great influence on the production of *Qi* resulting from digestion of food.

For Lung Qi Deficiency

TCM herbal formula A: Yu Ping Feng San (Jade Screen formula) (WEI Yilin (1345) Shi Yi De Xiao Fang, Generations Collection of Effective Herbal Formulas).

Herbal ingredients: Huang Qi, Bai Zhu, Fang Feng.

The formula is designed to improve the *defensive Qi* to form a solid protection front line to fend away potential invasion of the body. Huang Qi is the main ingredient for its power of enhancing the *Qi* in the *Lung* and *Spleen*. Bai Zhu can generate more *Qi* from the *Spleen*, and the *Qi* generated should be directed to the body surface which needs Fang Feng to guide the *Qi* to join the *defensive Qi*.

TCM herbal formula B: Bao Yuan Tang (LUO Fu (1675) Gu Jin Yi Tong Fang Lun, Ancient and Current Medical Formulas).

Herbal ingredients: Ren Shen, Huang Qi, Rou Gui, Gan Cao.

Different from Yu Ping Feng San, this formula employs another way to help the *Lung Qi*. In this formula, the *lung Qi* is supported by the *original Qi (Yuan Qi)* by choosing Ren Shen for the general promotion of *Qi*, particularly through the root of the *Qi (yuan Qi)*. The Rou Gui is a typical ingredient for entering the *Kidney* to warm up the *Qi* there. When the *Qi* in the *Kidney* is stirred by Gui Zhi, it is ready to reach out. The out-moving *Qi* is then joined by the *Qi* generated by Huang Qi, to be transported up to the *Lung*.

For Lung Yin Deficiency

TCM herbal formula A: Bai He Gu Jing Tang (ZHOU Zhi Qian (1774) Zhou Shen Zhai Yi Shu, Manuscripts Left by Zhou Shun Zhai).

Herbal ingredients: Bai He, Shu Di Huang, Sheng Di Huang, Dang Gui, Bei Mu, Mai Dong, Bai Shao, Jie Geng, Xuan Shen, Gan Cao.

This formula is the main prescription for all conditions of *Lung Yin* and *Fluid Deficiency*, after infection/fever or chronic damages in the *Lung*. Bai He is the chief herb to nourish the Lung and easy off the cough. Shu Di Huang, Xuan Shen, Mai Men Dong, and Bai Shao are working together to tonify the *Yin* of the whole body. The *Yin* generated needs to reach the *Lung*, so Jie Geng leads to the *Lung*. Bei Mu is a very effective herb for dry cough, mostly chronic. Besides, Sheng Di Huang can prevent empty heat from flaring up causing further weakness of *Yin*. Dang Gui is a helper as it nourishes blood which is a key accompaniment of *Yin* material.

TCM herbal formula B: Yang Yin Qing Fei Tang (ZHENG Mei Jian (1838) Chong Lou Yu Yue, The Jade Key to Throat Problems).

Herbal ingredients: Sheng Di Huang, Mai Dong, Xuan Shen, Bei Mu, Bai Shao, Mu Dan Pi, Bo He.

This formula is a variation of the Bai He Gu Jin Tang. The chief herb is different, but the combination of all *Yin* tonics is the same. Mai Dong, Xuan Shen, Bai Shao, and Sheng Di Huang are the ingredients of the former formula playing the same roles of *Yin* boosting. Instead of Dang Gui, Mu Dan Pi is used here to support the *Yin*. Mu Dan Pi is cool in nature and would fit into the overall purpose of the *Yin* tonifying better. Bo He is the herb leading to the *Lung* and is also a cool-natured herb. This role belonged to Jin Jie in the previous formula.

Spleen Qi Deficiency

In many cases of COVID-19, the digestive system is affected in two ways: one is the virus infection in the digestive tract leading to nausea and diarrhoea and another is the intake of drugs, typically painkillers as recommended, which causes side effects in the digestive system. In TCM, the *Spleen* system is responsible of the whole digestive function from ingestion to discharge. The *Spleen* system is also the main supporter/supplier to the *Qi* to the whole body. The direct damage from both SARS-II virus and the ingestion of non-food can cause damage to *Spleen Qi*, and the excessive demand of *Qi* supply during the infection could also dry up the *Spleen* function, leading to the shortage of *Qi* in the supplier itself. When *Spleen Qi* is weak or exhausted, the *Qi* level of the whole body is lower, and the physical performance is affected by the lack of support in the muscles. From a biological point of view, the stress status of COVID-19 could trigger the adrenaline reaction, causing a redistribution of the blood supply, wherein the digestive system is the looser in this resource redirection. The steroid response is also detrimental to the digestive system. From TCM's classic of Cold Attack Discussion (Shang Han Lun), the importance of protecting the digestive function was emphasised. It was recognised that the interruption in the digestive/*Spleen* System could be the main pathological mechanism after an acute stage of infection; hence, good attention and care are required for recovery.

The characteristic of *Spleen Qi Deficiency* is the lack of physical strength, dizziness when standing up or blacking out, poor appetite and indigestion, and weight gain.

Treatment principle in TCM: Tonifying *Qi* in Spleen and Stomach.

Acupuncture points: ST36, SP3, RN12, BL20, BL21.

ST36 is one of the commonly used acupuncture points and is titled "general point" suggesting its broad application and effectiveness in boosting the *Qi* and *Blood* for maintaining good health and treating weakness. It is used for all digestive conditions and helps the spleen to generate more *Qi* from good digestion of food.

SP3 is the major tonifying point for the *Qi* and *Yang* aspect.

RN12 is the front-Mu point of the *Stomach*, with a direct influence on the organ of the stomach. The point is very often used to boost the function of all digestive functions and, therefore, to improve the *Qi* of the *Spleen* and *Stomach.*

BL20 is the Back-Shu point of the *Spleen* while BL21 is the point of the *Stomach.* The two are next to each other and used together to support each other in improving the conditions of the *Spleen* and *Stomach.* The *Spleen* and *Stomach* are paired organs and always work together. Based on this understanding, the treatment requires the two points to be used at the same time to maximise the clinical outcomes.

TCM herbal formula A: Bu Zhong Yi Qi Tang (LI Gao (1247) Nei Wai Shang Bian Huo Lun, Answering the Confusion of Internal and External Impairment).

Herbal ingredients: Huang Qi, Ren Shen, Bai Zhu, Dang Gui, Chen Pi, Sheng Ma, Chai Hu, Gan Cao.

This formula is an enhanced prescription based on the classic formula of Si Jun Zi Tang consisting of Ren Shen, Bai Zhu, Fu Ling, and Gan Cao. For the worst cases of *Spleen Qi Deficiency* and its further development into *Spleen Sinking* (failure to move upwards to reach the head), the powerful uplifting Huang Qi is employed. Huang can tonify *Qi* of the *Spleen* and *Lung*; however, its characteristic of lifting *Qi* or moving *Qi* upwards is much needed here for the dizziness. In this formula, Huang Qi requires a daily dosage of 30 g while others are just within the usual daily dosage. Sheng Ma and Chai Hu are called into the formula to confirm the upwards movement of *Qi.* Dang Gui is used to support the formula by warming up blood which is the carrier of *Qi* and Chen Pi is a general *Qi* movement promoter. Together, the formula is efficient in generating *Qi* for the *Spleen* and facilitating the upwards movement to support the head.

TCM herbal formula B: Liu Jun Zi Tang (YU Tuan (1515) Yi Xue Zheng Zhuan, The Authentic Records of Medicine).

Herbal ingredients: Ren Shen, Bai Zhu, Fu Ling, Gan Cao, Chen Pi, Ban Xia, Gan Jiang Da Zao.

Similar to the former formula, this formula is also based on the classic *Qi* tonifying one of Si Jun Zi Tang, with two added ingredients of Chen Pi and Ban Xia. Ren Shen is the chief herb for *Qi Deficiency.* The combination of Chen Pi and Ban Xia is commonly seen in many formulas for treating *Dampness* and *Phlegm* retention. When *Spleen Qi* is weak, untreated food nutrients might not be utilised and become dampness.

Heart Yin/Blood Deficiency

Circulatory system impairments are the second most reported issues in post-COVID-19 syndrome. From early reports, it was recognised that the SARS-II virus has an easy entrance to the heart and blood vessels through the ACE-II receptor which is part of the regulatory/feedback structure for maintaining normal blood pressure and circulation functions, and the ACE-II is on the surface of all circulatory system structures. This explained the main reason for the circulation failure and clots. In many cases, the damage after the acute stage remains a long-lasting problem in the heart and blood vessel.

When the damage is more on the *Yin* aspect of the *Heart* system in TCM which is for the stabilisation of circulation and mental calmness, *Heart Yin Deficiency* is established.

The *Heart* System in TCM has another major function which is maintaining of consciousness and mental activity, in the term of *Shen* (mind). When the supply of blood and nutrition to the brain in biological terms is damaged as a consequence of the circulatory insufficiency, the TCM *Heart Blood Deficiency* is the representing pattern.

The characteristics of *Heart Yin Deficiency* are palpitation, anxiety, hot flushes, panic attacks, and difficulty in falling asleep. A red tongue and a rapid/thin pulse are the TCM indicators.

The characteristics of *Heart Blood Deficiency* are poor memory, poor concentration, and poor sleep featuring shallow sleep, being easily woken up, and difficulty in falling asleep again. Some patients experience a feeling of confusion about the information received, while some others find a lack of mental stamina which is expressed as the loss of an idea in the middle of a task. The tongue is pale and the pulse is thin.

Treatment principle in TCM: Tonifying *Heart Yin* and *Blood*.

Acupuncture points: HT7, HT6, SP6, KI3, BL15, BL14, PC5, SI3.

HT7 is the Yuan/source point of the *Heart* channel. The classic application of this acu-point is to support the *Heart* system in TCM, including all deficiency conditions featured in poor mental performance to insomnia.

BL15 is the direct connecting point to the *Heart* organ, while BL14 is connected to the *Pericardium* which is part of the *Heart* system as a protective shield. When the two are used together, the treatment effect is stronger. SP6 is a major *Yin* point for its combined power with three *Yin* organs. HT6 is a supporting point for HT7. PC5 supports the *Heart* by providing better support in the *Pericardium*. SI3 is the source point on the *Small Intestine* which is the paired organ of the *Heart*.

TCM herbal formula A: Zhi Gan Cao Tang (ZHANG Ji (unknown publication year) Shang Han Lun, discussion on Cold Attack Diseases).

Herbal ingredients: Zhi Gan Cao, Ren Shen, Sheng Di Huang, E Jiao, Mai Men Dong, Huo Ma Ren, Gui Zhi, Sheng Jiang, Da Zao, rice wine.

The formula was the classic example of how the weak *Heart*, particularly weak *Heart Yin/Blood*, was treated. The *Yin* and blood tonifying herbs are lined up here for the main purpose, including Sheng Di Huang, E Jiao, Mai Men Dong, and Huo Ma Ren. The blood could not be produced without *Qi*, so Ren Shen, Zhi Gan Cao, and Da Zao are called in to provide crucial support. However, they still need a direction to go to the heart, which is indicated by Gui Zhi, Huo Ma Ren, and wine. The formula has shown its clinical effectiveness in managing anxiety and mental weakness.

TCM herbal formula B: Du Shu Wan (Book Readers' Pill) (WANG Ken Tang (1602) Zheng Zhi Zhun Sheng, The Standards of Syndrome and Treatment).

Herbal ingredients: Ren Shen, Yuan Zhi, Chang Pu, Tu Si Zi, Sheng Di Huang, Di Gu Pi, Wu Wei Zi, Suan Zao Ren, Chuan Xiong.

The formula is not well known and is not selected in most textbooks. Nevertheless, it fits the purpose of treating "brain fog" well. From its name, it is easy to figure out that the purpose of this formula is to maintain good mental capacity and efficiency especially for a person using their mental power for their daily job. The indication of the formula includes poor concentration, poor memory, lost thread during work, slow thinking, and day dreaming. The key ingredients are Suan Zao Ren, Tu Si Zi, Sheng Di Huang, and Wu Wei Zi for tonifying the *Blood* in the *Heart.* Ren Shen is used for supplying *Qi* to generate *Blood.* The pair of Yuan Zhi and Chang Pu is famous for calming and sharpening the Mind (mental power). Di Gu Pi in combination with Sheng Di Huang could prevent *Empty Heat* which is the main cause of sleeping difficulty. And Chuan Xiong is for the blood to move, preventing stagnation.

According to observations of the authors, this formula should be administrated in the afternoon and before bedtime. The formula shows a clear tranquilising effect and helps in sleeping. If used in the morning, it may influence daily performance.

Kidney Deficiency

Kidneys are susceptible to COVID-19 impairment because of the richness of the ACE-II receptor in their blood vessel-dominated structure. The *kidney* is essential in maintaining the balance of blood volume by controlling the total amount of body fluid. When this function is damaged, the most likely consequence is the increased retention of body fluid. In TCM, this is the *Kidney* system weakness/deficiency. The *Kidney* system in TCM is also the pivot of reproductive function providing the driving force of sexual activity, the basic condition of fertility, and maintaining the stable body condition of pregnancy. If the *Kidney* system is unstable, then related problems can occur. One of the TCM *Kidney* functions is unique or not known in biological medicine, which is the rooting or deep inhaling function to facilitate a very slow and deep breath. In TCM, the deep and slow breath is the most beneficial part of the breathing function as it can connect the chest to the lower abdomen forging a deep relaxation to aid sleep. This function is also damaged in many sufferers.

The characteristics of Kidney deficiency are general weakness, lack of libido, miscarriage, low back pain, difficulty in holding breath for demanding physical performance, frequent urination, and oedema in the ankle area.

Treatment principle in TCM: Tonifying Kidney.

Acupuncture points: KI3, KI6, KI7, SP6, RN4, BL23, BL52, LU7.

KI3, KI6, and KI7 are the three main points on the *Kidney* channel for all weaknesses. According to many practitioners, the combination of KI3 and KI6 is the best for *Kidney Yin Deficiency* as the KI6 is a master point of the *Yin Qiao* vessel bearing a nature of yin influence. The combination of KI3 and KI7 can benefit the *Kidney Yang.*

BL23 and BL52 are both located at the lumber spine particularly L2 level and directly above the kidney organ. The BL23 is therefore the back Shu point of the *Kidney* and the BL52 is the helper. RN4 is the front point of *Ming Men* (gate of life) which has been the main acu-point for all weaknesses related to the essence in the *Kidney.*

LU7 is used according to the five-element theory. The Lung is a Metal organ and Kidney a Water organ. Attuned to their organ, the lung channel is a metal channel, while the kidney channel is a water one.The relationship between the two is that Metal/Lung promotes Water/kidney, translating into organ system as the *Lung* promoting the *Kidney*. The LU7 is linked with KI6 for this promoting pathway.

TCM herbal formula: Liu Wei Di Huang Wan (QIAN Yi (1119) Xiao Er Yao Zheng Zhi Jue,The Simple Guidance of Children' Disease and Medicine).

Herbal ingredients: Shu Di Huang, Shan Yao, Shan Zu Yu, Fu Ling, Ze Xie, Mu Dan Pi.

Shu Di Huang is the chief herb in this formula and it tonifies the *Yin* in the *Kidney*. The dosage is usually 30 g per day. Shan Yao is the herb directed at the *Spleen* which is the main supplier of *Kidney Yin* from digesting food and generating quality nutrition for the Kidney. Shan Zhu Yu is a *Yin* nourisher for the *Liver.* The *Kidney*, *Spleen*, and *Liver* are all *Yin* organs sharing the foot channels, and they are joined at SP6. So, working on all three *Yin* organs can make the total effect stronger. The other three ingredients, Fu Ling, Ze Xie, and Mu Dan Pi, are the balancers of the first three ingredients. Ze Xie prevents the accumulation of water in the *Kidney*, Fu Ling is used for *Dampness* in the *Spleen*, and Mu Can Pin for keeping the liver free of stagnation. Together, the formula can work smoothly and focus all effort on the *Kidney.*

Liver Qi Stagnation

Liver damage is frequently mentioned in the studies of post-COVID-19 conditions. In biological medicine, liver damage is considered to be caused by both the viral infection and as a side effect of drugs since liver is the main organ for detoxification/decomposing of the toxic materials from the blood stream. The extra burden could pile up to a high level of damage. TCM understands this damage in a similar way. The impairment in TCM is the result of accumulation of too much waste in the body, mostly the dampness or phlegm. Eventually, the accumulation will lead to a congestion in the liver system, forming a pattern of stagnation in the liver.

The TCM *Liver* system helps the emotional and physical coordination of the various parts/organs there by upholding orderly life activities. This could be described as regulating mental/emotional aspects, regulating the digestion, and the *Qi* and *Blood* flow. When patients of COVID-19 were treated in a hospital, or at home, their life activities were altered by the external environment and the illness itself was stressful, in addition, to there being no cure and being isolated from usual social connections. Thereafter, bad mental moments accumulated which eventually led to the *Liver* being overstretched to an abnormal level. This is most recognised in TCM as *Liver Qi Stagnation* in its early stages and could well be developing into a severe form of *Liver Qi & Blood Stasis*. This is the status of a patient who has recovered physically but not mentally and emotionally.

The characteristics of *Liver Stagnation* are emotional fluctuation, irritability, chest tightness, irregular bowel movement, irregular menstruation or amenorrhea (missing menses), tension headache triggered by emotion, lost interest in many previously loved activities, and wiry/taut pulse.

Treatment principle in TCM: Promoting *Qi* flow and soothing the *Liver.*

Acupuncture points: LR3, GB34, LI4, PC6, Yin Tang, DU20.

LR3 is one of the most used acupuncture points in daily practice and is the main acu-point for *Liver Qi Stagnation*. LR3 is the source point of the Liver channel, and thus can drive the *Qi* and *Blood* flow with its power/source. Needling LR3 with a tonifying method could release the energy of the channel to quicken the *Qi* and blood flow, and eventually eliminate the stagnation. LR3 could be used in combination with LI4, which forms the famous “four gates” point combination. When four gates are opened, free movement is then easy to reestablished.

LR3 is also commonly used with GB34. The GB channel is the one to inject *Qi* and *Blood* into the *Liver* channel at the foot. If the GB channel can pass its normal flow into the *Liver* channel, the *Qi* and *Blood* flow in the liver channel is naturally faster. The GB34 is the right one to pair with LR3 for this purpose.

PC6 and Yin Tang are for the calming down of emotions, particularly anger or frustration. They are useful to relieve symptoms but not help the overall *Liver* distress.

DU20 is the point of the DU channel; however, it is also the ending point of the *Liver* channel's internal pathway. Hence, DU20 is providing an upper opening for *Liver Qi* to move. According to the experience of the authors, this acu-point is one of the most popular ones for stress management among all patients.

TCM herbal formula A: Si Ni San (ZHANG Ji (unknown publication year) Shang Han Lun, Discussion on Cold Attack Diseases).

Herbal ingredients: Chai Hu, Zhi Ke (Qiao), Bai Shao, Gan Cao.

Chai Hu is the main ingredient of the formula, and it promotes the flow of *Qi*, releasing tension in the *Liver* by spreading the *Qi* upwards and outwards. Zhi Ke is the deputy in exercising the *Qi* spreading function, but it is lightly downwards directed. The two form a beautiful partnership in moving the *Qi* in the *Liver* to all directions. Bai Shao is a *Yin* protector used here to prevent any possible damage of the Liver from other herbs, because the two main herbs could potentially dry up the *Yin* or Blood. Gan Cao is the harmoniser of all herbs.

TCM herbal formula B: Chai Hu Shu Gan San (YE Wen Ling (1535) Yi Xue Tong Zhi, General Principles of Medicine).

Herbal ingredients: Chai Hu, Zhi Ke (Qiao), Bai Shao, Gan Cao (Same in formula A); Xiang Fu, Chuan Xiong, Chen Pi.

From long clinical practice, many practitioners found that Si Ni San might not be suitable in the longer term. Its effects on mental distress are not enough. Afterwards, an enhanced formula was introduced. This formula has all four ingredients from Si Ni San, plus a pair of herbs, Xiang Fu and Chuan Xiong. Xiang Fu works on *Qi* movement in the chest and coastal area where the *Liver Qi* is most active, and Chuan Xiong works on blood movement. The two together can promote *Qi* and *Blood* movement in a mutually supportive way. Hence, the overall *Qi*-spreading function of the formula is much better. Chen Pi is also a good supportive herb in the formula.

Damp-Phlegm accumulation

During an acute COVID-19 episode, the body function changes could lead to significant adjustment in the hormones and metabolism. There are reports of diabetes and related changes. Corresponding to such observation, TCM considers that the abnormality in metabolism is the result of dampness invasion of the body. This is drawn from the consensus from Wuhan, China, in 2020 where the initial cases of COVID-19 were reported and the area is well known for the environmental character of damp-heat in summer and damp-cold in winter when most cases were reported. Dampness was reflected as part of the nature of the new virus. The key identification of dampness is its lingering clinical manifestation of fever and blockage of the chest which is much longer than a flu in most cases. Accordingly, it is understood that the dampness was brought into the body when the illness started.

Dampness is difficult to clear up by our own defensive function or helped by Chinese herbs or acupuncture. This has been agreed upon since the era of Internal Classic. The reason is that dampness is like fog and can spread slowly into every part of the body, from the upper to lower part, from skin to deep located internal organs. The dampness is a *Yin* pathogenic factor with little or no moving power inside. Its ability to be widespread is still unclear, but what has become clear is that the task to remove the dampness requires time and patience.

On the other hand, the dampness could be generated inside the body when some organ systems are functioning poorly. The *Spleen*'s weakness could lead to the nutrients being static, not arriving to the organs and tissues in need. The static nutrients then become unused and wasted, finally turning into dampness. The dysfunction of the *Kidney* could also allow too much unwanted water to stay inside our body, in the form of either water retention or dampness. Heavy food or rich food which is full of nutrients and fat could be a major trigger factor for internally generated dampness as it demands high performance of the *Spleen* to digest and distribute it to the right place for the right purpose. When the rich food is constantly oversupplied, the system will fail to utilise it, and the surplus will become a burden and go to waste. The surplus could stay within the digestive system in the form of food retention and could also be concealed in the whole body as dampness.

Phlegm is a condensed form of water or dampness. It could be the mucus coming out of the chest when a cough occurs, which is the visible form of phlegm. It can also be hiding inside organs and channels in the form of lumps without pain and colour change. This lump could be retained anywhere. Regarding the fibrosis in the lungs caused by the deposit of fibres, TCM understands that the process is driven by the phlegm in the lungs becoming solid and hard to remove. *Phlegm* is stubborn, meaning more difficult than dampness to remove.

The characteristics of dampness/phlegm are lack of a fresh feeling in the head, face, and all over (like the feeling of waking up but not cleaning the face and not stretching the body); heaviness or tightness in the body; aching in the morning and less in the afternoon; poor appetite; loose stools; increased mucus in the mouth; a greasy tongue coating, and a loss of smell and taste.

The characteristics of phlegm are large amounts of phlegm introduced with cough, chest fullness, nodules, lumps, mental confusion, and a greasy coating.

Treatment principle in TCM: Resolving the dampness and phlegm.

Acupuncture points: SP9, ST40, ST25, ST28, RN9, SJ6, BL22.

SP9 is the most quoted acu-point for clearing dampness. It is located on the *Spleen* channel, making it the point for keeping the *Spleen* function of transporting body fluid in a good status.

ST40 is the number one point for *Phlegm*, both visible and invisible. The two always work together well.

ST25 and ST28 provide a way for the *Dampness/Phlegm* to be discharged through the *Large Intestine*, the biggest discharging organ. RN9 is the switching acu-point on the *Small Intestine* for its function of separating the water parts in its content from the solid parts and sending the water directly to the *Bladder* for discharge.

RN9 could increase the discharge of water from the *Bladder*. SJ6 and BL22 both stimulate *San Jiao* (Triple Burner, Triple Energiser) to allow water to pass through it easily, not retaining it inside the body.

TCM herbal formula A: Er Chen Wan (Royal Medical Office, Song Dynasty (1078) Tai Ping Hui Min He Ji Ju Fang, Formulas of Great Peace and People's Benefit Pharmacy).

Herbal ingredients: Ban Xia, Chen Pi, Fu Ling, Gan Cao.

Er Chen Wan is the basic formula for all other *Damp/Phlegm* clearing formulas. The principal herb is Ban Xia. It can resolve *Phlegm* and *Dampness* from the *Lung* and *Spleen*, on both visible *Phlegm*, which can be coughed out as sputum, and invisible *Phlegm* in the form of confusion in the mind and lack of understanding. Chen Pi moves *Qi* around, and therefore does not lead to the retention of *Dampness* or *Phlegm*. Fu Ling promotes the discharge of extra water/body fluids by way of urination. The three herbs work in different ways to clear the Dampness/Phlegm.

TCM herbal formula B: San Zi Yang Qin Tang (Tamba Motoyasu 丹波元坚 (1800) Jie Xiao Fang — All Effective Formulas, recorded in Za Bing Guang Yao, Extended Briefing of Misalliance Diseases).

Herbal ingredients: Su Zi, Bai Jie Zi, Lai Fu Zi.

This formula explores the combination of three seeds for the purpose of reducing the phlegm/mucus in the *Lung* and then relieving breathing difficulty. Su Zi is the one entering the *Lung* and sending the *Lung Qi* downwards. It is the chief herb for breathlessness and asthma. Bai Jie Zi is hot in nature and is used for heating the mucus and promoting mobility. *Phlegm* is a *Yin*-natured material and it is sticky and holds onto its position. Bai Jie Zi can make it move, allowing it to reach the windpipe to be coughed out. Lai Fu Zi addresses the source of water, which is the *Middle Jiao*. When the *Middle Jiao* works in the normal condition, the production of useful body fluid is increased and the useless water is minimised.

TCM herbal formula C: Wu Ling San (ZHANG Ji (unknown publication-year) Shang Han Lun. Discussion on Cold Attack Diseases).

Herbal ingredients: Fu Ling, Zhu Ling, Ze Xie, Bai Zhu, Gui Zhi.

Wu Ling San is a classic formula for all water and dampness retention mild cases. Among the five ingredients, three are shown to increase urination, causing a diuretic effect. They are Fu Ling, Zhu Ling, and Ze Xie. Bai Zhu is the herb that can dry up the *Dampness* from the source, which is the digestive system, although TCM views it as the *Spleen* system. Gui Zhi is hot in nature and used here for leading the other herbs to the areas where they should be working, along with warming up the dampness or water, allowing changes to happen.

TCM herbal formula D: Er Miao San (ZHU Zhen Hen (1347) Dan Xi Xin Fa, Mind Understanding of Medicine by Dan Xi).

Herbal ingredients: Cang Zhu, Huang Bai.

Er. Miao San is the best, concise example of how *Damp-Heat* could be treated. Cang Zhu is hot and drying. It is used here to dry up the *Dampness.* Huang Bai is cold and dry. It can cancel the hot nature of Cang Zhu and help Cang Zhu to dry the dampness. The dosage is always the key as an overall cold nature of the formula should be maintained for the treatment of *Damp-Heat.* Therefore, Huang Bai should always be the larger partner in the formulas.

Principle of Treatment Plan, the Priority, and Treatment Focus Point

Post-COVID-19 syndrome is a chronic condition, and the condition is usually stable for a while. In TCM, the condition is considered more or less in a deadlock position. The pathogenic factor, SARS-II virus, is cleared from the blood stream. Nonetheless, a secondary pathology remains and will not go away quickly or easily. There are many treatment strategies used by practitioners in dealing with a situation like the one in discussion. From very ancient times, the protection of *Stomach Qi*, the restoring of *Qi* and *Yin* (mostly lung), and promoting the discharge of dampness and *Phlegm* were all discussed according to clinical observations. Among all mentioned doctrines, the common point in terms of management of treatments is that the treatment plan should be maintained for around 4 weeks, namely, a treatment course of 4 weeks. And another agreed point is to avoid heavy intake of herbs, or powerful acupuncture stimulations, to protect the impaired or exhausted organs from further damage. Heavy intake of medicine and herbs can easily further damage the digestive system. Although no clear signs of existing damage could be found, the protection of the *Spleen* and *Stomach* is still a principle applicable to most cases.

Many may argue that the common methods are to tonify the systems and should be considered for improving the functions of those organs. Indeed, those tonifying herbs are less likely to cause new damage compared to those powerful *Heat-Clearing* and *Stasis-Removing* herbs. Nevertheless, before they work on the tonifying action, they are still required to be accepted by the digestive system, and most ancient practitioners had made great contributions in mitigating this potential problem. For example, their herbal formulas included some herbs to prevent the problems that might be caused by the main tonifying herbs.

Another point worth mentioning is that fluctuation of the situation is common. With no new condition or pattern added, the treatment principle and the acupuncture and herbal treatment prescription should be consistent.

In terms of acupuncture treatment, to avoid heavy intervention, two precautions should be put in place. The first one is not relying on some major powerful acu-points. They can produce strong reactions and achieve visible changes. However, they could move the *Qi* and *Blood* too much, and the strong reaction to needling can then consume the *Qi* and *Blood*. This could be managed with more acu-points to be used, each with less intensive stimulation. Another way to manage the level of intervention is to avoid repeating the same acupuncture points too many times. Using alternative acu-points is the strategy. Many acupuncture points share the same action when they are on the same channel. For example, PC3, PC5, PC6, and PC7 are all similar in their clinical applications, for clearing *Heat* from the *Heart*, calming down the mind (*Shen* in TCM), relieving heart pain, treating nausea, etc. If PC6 is used several times, it could be replaced by PC5 or PC3. The total treatment result from this needling session might not be as powerful, but it allows the channel and the organ to response differently, and that can minimise the overconsumption of the *Qi* and *Blood* in the channel and corresponding organs.

TCM Lifestyle Advice

Food advice principles

Whenever the treatment of acupuncture and/or TCM herbal medicine is given to patients, the main therapeutic intervention is applied to the patients. Then, food advice should be in line with the principle of treatment. The principle of treatment should be according to syndrome pattern and the diseases.

In this context, the disease aspect is relatively simpler. The post-infection stage is a recovery stage, not a new disease. In this stage, the ancient discussion was focused on two main issues: The first was that the damaged digestive system might be overloaded if too much nutritious food containing too much meat and fat is ingested; therefore, balanced and easily digestible foods are advised. The second is about too much food in one nature, particularly hot-natured food. For example, hot spicy food has the capacity to wake up the appetite allowing for the ingestion of more food, but it can flame up the residual heat in the acute stage when the *Yin*/blood is weak.

Therefore, in terms of food advice corresponding to disease, one needs to stick to the principle of healthy eating with a balanced structure of all nutrition and avoiding stimulants in food, such as hot spicy food, strong alcohol, fermented foods, and cheeses of hard textures.

Regarding food, according to syndrome pattern differentiation, the deficiency patterns require good diet more than excess patterns. The reason is that quality food contains the essential elements to generate *Blood* and *Yin*, and *Qi* as well.

For *Blood Deficiency*, well-stewed meats of all kinds are extremely beneficial. They provide the dense/heavy food *Qi*, to be transformed by the *Spleen* into nutrient *Qi*, which can then be converted into blood. For *Yin Deficiency*, white meats, chicken, fishes, and duck are the source of yin nutrient for the *Spleen* to take into the body.

For *Qi* and *Yang Deficiency*, warm-natured food is advised. A balanced food structure containing eggs, soft cheeses, and herbs like ginger powder and cinnamon is advised. Mushrooms are very important if the patient does not enjoy vegetables.

However, when no TCM diagnosis is established, the general principle of TCM lifestyle should be followed, which is very similar to what is recommended by the National Health Service (NHS). Firstly, COVID-19 is a very consumptive disease and the damage left in the body will need a higher than normal supply of key nutrients to produce new tissue, replenish the lost antibodies and immune cells, and rebalance the different parts of the body after the stress response. The key nutrients are proteins and vitamins, plus essential oils, which can only be directly supplied from foods containing them (NHS, 2022). When a good balance of food or meat, nuts/seeds, vegetable, and fruits is served, there is no need for the extra supply of food. For those who are vegetarians or vegans, the supply of protein should be well adjusted by increasing the number of nuts and seeds discussed below which contain high-quality proteins and essential oils.

Food supplement, vitamins, and minerals

Vitamins are essential nutrition for all human life functions. Generally, when a person has a balanced diet and is in a healthy condition, there is no need to take extra vitamins.

During an infection, the body is mobilised to support the defensive system or immune function, and there is increased demand for clearing the harmful materials, which will have a higher demand for vitamins and minerals. The national guideline from the NICE supports this practice.

Nuts and fruits for restoring body functions

Nuts are a rich source of proteins and minerals. They contain a full spectrum of nutrients to meet the needs of a new life (a sprout of plant) from its germinating onwards. This is similar to the full nutrients in an egg being enough for a new animal life. Based on such observations, TCM recorded many nuts and seeds as being very nutritious and can tonify the essence in the *Kidney*, *Spleen*, and other important organs. One of the best examples is that the walnut is considered to be a good tonifying food for the *Kidney*, and peanut for the *Spleen*, almond for the *Lung*, pistachio for the *Liver*, and pine nut for the *Heart.*

Hazel nut, chestnut, sunflower seeds, and pumpkin seeds are all good sources of nutrition and good for supplying a broad spectrum of nutrition.

Blended nuts are more useful than a single nut in TCM nutrition. Although all nuts are well balanced for the needs of plants life, none of them could provide all the nutrients a human life needs on its own, for the reason that a human life's yin/yang balance is different to a plant. However, they are complementary to each other, and when nuts are blended, they can meet all nutrition needs of human life, and reach a higher level of balanced supply of food nutrients. In biological terms, blended nuts will provide proteins offering the complete essential amino acids and essential lipids required along with minerals.

Many people are not sure if they can take nuts because of their concern of the high percentage of oil contained in nuts, particularly among those suffering from cardiovascular diseases or hyperlipidaemia. Nevertheless, all research suggests that the intake of nuts would not cause a higher risk of raised blood sugar and cholesterol.

Hemp seed has been the new topic in the last 20 years. It is not a TCM food but is of great interest for many patients suffering from ME, MS, and fibromyalgia. The potential benefits range from energy endurance, mood enhancement, and relieving depression, pain, and inflammation. In TCM, a similar seed called Huo-Ma-Ren (cannabis seed) is used for treating *Blood Deficiency* and to support the *Heart* for poor memory and poor concentration and to support the *Large Intestine for* constipation. The problem is the cannabis seed is limited to medicinal use. So, it cannot be suggested as a food supplement. This is because the cannabis seed contains a tiny amount of THC, a psychoactive compound which is still subject to legal review for broad use. Although hemp seeds contain a trace amount of THC, they are fully legal for food purposes. From the experience of patients suffering from ME and many other chronic illnesses, it is clear that a small amount of the seed every day (10–20 g) blended into other nuts or seeds will bring benefit.

There are many other seeds trending now as a supply of good plant-sourced oils which are rich in unsaturated oil and good-quality proteins. Both are essential for repair of tissue damage. Therefore, adding those seeds into food will help recovery. The seeds in this range include sesame seeds, chia seeds, flax seeds, and sunflower seeds. Generally, their total amount needs to be controlled to within 50 g a day, and when they are added other sources of calorie-rich food should be reduced accordingly to avoid putting on weight unnecessarily.

Fruits are the best source of some vitamins and fibres. The information regarding healthy eating of fruits is available in most public health sources. In TCM, some fruits possess therapeutic values and should be consumed according to the health conditions.

Plums are cool in nature in TCM and are one of the best fruits to keep bowels functioning well. If constipation happens due to a lack of body fluid or lack of exercise, 2–3 portions of fresh or tinned plum a day will be enough for most patients. It is safe to continue for a few weeks.

Contrary to plums, steamed apples, pomegranates, and papayas are the three fruits for improving the function of the digestive system and relieving diarrhoea.

For a dry cough, steamed/boiled pears, pomegranates, Sharon fruits, and boiled orange juice could be mixed to produce a cough-relieving juice. It should be bottled and sipped frequently or when a tickling feeling in the throat triggers a cough.

Tea and coffee in consideration

Tea and coffee are both daily stimulants and considered to be essential to many people's daily life. They can help people refresh their mind in the morning and stay alert during the day.

When brain fog is a symptom of patients, an instinctive reaction is to use tea or coffee to sharpen the mind. However, many patients have tried this method and failed.

In TCM, tea and coffee are both yang-bursting materials causing the yang/*Qi* to be released from the internal organ for a temporary high performance. If the stimulants are used in the correct way and incorporated with other lifestyle measures, they could help with the generation of *Qi* and *yang*.

The common recommendation in TCM is that the tea and coffee should be consumed when the *Yang* is rising, or when a further stretching of *Yang* is needed. This is a suggestion of morning or midday. They should be served with some food which can provide energy quickly, for example, snacks, because when the yang is lifted by the tea/coffee, it needs the *Qi* to follow. Otherwise, the *Yang* is an empty *Yang* without root, and exhaustion happens very quickly.

TCM mind–body exercises (Taiji, Yoga, Qigong, Dao Yin, physical exercise)

Because mental and emotional suffering is so common among post-COVID-19 syndrome patients, the need for whole-system care is important. Treatment using acupuncture and herbs is essential, but self-improvement is equally important, along with social and family support. Among self-improvement, mind–body exercise in TCM has an advantage and was proven to be effective.

Mind and body exercises connect the three energy centres known as Dantian, using the energy of air-*Clear Qi* in TCM for the energy exchange. When the connection is maintained, the mind is established because of the lower-energy centre which has a greater power of rooting the mind and spirits into the essence stored in the lower Dantian. Depending on the clinical need, if a patient has a weak mind, leading to depression, and a lack of confidence, then the middle centre that supplies *Qi* and *Blood* to the whole body could become the centre point of focus and attention to provide the support required for the mind (Deadman, 2016).

Individualised exercise prescription is the key for success. Taiji or Qigong can be performed for the same. Generally speaking, for anxiety, restlessness, insomnia, and anger, the focus should be on the centre at the lower Dantian. When the symptoms are poor concentration, poor understanding and planning, and lack of confidence, the centre of connection is the middle Dantian. When the emotional fluctuation and dizziness are the main symptoms, the arms and legs should be used to assist the communication.

Taiji

Taiji has three levels, the physical moves, the combined physical moves and breathing techniques, and the highest level of mind leading the breath and body. It is impossible for a beginner who starts the exercise to do the second level and third level, although they might be most beneficial.

It is always advised to start with a group of people under the guidance of an experienced coach/teacher. Available evidence suggests that group exercise could maximise the effect of improving functions of the lung and heart, and also relieve mental illness from depression to anxiety.

If the very basic 24 moves style of Taiji could be learnt and performed in a group within 3 months, the physical movements will help the channels to open and this will reduce liver *Qi* stagnation a great deal.

Qigong

For those who cannot join a Taiji group or find it difficult to physically learn and perform the movement due to extreme weakness, Qigong would suit the purpose, as the standing and sitting styles are well developed for modern life.

Again, to start Qigong, a tutor/instructor will be essential, although many could learn it from online courses. The exercise of Qigong at the beginner stage requires one to fix the attention on one point to clear the mind of any other mental activities. This is a common method used by most people. To choose this fixing point, the principles mentioned above apply. For restlessness, the lower abdomen is the obvious focus point, while for a weak mind, the middle-chest Dantian is the point. If the mental problem has no fixed pattern, then the palm centres can fix the mind with gentle circular movements.

Overall, whatever the Qigong style is chosen, one must make sure that the finishing point is relaxed and all fixing points should be released, allowing the body to re-adjust the *Qi* and *Blood* to daily life and a good working condition.

Self-massage according to channels (*Dao Yin*)

Self-massage in TCM is not applying touch over the body in circular motion. It requires knowledge of channels and *Qi/Blood* moving directions. Based on an understanding of the direction of *Qi* and *Blood* movement, the patients then warm up the palms and get the mind fixed on the palm, touching and rubbing the body part according to the *Qi* and *Blood* direction.

This produces two therapeutic effects: The focusing of the mind leads to clearing the mind of disturbing ideas and the physical sliding/touching over the body part can relax the muscles and the nerves controlling them. Together, a relaxing and regenerating effect can be achieved.

Physical exercise

The principle of exercise is about physically promoting the *Qi* and *Blood* flow, but not causing them to become exhausted. *Qi* and *Blood* only maintain their normal function through movement. Static *Q*i and *Blood* will lose their energy and becoming useless *Qi* needing to be exhaled. Physical exercise applies force to let the *Qi* and *Blood* move. Additionally, new blood can be converted from *Nutrient Qi* in circulation.

For *Yang Deficiency* sufferers, the best physical exercise will be short bursting-type exercise, which requires using 70–80% of physical strength for about 2–3 min. Then, one should rest for 3 min and repeat this until the heartbeat is fast but not wild, and the body is feeling hot, prompting sweating to start. For a patient of yang deficiency, it might only take three such repeated exercises to reach the requirement. The exercise could be climbing upstairs, fast bicycling in the gym or on a cycling machine, running, standing up/squats, etc. This is often in the categories of anaerobic exercise. It digs into our storage of energy without the use of air/oxygen, and consequently it changes the way the energy is released and fundamentally builds strong bones and muscles for *Qi* and *Blood.*

For the patients of *Qi*, *Yin*, and *Blood Deficiency*, gentle and enduring exercise will be more useful. This allows the body to adjust the physical capacity and mobilise the *Qi* from those organs not damaged yet to support the whole body. Walking is a typical example. The exercise is usually called aerobic exercise, which improves the function of respiratory system/lung and the circulation system, and energy efficiency.

With regard to excess syndrome patterns like *Liver Qi Stagnation* and *Damp/Phlegm* patterns, expansive, shape-forming exercises will be most appropriate. Opening the tissues allows every part of the body to yield its tension. In TCM, this allows the free flow of *Qi* and *Blood*. Stagnation is cleared due to the encouragement of fluid mobilisation. For *Dampness*, expansion of the tissue drives *Yang* and *Qi* to every edge, leaving nowhere for the *Dampness* to go. When *Yang* can warm the body up, the dampness can then be heated to move and mobilise, allowing the *San Jiao* to promote it to the *Lung*, *Spleen*, or *Kidney*, who could then convert the waste to disposable water, and discharge it. When doing this type of exercise, it is essential to join a training course under guidance in addition to paying attention to the gradual progress.

Reference

Deadman, P. (2016). *Live Well Live Long: Teachings from the Chinese Nourishment of Life Tradition.* Journal of Chinese Medicine Limited.

NHS (National Health Service) (2022). Covid recovery-eating well. NHS-Your COVID Recovery. Available at: https://www.yourcovidrecovery.nhs.uk/your-wellbeing/eating-well/#:~:text=Meat%2C%20fish%2C%20eggs%2C%20beans,and%20maintains%20your%20muscle%20strength.&text=Aim%20for%20three%20thumb%2Dsized,soya%20milk%20fortified%20with%20calcium.

Chapter 4

Impaired Lung System (Interstitial Lung Disease, ILD)

Post-COVID-19 Interstitial Lung Disease (ILD)

The primary organ/tissue of COVID-19 infection is the lung and respiratory system. During the acute attack phase, mild to severe inflammation happens in the lung, although this is not limited to the lung and can include the bronchi, throat, and nose, and usually develops into the whole respiratory system.

The SARS-CoV-2 virus enters primarily into the alveolar epithelial cells, which triggers a series of immune responses locally that are supported by the whole immune system. The immune response is exhibited in the presenting of macrophage infiltration and induces a localised hyper-inflammatory cell state that causes the damage in the lungs in the acute stage. These are then followed by increased quantity of mesenchymal cells plus fibroblasts in the lungs and the space among the cells is filled with fibres as repair of the tissue takes place (Rendeiro *et al.*, 2021).

Another problem in COVID-19 is that the virus somehow changed the modelling in the lung epithelial during and after infection, which leads to failure of lung tissue regeneration which is essential to replace the damaged cell/tissue. Instead of normally shaped functional tissues, fibroblasts are increased, thus stimulating the production of more fibres which is counterproductive to the functioning of the lungs' gas exchange. This was not observed with bacterial pneumonia.

The combination of cell damage, failed replacement, newly deposited fibres, and congestion with immune cells in the local area becomes a causative factor permitting a barrier within the tissue between inhaled air and the blood flow, creating a foundation, a thicker and impermeable layer. Consequently, the gas exchange function becomes lowered. This could result in acute respiratory distress syndrome, requiring oxygen supply and ICU treatment and care.

When the acute stage is over, a person has the potential to return to their normal constitution and function of the lungs, if full recovery succeeds. However, many will continually suffer because of normal lung cell loss and increased fibrous tissue formation. The main function of the lungs, the gas exchange, is weakened. The oxygen supply is not ideal; thus, the patients are struggling, particularly when high demands of oxygen are made during physical or immense mental activities. During this stage, the most common symptoms of fatigue, breathlessness, cough, and chest tightness, are all a consequence of weakened lungs, in the context of academic discussion with regard to ILD.

Since this pandemic is a relatively new clinical condition, there has not been sufficient time and opportunity to study how long the normal lung structure takes to be rebuilt, or if this extra fibre will eventually be replaced by functional alveolar epithelial cells and would allow for the easy exchange of oxygen and carbon dioxide, the diffusing capacity of the lungs (DLCO). Therefore, proactive approaches are considered by the authors to be very important, in the hope of early treatment calming down the hyper-immuno-reaction, "cytokine storm", allowing for a restructuring without the influence of the virus or hyper status of the immune system.

In this context, acute respiratory distress syndrome (RDS) (acute lung failure) is not discussed since the patients need ICU treatment. The prolonged respiratory RDS could be presented to complementary medicine practitioners including TCM practitioners when they are discharged from the hospital, when circumstances continue in a relatively stable condition.

The Key Identifications of the Lung Impairment

Symptoms are breathlessness (short breath, shallow breath, choked sensation during exercise), intolerance to exertion (not able to perform some physically demanding tasks, i.e., climbing stairs), cough (dry cough), and chest tightness. The face, lips, and tongue are bluish (cyanosis). The blood oxygen saturation level is often lower than 95% and considered a warning sign for otherwise healthy children and adults.

The lung fibrosis could be established by positive emission computed tomography (PECT) and MDCT reports (Ali and Ghonimy, 2021; Han *et al*., 2021). However, since histologic analysis was not performed with

CT scanning, a pathological confirmation of lung fibrosis is not possible at this stage (Well *et al.*, 2021). There are no well-established biomarkers for diagnosis of ILD or lung fibrosis yet.

Cancer/tumour should be excluded by CT or MRI scanning. In addition, heart failure could also be present causing a shortage of oxygen and similar symptoms. It is important that differential diagnosis is cleared using blood test, chest images of CT/MRI, and other heart diagnosis tests.

Syndrome Patterns and Treatment of TCM

The post-COVID-19 ILD is mostly a clinical condition present for long COVID-19 or post-COVID-19 stages, where the temperature is normal and most patients are living at home. This profile suggests that the syndrome patterns are present for most cases in the chronic/recovery stages, and therefore the Zang-Fu syndrome pattern system would be the most appropriate approach for TCM diagnosis and treatment, although in the Warm-Disease Syndrome Pattern system, the recovery stages were also discussed.

At present, there is insufficient data to generate a statistical profile to encompass all syndrome patterns the ILD patients might present with. Syndrome patterns were visibly observed by the authors and their colleagues, condensed into the following syndrome patterns alongside of real-life clinical case records and outcomes.

Phlegm and Heat accumulation in the Lungs

Clinical features and signs: Signs are cough with phlegm that is white or yellow or a mixture of colours, tenderness or pain in the chest, recurrent minor fever occasionally, thirst, constipation or sluggish bowels, sore throat, a red tongue with a thin or thick greasy coating, and a rolling and rapid pulse.

Treatment principle in TCM: Clearing excessive heat and accumulated phlegm in the lung.

Treatment: Herbal prescription.

Pinyin: Variated Qingfei Paidu Decoction.

English name for decoction: Variated Decoction of Clearing Lung and Eliminating Toxicity Decoction.

Role in formula	Name/ Pinyin	Name/Latin	Dose (g)	Function
Chief herb	*Ma Huang	Herba Ephedrae	10	*Ma Huang is replaced by Ting Li Zi due to legal restrictions.
	Ting Li Zi	Semen/Descurainiae seu Lepidii	10	Ventilates the lung and releases the external wind-heat.
Deputy herb	Shi Gao	Gypsum Fibrosum	10–30	Clears excessive heat in the upper burner.
Assistant herb	Xing Ren	Semen Pruni Armeniacae	10	Ventilates the lung and eases cough.
	Gui Zhi	Ramulus Cinnamomi Cassiae	6–10	Warms and releases external wind and promotes the *Qi* flowing through the upper burner.
	Jiang Ban Xia	Rhizoma Pinelliae Ternatae	10–15	Eliminates excessive dampness and phlegm.
	Sheng Jiang	Rhizoma Zingiberis Officinalis Recens	10	Promotes warming and eliminates cold-damp accumulation in upper and middle burners.
	Chen Pi	Pericarpium Citri Reticulatae	10	Eliminates excessive dampness and phlegm.
	Huo Xiang	Herba Agastaches seu Pogostemi	10	Eliminates the external wind and dampness, harmonies the stomach.
	Zi Yuan	Radix Asteris Tatarici	10	Eliminates the external wind and promotes ventilation of the lung.
	Kuan Dong Hua	Flos Tussilaginis Farfarae	10	Releases wind-heat in the lung and stops cough by eliminating phlegm.
	Zhu Ling	Sclerotium Polypori Umbellati	10–30	Clears excessive dampness and fluid, pushes urine to pass easily.
	Bai Zhu	Rhizoma Atractylodis Macrocephalae	10–30	Replenishes the general and middle burners' *Qi* and dries the excessive dampness.
	Gan Cao	Radix Glycyrrhizae Uralensis	5	Harmonises all the herbs to work well together and regulates the stomach.
Guiding herb	Jie Geng	Radix Platycodi Grandiflori	10	Leads all the herbs to the lung and the upper burner.

Method: The instructions for both raw herbs and concentrated herbs are available in the appendix. This formula is a reducing herb combination.

Analysis:
Ma Huang is replaced with Ting Li Zi; Xing Ren, Shi Gao, and Gan Cao form the complete composition of MXSG decoction (Ephedra, Apricot Kernel, Gypsum, and Liquorice Decoction) as the main formula to dispel excessive lung heat and release the external wind-heat. Jiang Ban Xi, Chen Pi, and Fu Ling are the complete composition for Er Chen decoction (Decoction of two old (cured) drugs) to eliminate excessive *Dampness* and *Phlegm.* Huo Xiang and Gan Jiang expel the external *Cold-Damp.* Zhu Ye and Zhu Ling dispel accumulated fluid. Gui Zhi agitates yang *Qi* in general.

For other herbal formulas for consideration, please refer to relevant sources:

- *Huo Ling Shuang Hua Yin* (Agastaches, Poria, and Japonicae Decoction) is used for the heat still accumulated at the exterior and inside the lung, but it is quite a moderate prescription that can be given to patients in all styles.
- *Lian Hua Qing Wen* (Clear Heat and Detoxify Capsules) is used for some excessive heat accumulated in the lung with a good condition in the stomach which can be given to a patient with an excessive heat pattern.
- *Xiao Qing Long* (Minor Blue Green Dragon Decoction) is used for some *Cold-Phlegm* accumulated in the lungs which can be given to the patient with cold or deficiency style.

Advice: This pattern can be seen in patients with post-COVID-19 interstitial syndrome. However, recurrent inflammation remains in the lungs due to the incomplete healing. This syndrome pattern can exist alone or in combination with deficiency syndrome patterns.

Lung and Spleen Qi Deficiency

Clinical features and signs: Signs are weak breathing, breathlessness, tenderness of chest, recurrent cold/flu, aversion to cold, tiredness, difficulty in moving (difficulty in walking distances, including climbing stairs), coughing or wheezing when participating in activities, loose bowels or diarrhoea, bloated stomach and abdomen, no appetite, and a pale tongue with teeth marks and less white coating.

Treatment principle in TCM: Replenishing *Lung and Spleen Qi.*

Treatment: Herbal prescription.

Pinyin: *Yu Ping Fen* variated with *Bu Zhong Yi Qi* Decoctions.

English name for decoction: Jade Windscreen Powder variated with Tonify the Middle and Augment the *Qi* Decoction.

Role in formula	Name/ Pinyin	Name/Latin	Dose (g)	Function
Chief herb	Huang Qi	Radix Astragali Membranacei	10–30	Strengthens the defensive *Qi* and general *Qi*.
Deputy herb	Bai Zhu	Rhizoma Atractylodis Macrocephalae	10–30	Promotes strengthening of general *Qi* and middle *Qi*.
Assistant herb	Fang Feng	Radix Ledebouriellae Divaricatae	10	Eliminates the external wind.
	Dang Shen	Radix Codonopsis Pilosulae	10	Supports strengthening of general *Qi* and post-heaven *Qi*.
	Fu Ling	Sclerotium Poriae Cocos	10	Supports strengthening of general *Qi* and dries the excessive dampness.
	Chen Pi	Pericarpium Citri Reticulatae	10	Supports strengthening of the lung and stomach *Qi* and dries excessive dampness to stop cough.
	Dang Gui	Radix Angelicae Sinensis	10	Nourishes *Yin* and blood.
	Chai Hu	Radix Bupleuri	10	Dredges the stagnated *Qi* for general relaxation.
	Zhi Gan Cao	Radix Glycyrrhizae Uralensis	5	Harmonises all of herbs to work well together and regulate the stomach.
Guiding herb	Sheng Ma	Rhizoma Cimicifugae	10	Leads all the herbs in the prescription to affect the lung and spleen.

Method: The instructions for both raw herbs and concentrated herbs are available in the appendix. This formula is a tonifying herb combination.

Analysis: Huang Qi, Bai Zhu, and Fang Fen strengthen the defensive *Qi* and release external *Wind-Cold* pathogenic *Qi* as a complete composition of Yu Ping Feng San. Dang Shen, Fu Ling, and Bai Zhu reinforce the *Spleen Qi* in the middle burner. Chai Hu and Sheng Ma ascend the three burners' *Qi* up and spread it throughout general body. Dang Gui nourishes *Yin* and *Blood.* Gan Cao harmonises the *Stomach* and adjusts all herbs as a complete composition of Bu Zhong Yi Qi Tang. Both formulas are used together to replenish external and internal *Qi*, and strengthen *Lungs* and *Spleen.*

Advice: This treatment is suitable to be given to the patients with post-COVID-19 syndrome in a gentle pattern, initial stage, simple styles of lung inefficiency, or general weakness only.

Lung Qi and Heart Yin Deficiency

Clinical features and signs: Signs are weak breathing, breathlessness, soreness, dry throat, wheezing and cough with coarse laboured breathing sound, feeling thirsty, palpitations, insomnia, anxiety, hot flashes during the night with sweating, and tongue is red in colour and slim with a plump tongue body without a coating.

Treatment principle in TCM: Replenishing *Lung Qi* and nourishing *Heart Yin.*

Treatment: Herbal prescription.

Pinyin: *Bu Fei Tang* variated with *Sheng Mai Yin* Decoctions.

English name for decoction: Tonify the Lungs Decoction variated with Replenish Pulse Decoction.

Role in formula	Name/ Pinyin	Name/Latin	Dose (g)	Function
Chief herb	Ren Shen Mai Men Dong	Radix Ginseng Tuber Ophiopogonis Japonici	10 10	Replenishes the lung and spleen *Qi*, nourishes the lung and heart *Yin*.
Deputy herb	Huang Qi	Radix Astragali Membranacei	10	Supports replenishing of the lung and heart *Qi* and general *Qi*.
Assistant herb	Shu Di Huang	Radix Rhemanniae Glutinosae Praeparata	10	Supports replenishing of the lung and general *Yin*.
	Wu Wei Zi	Fructus Schisandrae Chinensis	10	Nourishes *Yin* and harmonises sourness and sweat to cultivate the lung and stomach *Yin* with Dazao.
	Sang Bai Pi	Cortex Mori Albae Radicis	10	Dredges through lung *Qi* and eliminates excessive phlegm to stop cough.
	Kuan Dong Hua	Flos Tussilaginis Farfarae	10	Nourishes the lung, eases cough, and dispels phlegm.
	Ziyuan	Radix Asteris Tatarici	10	Releases external wind, eases cough, and dispels phlegm.
	Da Zao	Fructus Zizyphi Jujubae	10	Harmonises the stomach and nourishes the lung in its sweat mixed with Wu Wei Zi's sourness.
Guiding herb	Sheng Jiang	Rhizoma Zingiberis Officinalis Recens	10	Leads all the herbs in prescription to go to lung and stomach.

Method: The instructions for both raw herbs and concentrated herbs are available in the appendix. This formula is a tonifying herb combination.

Analysis: Ren Shen and Huang Qi strengthen the *Lung* and *Spleen Qi.* Mai Men Dong and Shu Di Huang nourish Lung *Yin*. Sheng Jiang warms the middle burner and releases what is left of the pathogenic *Wind.* Sang Bai Pi dredges through *Lung Qi*, plus Kuan Dong Hua and Zi Yuan nourish the *Lung*, ease cough, and dispel *Phlegm*. Wu Wei Zi and Da Zao harmonise the sourness and sweat to cultivate *Lung Yi* and the *Stomach.* Ren Shen, Mai Men Dong, and Wu Wei Zi reinforce *Qi* and nourish *Yin* together to promote the *Lung* and *Heart* as a full composition of Sheng Mai Yin.

Advice: This pattern is seen in patients with post-COVID-19 syndrome in which the lungs are involved and the heart may also be affected, or some mental disorders can appear, so both *Qi* and *Yin* should be treated.

Lung and Kidney Yang Deficiency

Clinical features and signs: Signs are breathlessness, wheezing, difficulty breathing, cough with phlegm, occurrence of breathing distress which worse while moving, dry or wet rales in the lungs when listening with a stethoscope, oedema of the lower legs, ankles, hands, or fingers, a pale and swollen tongue with slippery or white coating, and a rolling or fine pulse.

Treatment principle in TCM: Warming and strengthening *Lung* and *Kidney Yang*, releasing excessive fluid.

Treatment: Herbal prescription.

Pinyin: Zhen Wu variated with Jin Kui/Gui Shen Qi Decoction.

English name for decoction: True Warrior Decoction variated with Kidney *Qi* Decoction from Golden Cabinet.

Role in formula	Name/Pinyin	Name/Latin	Dose (g)	Function
Chief herb	*Fu Zi	Radix Lateralis Aconiti Carmichaeli Praeparata	5–10	*Fu Zi is replaced by Rou Gui due to legal restrictions.
	Rou Gui	Cortex Cinnamomi Cassiae	5–10	Warms and agitates the kidney and general yang *Qi*.
Deputy herb	Bai Zhu	Rhizoma Atractylodis Macrocephalae	10–30	Promotes strengthening of yang and *Qi* in upper and middle burners.
	Shu Di Huang	Radix Rhemanniae Glutinosae Praeparata	10–30	Promotes nourishing of the kidney and general *Yin*.
Assistant herb	Bai Shao	Radix Paeoniae Lactiflorae	10	Nourishes general *Yin* in three burners.
	Gui Zhi	Ramulus Cinnamomi Cassiae	6–10	Warms and agitates yang *Qi* and dredges the stagnated *Qi*.
	Shan Zhu Yu	Fructus Corni Officinalis	10	Supports nourishing of the kidney *Yin* and *Qi*.
	Shan Yao	Radix Dioscoreae Oppositae	10	Supports replenishing of the kidney and spleen *Qi*, and dries excessive dampness.
	Mu Dan Pi	Cortex Moutan Radicis	10	Clears remaining heat in the three burners.
	Ze Xie	Rhizoma Alismatis Orientalis	10	Supports release of excessive dampness.
	Xiang Fu	Rhizoma Cyperi Rotundi	10	Dredges the stagnated *Qi*.
	Fu Ling	Sclerotium Poriae Cocos	10	Promotes elimination of excessive dampness and accumulated fluid.
	Gan Cao	Radix Glycyrrhizae Uralensis	5	Harmonises all the herbs to work well together and regulates the stomach.
Guiding herb	Sheng Jiang	Rhizoma Zingiberis Officinalis Recens	10	Leads all the herbs in the prescription to go to the lung and stomach.

Method: The instructions for both raw herbs and concentrated herbs are available in the appendix. This formula is a reducing herb combination.

Analysis: The main herbs, like Fu Zi which we have to replace with Rou Gui, warm the *Kidney Yang*. Shu Di Huang, Shan Zhu Yu, and Shan Yao replenish the *Kidney* and *Spleen Qi* as three tonifications. Mu Dan Pi, Ze Xie, and Fu Ling clear *Empty Heat* and release excessive fluid as three reductions. Bai Shao and Gui Zhi increase the drying of *Damp* and agitate *Yang Qi* to emphasise the eliminating fluid effect as Zhen Wu Tang is added in, so the mixed formulas can reinforce *Kidney Yang* deficiency with excessive fluid accumulation.

Advice: This pattern is seen in the patients with post-COVID-19 syndrome in the form of lung failure with some fluid accumulated in the lungs or in the circulation at the chest and the extremities along with insufficient lung and weakness at the chronic and severer stages.

Blood Stasis in Lung and Heart

Clinical features and signs: Signs are breathlessness, tenderness or soreness of the chest, breathing distress accompanied by a recurrent pain in the chest, palpitations, laboured breathing, difficulty breathing along with a sharp sound when listening with a stethoscope, difficulty breathing when lying flat during the night time, a dark red or light red tongue colour with many blue stasis marks along with less tongue coating, and a deep, fine, or irregular pulse.

Treatment principle in TCM: Activating blood and removing blood stasis.

Treatment: Herbal prescription.

Pinyin: Xue Fu Zhu Yu Decoction.

English name for decoction: Drive Out Stasis in the Mansion of Blood Decoction variation.

Role in formula	Name/ Pinyin	Name/Latin	Dosage (g)	Function
Chief herb	Tao Ren	Semen Pruni Persicae	10	They activate the blood and remove stasis.
	Hong Hua	Flos Carthami Tinctorii	10	
Deputy herb	Dang Gui	Radix Angelicae Sinensis	10	Nourishes the blood and keeps the blood moving.
	Chi Shao	Radix Paeoesniae Rubrae	10	Moves blood, with a cool nature, prevents heat.
	Chuan Xiong	Radix Ligustici Wallichii	6	Moves blood.
Assistant herb	Sheng Di Huang	Radix Rehmanniae Glutinosae	10	Cool in nature to balance the other hot-natured herbs.
	Chuan Ni Xi	Radix Cyathulae Officinalis	6	Moves blood downwards.
Guiding herb	Jie Geng	Radix Platycodi Grandiflori	6	Leads the herbs to the chest and lung.
	Chai Hu	Radix Bupleuri	6	Spreads the *Qi* to help the blood.
	Zhi Qiao	Fructus Citri Aurantii	6	Spreads the *Qi* to help blood move.

Method: The instructions for both raw herbs and concentrated herbs are available in the appendix. This formula is a reducing herb combination.

Analysis: Sheng Di Huang, Dang Gui, Chi Shao, and Chuan Xiong form a full composition of Si Wu Tang for nourishing blood. Tao Ren and Hong Hua invigorate blood circulation, ease pain, and soften solid stasis. Chuan Niu Xi removes the *Blood Stasis*. Jie Geng leads all the herbs to the *Lung* meridian and removes *Lung Qi* circulation. Gan Cao harmonises all the herbs and calms the *Stomach*. These formulas can remove blood stasis from the *Lung* and whole body.

Advice: This treatment can be used alone or in combination with other prescriptions for treating lung failure with signs of blue stasis at the extremities, along with lungs fibrosis. Some herbs, such as Huang Qin, Da Huang, and Dan Shen which have proved to be anti-fibrosis substances by laboratory research, can be used in the prescription as well.

Acupuncture point selection and rationale

Body acupuncture:
Main points: Shanzhong (REN17), Zhongwan (REN12), Qihai (REN6), Guanyuan (REN4), Kongzui (LU6), Lieque (LU7), Taiyuan (LU9).

Assistant points:

- More cough: Yuji (LU10), Shaoshang (LU11).
- Chest pain: Zhongfu (LU1).
- Recurrent fever: Quchi (LI11), Hegu (LI4).
- Fatigue: Yinlingquan (SP9), Sanyinjiao (SP6), Zusanli (ST36).
- Constipation: Zhongfu (ST25), Diji (SP8).
- Palpitation: Neiguan (P6), Shenmen (HE7).

Explanation: Shanzhong, Zhongwan, Qihai, and Guanyuan are the main points along the conception vessel for strengthening and agitating *Vitality Qi* which is sourced for promoting all the organic *Qi.* Kongzui and Lieque emphasise replenishing of the *Lung Qi.* Yuji and Shaoshang as Jing-well and Ying-spring points of the *Lung* meridian ease cough. Zhongfu as the first point of the *Lung* meridian can ease chest pain. Quchi and Hegu decease fever and clear excessive *Heat.* Yinlingquan and Sanyinjiao replenish *Spleen Qi* to reduce fatigue. Zusanli reinforces the *Spleen* and *Stomach Qi* to consolidate *Qi* in the middle burner and general body. Zhongfu and Diji make bowel movement easy. Neiguan and Shemen stabilise the *Heart Qi* and calm the mind down. An acupuncture group should be formed according to the individual case for regulating his/her balanced state and promoting self-healing.

Analysis: REN17 is a point of the sea of *Qi*; therefore, it is extremely influential in regulating *Qi* in the chest, and it is located in the middle of the sternum. REN12 is a front Mu point on the conception vessel that converges with the *Small Intestine*, *San Jiao*, and *Stomach* channels, giving rise to harmony in the middle *Jiao* and regulating *Qi.* REN6 is the sea of *Qi* and able to fortify *Yang*, along with REN4 being the sea of blood; these points on the conception vessel are used for agitating *Vital Qi* and sourced from the promotion of the *Original Qi.* LU6 and LU7 as a *Lung* source point accentuate the replenishment of *Lung Qi.* LU10 the *Ying-Spring* and LU11 the *Jing-Well* points of the *Lung* meridian are used to ease cough. In addition, LU1 is used, and the first point of the *Lung* meridian is known to ease chest pain. LI11 and LI4 decrease fever and clear excessive *Heat* accumulation and complement the *Zang Fu* relationship with the *Lung*. On the lower medial leg, SP9 and SP6 reside acting to replenish *Spleen Qi* to reduce fatigue; in addition, ST36 reinforces the *Spleen* and *Stomach Qi* and promotes the consolidation of *Qi* in the middle burner and general body. Furthermore, ST25 and SP8 promote bowel function. The *Shen* disturbance requires the support of PC6 and HT7 to stabilise the *Heart Qi* along with calming the mind down. Acupuncture points are selected according to the presentation of an individual case, complementing the promotion, and regulation, of a person's self-healing to achieve homeostasis.

Case Study

Lungs and heart impairments after a COVID-19 suffered

A 71-year-old male retired engineer had been diagnosed with COVID-19 due to an increased body temperature of 38°C, classified as fever. He also had a cough, breathlessness, and chest pain. The patient and his partner visited their daughter's family in London during March 2020 causing him to be admitted to the ICU. Since the post-COVID-19 attack, he has manifested difficulty breathing, along with wheezing, and even dyspnoea. His arterial oxygen saturation (SaO_2) reduced during the previral infection; healthy oxygenation levels range from 95% to 98% but in this case the male exhibited a lower SaO_2 of 83%. He was discharged from hospital following a week in intensive care, with the use of a continuous positive airway pressure (CPAP) to promote oxygenation with minimal effort on his behalf. In addition, antibiotics and other relevant treatments were administered. However, he further reported difficulty in breathing accompanied by wheezing, cough, and tenderness located in the chest area when attempting to become mobile. Furthermore, difficulties continued for him with breathing during sleep, coupled with bad dreams. All his symptoms became aggravated when he attempted to participate in gentle activity, including an attempt to walk 10 m indoors. His arterial oxygenation lingered around 89–91% with lower readings on his left wrist as opposed to his right. Observations included a red and plump tongue, with teeth marks, and a greasy-dry-thick coating.

Clinical features and signs: Signs were wheezing and breathlessness, difficulty walking, unable to even walk 10 m in his flat, keeping his mouth open while sleeping, tiredness, lethargy and poor spirit, no appetite with minor constipation, alight red tongue with white greasy coating, and SaO_2 of 89–91.

Differentiation syndromes of TCM: *Qi* and *Yin* deficiencies with unclear *Heat* and *Dampness* accumulation in the *Lungs*.

Treatment principle in TCM:

1. Reinforcing *Qi* and nourishing *Yin* to *Lungs* and *Heart*.
2. Releasing *Heat* and expelling *Dampness*.

Treatment: Herbal prescription.

Pinyin: Er Chen Tang variated with Bu Fei Decoction.

English name for decoction: Decoction of Two Old Drugs variated with Tonify the Lungs Decoction.

Herbal powders (g):

Jiang Ban	Xia Rhizoma Pinelliae Ternatae 15 g
Chen Pi	Pericarpium Citri Reticulatae 10 g
Fu Ling	Sclerotium Poriae Cocos 10 g
Huang Qin	Radix Scutellariae Baicalensis 10 g
Da Qing Ye	Folium Isatidis 10 g
Xuan Shen	Radix Scrophulariae Ningpoensis 10 g
Bei Sha Shen	Radix Glehniae Littoralis 10 g

Mai Men Dong	Tuber Ophiopogonis Japonici 10 g
Chuan Lian Zi	Fructus Meliae Toosendan 10 g
Gua Lou Ren	Semen Trichosanthis 10 g
Bai He	Bulbus Lilii 10 g
Tai Zi Shen	Radix Pseudostellariae 30 g
Gan Cao	Radix Glycyrrhizae Uralensis 5 g

The above-mentioned herbs were decocted as herbal juice and taken twice daily.

Treatment result and analysis:
After the treatment dose and modified herbal prescription, he reported improvement week by week, for a month. He could participate in activities that he previously reported were not available to him, such as walking 10 min indoors. Furthermore, he had progressed to walking outside daily, including climbing up flights of steps up to four floors in his residential flat. His SaO_2 increased to a near normal range of 94–95%. This progression concluded he was recovering.

This case highlights many implications because of long COVID-19 syndrome. The lung collapse and heart impairment are because the pneumonic infection of COVID-19 escalated to a serious, critical stage. After medical attention and intensive treatment in the ICU for a week, the patient had not completely healed from COVID-19, although he was discharged. The symptoms he suffered from included a lower SaO_2 which indicates the substandard function of breathing and gas exchange in lungs, with the SaO_2 on the left wrist being lower than the right wrist, which emphasises an insufficiency of oxygen supply to the cardiological musculature. Therefore, herbs were chosen to release the excessive heat and expel the remaining dampness in the body, eliminating any residual external pathogenic factors of COVID-19 from the lungs. Herbs for reinforcing *Qi* and nourishing *Yin* to promote self-healing cascade to the lungs and heart and prevent the occurrence of organ fibrosis.

References

Ali, R. M. M. and Ghonimy, M. B. I. (2021). Post-COVID-19 pneumonia lung fibrosis: A worrisome sequelae in surviving patients. *Egyptian Journal of Radiology and Nuclear Medicine*, 52, 101. https://doi.org/10.1186/s43055-021-00484-3.

Bazdyrev, E., Rusina, P., Panova, M., Novikov, F., Grishagin, I., and Nebolsin, V. (2021). Lung fibrosis after COVID-19: Treatment prospects. *Pharmaceuticals*, 14(8), 807. https://doi.org/10.3390/ph14080807.

Delorey, T. M., Ziegler, C. G. K., Heimberg, G., *et al.* (2021). COVID-19 tissue atlases reveal SARS-CoV-2 pathology and cellular targets. *Nature*, 595, 107–113. https://doi.org/10.1038/s41586-021-03570-8.

Han, X., Fan, Y., Alwalid, O., *et al.* (2021). Six-month follow-up chest CT findings after severe COVID-19 pneumonia. *Radiology*, 299, E177–E186.

Rendeiro, A. F., Ravichandran, H., Bram, Y., *et al.* (2021). The spatial landscape of lung pathology during COVID-19 progression. *Nature*, 593, 564–569. https://doi.org/10.1038/s41586-021-03475-6.

Wells, A. U., Devaraj, A., and Desai, S. R. (2021). Interstitial lung disease after COVID-19 infection: A catalog of uncertainties. *Radiology*, 299, E216–E218.

Chapter 5

Impairments in the Heart/Circulation System

Cardiovascular Impairments in Post-COVID-19 Stages

When the SARS-CoV-2 virus comes into contact with a human, the initial pathway of invasion into the body is via the external barrier of the respiratory system and outer surface defence. There are abundant ACE-II (Angiotension-Converting Enzyme) receptors which are broadly distributed within the respiratory tract surface, in the alveolar epithelial cells as a defensive function. However, when the virus is released from the infected cells, it can be discharged by mucus coughed out into atmosphere, to infect other people; furthermore, it can be released into the blood stream as blood is constantly flowing through the lungs. The SARS-CoV-2 virus in blood will take the same pathway of ACE-II to get into any other cells with the receptor on their surface. The cardiac muscle cells and vascular endothelial cells, the inner wall of blood vessels, are also rich in ACE-II receptors, and consequently, the virus can easily enter the body's circulation system, including the heart. This inevitability leads to immune response and inflammation in the tissues, which could be described in pathological terms as lymphocytic infiltration in the myocardium, swelling of cardiac cells, and even death of cells. This can cause heart failure. This inflammatory pathology principally leads to the clinical diagnosis of myocarditis and is evidenced by finding CD3+ and CD8+ cytotoxic lymphocytes with CD68 macrophages in heart tissues (Maiese *et al.*, 2021; Mele *et al.*, 2021). Another way the heart is impaired is by the subsequent prothrombotic state that can be presented as coronary microthrombosis, which partially blocks the blood flow to the heart. It can produce a mild cardiac infarction (Maiese *et al*., 2021; Pellegrini *et al*., 2021). The former impairment is repairable, while the latter is difficult to fully recover.

In the NICE guideline and current CDC information, the sequelae of both myocarditis and cardiac infarction are considered, and the common symptoms typically include palpitation, pain at the centre of chest, and intolerance to exercise. The symptoms of most patients could be recognised by having an electrocardiogram (ECG) and Cardiological Magnetic Resonance Imaging (CMRI).

Nashiga *et al.* (2020) provided an early warning of the potential cardiac impairments through their study of SARS patients and suggested that those with preexisting cardiovascular conditions will have much worse outcomes, even death, compared to the general population. On the other hand, the damage could last very long and cause problems leading to chronic illnesses. This was soon confirmed by Dreck *et al.* (2020) with a global team from 1216 cases examined with echocardiograms. Among all those recording no preexisting cardiac conditions (901), 46% had abnormal echocardiogram results, with both myocardial infarction (3%) and myocarditis (3%) being diagnosed. Since then, there have been more and more clinical reports on this aspect.

From existing medical knowledge, young sufferers of the two conditions might recover to some degree, but middle and aged patients will find it difficult to fully recover, with potential for permanent damage. This is an overview of how the post-COVID-19 heart impairment is caused.

Key Clinical Identification

Main symptoms: Symptoms are palpitation (irregular heart beating), chest pain at the centre or left side, angina, chest tightness, intolerance to physical exercise, breathless when lying down, and oedema in the legs/ankles.

WM diagnostic tools: ECG, echocardiogram, and CMRI could provide key clinical diagnosis.

Blood tests: Cardiac troponin is the most reliable biomarker of heart tissue injury.

Red flag

When a foamy mucus, red/brown in colour, is produced, there is breathing difficulty when in a lying down position, and bluish tongue/lips/fingernails are noticed, it is very possible that a heart failure has happened. Medical examination should be carried out first before TCM treatment.

Syndrome Patterns and Treatment of TCM

When the diagnosis of acute heart failure is clear and the patients are advised by their medical professionals to manage the condition from home, TCM approaches should be introduced as early as possible. However, their medications should not be changed unless they were told by those who prescribed the medicines.

The impairment in the circulation system is internal damage, not caused by external pathogenic factors (EPFs), and the best syndrome pattern to use is the Zang-Fu pattern system. The patterns listed below are examples, reflecting the clinical observation of the authors and their discussion with colleagues.

Heart Qi Deficiency

Clinical features and signs: Signs are breathlessness, wheezing or cough during exertion, palpitation, irregular heartbeats, tiredness, fatigue, not wanting to talk, pale complexion, easily sweating, a pale tongue with teeth marks and less or thin white coating, and a weak-fine irregular pulse.

Treatment principle in TCM: Replenishing the *Vitality* and the *Heart Qi.*

Treatment: Herbal prescription.

Pinyin: *Bao Yuan Tang* variated with *Gan Mai Da Zhao Tang.*

English name for decoction: Preserve the Primal Decoction variated with Liquorice, Wheat, and Jujube Decoction.

Role in formula	Name/ Pinyin	Name/Latin	Dose (g)	Function
Chief herb	Ren Shen	Radix Ginseng	10	Replenishes the lung and heart *Qi*, and general *Qi*.
Deputy herb	Huang Qi	Radix Astragali	10–30	Supports replenishing of general *Qi* in the upper and middle burners.
Assistant herb	Da Zao	Fructus Zizyphi Jujubae	10	Nourishes stomach yin and heart yin.
	Gan Cao	Radix Glycyrrhizae Uralensis	5	Nourishes heart yin and replenishes heart *Qi*, harmonises the stomach and adjusts all formulas.
Guiding herb	Rou Gui	Cortex Cinnamomi Cassiae	3–5	Agitates original *Qi* to support the heart yang and *Qi*.

Method: The above-mentioned herbs are collated as a herbal formula of dry herbs, boiled into herbal juice, and taken twice daily, or made into a concentrated herbal powder of which 6 g is taken with warm water twice daily.

Analysis: Ren Shen and Huang Qi replenish Vitality *Qi* and *Heart Qi* as the main herbs. Rou Gui agitates the original *Qi*, along *with Heart Yang* and *Qi*. Da Zhao nourishes the *Heart* and *Stomach Yin*. Gan Cao harmonises the *Stomach* and adjusts all formulas. If using Sheng Mai Yin, Mai Men Dong and Wu Wei Zi are added to nourish *Heart Yin* for replenishing both *Qi* and *Yin* together.

Advice: This pattern can be seen when the heart is weaker and in the gentle stage of *heart* failure in the long COVID-19 syndrome.

Heart Qi and Yin Deficiency

Clinical features and signs: Signs are breathlessness, wheezing on exertion, palpitation, chest pain or recurrent angina, dry mouth and thirst, recurrent feeling of heat, red face, hot flashes during the night with sweating, restlessness, insomnia, and a red tongue with less coating or without coating.

Treatment principle in TCM: Replenishing *Heart Qi* and nourishing *Heart Yin.*

Treatment: Herbal prescription.

Pinyin: *Sheng Mai Yin* variated with *Tian Wang Bu Xin Tang.*

English name for decoction: Generate the Pulse Decoction variated with Emperor of Heaven's Special Pill to Tonify the Heart.

Role in formula	Name/ Pinyin	Name/Latin	Dose (g)	Function
Chief herb	Ren Shen	Radix Ginseng	10	Replenishes the vitality *Qi* and heart *Qi.*
	Mai Men Dong	Tuber Ophiopogonis Japonici	10	Nourishes the heart and lung yin.
Deputy herb	Wu Wei Zi	Fructus Schisandrae Chinensis	10	Promotes nourishing of heart yin and general yin.
Assistant herb	Sheng Di Huang	Radix Rehmanniae Glutinosae	10–30	Emphasises nourishing of heart yin and original kidney yin.
	Xuan Shen	Radix Scrophulariae Ningpoensis	10	Emphasises nourishing of the heart and lung yin.
	Bai Zi Ren	Semen Biotae Orientalis	10	Cultivates the heart and calms the mind down.
	Suan Zao Ren	Semen Zizyphi Spinosae	10	Cultivates the heart and liver, calms the mind down, and promotes relaxation.
	Yuan Zhi	Radix Polygalae Tenuifoliae	10	Cultivates the heart and calms the mind down to promote relaxation.
Guiding herb	Gan Cao	Radix Glycyrrhizae Uralensis	5	Nourishes heart yin and replenishes heart *Qi*, harmonises the stomach, and adjusts all formulas.

Method: The above-mentioned herbs are collated as a herbal formula of dry herbs, boiled into herbal juice, and taken twice daily, or made into a concentrated herbal powder of which 6 g is taken with warm water twice daily.

Analysis: Ren Shen replenishes *Vitality Qi* and *Heart Qi* as the main herb. Mai Men Dong and Wu Wei Zi nourish *Heart Yin* as assistant herbs as part of the full composition of Sheng Mai Yin, which has been proven to manage various states of heart issues by research. Sheng Di Huang and Xuan Shen emphasise nourishing of *Heart* and *Lung Yin.* Bai Zi Ren and Yuan Zi cultivate the *Heart* and calm the mind down. Suan Zao Ren nourishes *Heart* and *Liver Yin.* All of these herbs together replenish *Heart Qi* and nourish *Heart Yin* to promote *Heart* recovery. This pattern can be seen in cases with *Heart* inefficiency and the early stage of heart failure, accompanied by some psychological symptoms.

Advice: This pattern can be seen in the cases where the patients have a weaker *Heart* and are in the gentle stage of heart failure, accompanied by some psychological symptoms.

Heart Yang Deficiency and Fluid accumulation

Clinical features and signs: Signs are palpitation, chest pain or recurrent seizures of angina, breathlessness with coarse breathing sounds, tenderness of chest, difficulty breathing when lying down, cough with pink or foamy mucus, abdominal distension, swelling of legs, ankles, and feet, cold hands and feet, aversion to cold, pale and puffy face, weak spirit, pale and plump tongue with white or greasy coating, a deep-fine-irregular pulse.

Treatment principle in TCM:

1. Warming and reinforcing heart yang.
2. Dredging accumulated fluid.

Treatment: Herbal prescription.

Pinyin: Gui Zhi Gan Cao Tang variated with Zhen Wu Tang.

English name for decoction: Cinnamon and Liquorice Decoction variated with True Warrior Decoction.

	Name/ Pinyin	Name/Latin	Dose (g)	Function
Chief herb	Ren Shen	Radix Ginseng	10	Replenishes the heart *Qi* and original *Qi*.
Deputy herb	Gan Jiang	Rhizoma Zingiberis Officinalis	10	Warms the heart and middle yang.
	Gui Zhi	Ramulus Cinnamomi Cassiae	6–10	Warms and agitates the yang *Qi*.
Assistant herb	Fu Ling	Sclerotium Poriae Cocos	10	Eliminates excessive dampness and strengthens the spleen to pass fluid.
	Zhu Ling	Sclerotium Polypori Umbellati	10–30	Eliminates excessive dampness and strengthens the spleen to pass fluid.
	Bai Zhu	Rhizoma Atractylodis Macrocephalae	10–30	Replenishes the spleen *Qi* and general *Qi* to strengthen the passing of fluid.
	Ze Xie	Rhizoma Alismatis Orientalis	10	Eliminates excessive fluid.
Guiding herb	Zhi Gan Cao	Radix Glycyrrhizae Uralensis	5	Nourishes heart *Yin* and replenishes heart *Qi*; harmonises the stomach and adjusts all formulas.

Method: The above-mentioned herbs are collated as a herbal formula of dry herbs, boiled into a herbal juice, and taken twice daily, or made into a concentrated herbal powder of which 6 g is taken with warm water twice daily.

Analysis: Ren Shen replenishes the *Heart Qi* as a basic herb. Gan Jiang and Gui Zhi assist to warm and agitate *Heart Yang.* Zhu Ling and Fu Ling release accumulated fluid from the *Lung* and *Heart.* Ze Xie decoction eliminates the excessive fluid from the lower burner. Bai Zhu reinforces the *Spleen,* drying the *Damp* and complementing the effect of fluid elimination. Gan Cao complements the herbs in addition to supporting the *Stomach.*

Advice: This pattern can be seen in heart failure with fluid accumulation in the lungs or abdomen and lower body.

Heart Blood Stasis

Clinical features and signs: Signs are breathlessness; recurrent angina or chest pain; the occurrence of severe pain, on occasion radiating to the left arm or shoulder; tenderness of the chest; a dark red tongue with blood stasis marks on the tongue, stasis local to the ligament under the tongue, with a thin white coating; and a wiry-uneven pulse or knotted, intermittent, skipping pulse. These symptoms are triggered or aggravated by a bad mood.

Treatment principle in TCM:

1. Activating blood to remove blood stasis.
2. Removing obstruction in meridians to release pain.

Treatment: Herbal prescription and acupuncture.

Pinyin: Xue Fu Zhu Yu Tang.

English name for decoction: Drive Out Stasis in the Mansion of Blood Decoction.

	Name/ Pinyin	Name/Latin	Dose (g)	Function
Chief herb	Dang Gui	Radix Angelicae Sinensis	10	Replenishes and nourishes *Yin* and blood.
	Sheng Di Huang	Radix Rehmanniae Glutinosae	10–30	Nourishes the kidney and general *Yin*.
Deputy herb	Tao Ren	Semen Pruni Persicae	10	Invigorates blood circulation, eases pain, and softens solid stasis.
	Hong Hua	Flos Carthami Tinctorii	10	Invigorates blood circulation, eases pain, and softens solid stasis.
Assistant herb	Zhi Qiao	Fructus Citri Aurantiio	10	Removes general stagnated *Qi* and softens the solid stasis.
	Chi Shao	Radix Paeoesniae Rubraeo	10	Invigorates the blood stasis and removes stagnated *Qi* in the blood.
	Chai Hu	Radix Bupleuri	10	Dredges the stagnated *Qi*.
	Chuan Xiong	Radix Ligustici Wallichii	10	Invigorates the blood stasis, eases the pain, and removes stagnated *Qi* in the blood.
	Chuna Niu Xi	Radix Cyathulae Officinaliso	10–15	Releases stasis blood.
	Gan Cao	Radix Glycyrrhizae Uralensis	5	Harmonises all the herbs to work well together and regulates the stomach.
Guiding herb	Jie Geng	Radix Platycodi Grandiflori	6–10	Jie Geng leads all the herbs to the lung meridian and removes lung *Qi*'s circulation.

Method: The above-mentioned herbs are collated as a herbal formula of dry herbs, boiled into herbal juice, and taken twice daily, or made into a concentrated herbal powder of which 6 g is taken with warm water twice daily.

Analysis: Sheng Di Huang, Dang Gui, Chi Shao, and Chuan Xiong form a full composition of Si Wu Tang for nourishing the blood. Tao Ren and Hong Hua promote the blood circulation, ease pain, and soften solid stasis. Chuan Ni Xi removes the blood stasis. Jie Geng leads all the herbs to the upper burner and promotes *Qi* circulation. Gan Cao harmonises all the herbs and calms the *Stomach.* The formula can remove Blood Stasis from the *Heart* and the whole body.

Advice: This pattern can be seen when there is an angina attack and swelling in the limbs or lower body caused by the heart damage. The post-COVID-19 syndrome can be involved in either heart inefficacy or heart failure.

Acupuncture

Acupuncture point selection and rationale

Main points: Shanzhong (REN17), Baihui (DU20).

Assistant points: Jianshi (PC5), Daling (PC7), Shenmen (HE7), Shaohai (HE3); Gongsun (SP4), Xuehai (SP10), Yinlingquan (SP9), Sanyinjiao (SP6); Waiguan (SJ5), Zulinqi (GB41), Hegu (LI4), Taichong (LIV3); Jiuwei (REN15), Shangwan (REN13), Qihai (REN6), Guanyuan (REN4).

Analysis: REN17 regulates the collective *Qi*, which is the *Qi* united in the chest, and agitates the Heart *Qi*. DU20 governs general *Qi* in the whole body and relaxes the mind. P6 is the confluent point of the *Yin Linking Vessel, and also* the Jing-river point. PC7 is the *Shu-Stream* point of the *Pericardium* meridian can dredge the Heart *Qi*. HE7 is a *Shu-Stream* point, and along with HT3, the *He-sea* point of *Heart* meridian, it can nourish *Heart Yin* by leading all the points to the *Heart.* SP9 and SP4 reinforce the *Spleen Qi* to support the *Heart.* SJ5 and GB41 as the cross points promote stagnated *Qi* diffusion. LI4 and LR3 are the four gates and able to promote both stagnated *Qi* and clearing of excess *Heat.* REN15, REN13, REN6, and REN4 are points on the *Conception Vessel* and recognised to promote all organs and *Vitality Qi*. Depending on the individual case presentation, we should select a group of points specific to the patient.

Case Study

A 63-year-old policewoman presented with prolonged recurrent palpitation following the viral infection of COVID-19. She suffered from COVID-19 infection for 1 week. Her fever, cough, and chest pain subsided quickly; however, she was experiencing recurrent breathlessness, palpitation, and minor angina, which is a sharp pain at the central left chest lasting a few seconds to 1–2 min. On occasion, there were daily attacks following a negative polymerase chain reaction (PCR) test. An ECG was done by her GP and confirmed an irregular heartbeat demonstrating an atrial ectopic beat. Symptoms included feeling nervous, restless, and tired, leading to a diagnosis of an affected heart, which is consequently a part of the post-COVID-19 syndrome. No Western medicine is given, and she is advised to fully rest by her GP.

Clinical features and signs: Signs were stress, restlessness, breathlessness, minor angina attacks occasionally, disturbed sleep and waking up during the night with panic attacks, low mood, and worrying.

- Tongue: Light red tongue with less white coating.
- Pulse: Wiry pulse with irregular missing beat, with irregularity of 5–10 missing heartbeats per minute.
- ECG: Minor irregular heartbeat in atrial type.

WM diagnosis:

1. Long COVID-19 syndrome.
2. Stress with anxiety and depression.

Differentiation syndromes of TCM:

1. *Heart Qi Deficiency* and *Blood Stasis*.
2. *Liver Qi Stagnation*.

Treatment principle in TCM:

1. Replenishes the *Heart Qi* and *Yin*.
2. Smooth *Liver Qi Stagnation* and *Heart Stasis*.

Treatment: Herbal prescription and acupuncture.

Herbal prescription

Pinyin: Sheng Mai Yin plus Chai Hu Shu Gan Wan.

Method: The above mentioned herbs are made into a concentrated herbal powder of which 6 g is taken twice daily.

Acupuncture point selection and rationale

Main points: Baihui (DU20), Shanzhong (REN17); Taiyang (Ext), Zhongwan (REN12), Qihai (REN6), Guanyuan (REN4); Neiguan (P6), Gongsun (SP4), Waiguan (SJ5), Zulinqi (GB41), Shenmen (HE7), Tongli (HE5).

Treatment result and analysis: The patient reported feeling much better. The irregular heartbeats had reduced over a 4-week period, including the chest pain/angina attacks. A sense of relaxation, good sleep, and general well-being were reported. The patient continued regular acupuncture treatments to maintain an improved quality of life.

References

Dweck, M., Bularga, A., Hahn, R., Bing, R., and Lee, K. K. (2020). Global evaluation of echocardiography in patients with COVID-19. *European Heart Journal — Cardiovascular Imaging*, 21(9), 949–958. https://doi.org/10.1093/ehjci/jeaa178.

Maiese, A., Frati, P., Del Duca, F., Santoro, P., Manetti, A. C., *et al.* (2021). Myocardial pathology in COVID-19-associated cardiac injury: A systematic review. *Diagnostics*, 11(9), 1647. https://doi.org/10.3390/diagnostics11091647.

Mele, D., Flamigni, F., Rapezzi, C., *et al.* (2021). Myocarditis in COVID-19 patients: Current problems. *Internal and Emergency Medicine*, 16, 1123–1129. https://doi.org/10.1007/s11739-021-02635-w.

Nishiga, M., Wang, D.W., Han, Y., *et al.* (2020). COVID-19 and cardiovascular disease: From basic mechanisms to clinical perspectives. *Nature Reviews Cardiology*, 17, 543–558. https://doi.org/10.1038/s41569-020-0413-9.

Pellegrini, D., Kawakami, R., Guagliumi, G., Sakamoto, A., Kawai, K., *et al.* (2021). Microthrombi as a major cause of cardiac injury in COVID-19. *Circulation*, 143(10), 1031–1042. https://doi.org/10.1161/CIRCULATION AHA.120.051828.

Chapter 6

Liver Impairments

Liver Impairments During COVID-19 Infection

Early research has been carried out in Italy by Songzogni *et al.* (2020) to find out if the liver is another target of the SARS-CoV-2 virus, and if there is any damage to the liver. They checked biopsies from 48 patients who died of COVID-19 respiratory failure who had no previous clinical conditions of the liver. The findings suggest that the inflammation response was not obvious in liver tissue, the liver is not a major object of the virus, and no sign of liver failure was revealed. Nonetheless, other damage was found to be related, or similar, to that appearing in the cardiovascular system. One is the partial or complete thrombosis of blood vessels and the other one is the dilation of intrahepatic blood vessels. The two changes cause the liver to enlarge and become partially fibrotic. The endothelial layer of blood vessels might be attacked by the SARS-CoV-2 virus directly or simply one part of the overall damage in the whole blood vessel network and has been discussed in previous chapters.

Immune system overreaction is also considered as liver damage appears to be related to the increase of virus-induced cytopathic agents. It is also important to know that the liver impairment could be the result and manage the use of potentially hepatotoxic drugs, including antiviral agents (Cichoż-Lach & Michalak, 2021).

As the pandemic continues and larger patient numbers are reviewed, a better understanding of the relationship between liver conditions and COVID-19 will be achieved. This ranges from preexisting conditions leading to worse outcomes of the infection to the abnormal liver biochemistry function readings and their relationship with lifestyle changes.

Newly added liver problems, such as liver failure, remain rare as the clinical database is becoming bigger and bigger; however, functional damage is common in all COVID-19 patients lasting for months and years. A review on Chinese patients suggests that liver functional impairment happens to between 16% and 29% of patients and is manifested in raised reading of alanine aminotransferase (ALT) and aspartate aminotransferase (AST), which are the most used tools to assess the liver status. The damage might be linked to direct damage of the liver cells, the cytokine storm, or drugs/chemical liver damage (Du *et al.*, 2022). This is acknowledged by the CDC, stating that elevated levels of liver enzymes of alanine aminotransferase (ALT) and aspartate aminotransferase (AST) indicate at least temporary damage (CDC, 2021).

A Japanese study examined 60 patients, out of which 52% (31) showed high ALT. The raised ALT is linked to obesity, significantly higher D-dimer, high white blood cell count, and an increase of C-reactive protein, ferritin, and fibrinogen. Except for D-dimer, the others are all related to the infection and inflammation of COVID-19. The study suggested that the raised ALT might be caused by microvascular thrombosis in addition to systemic inflammation (Trutrumi *et al.*, 2021).

Marjot *et al.* (2021) narrated a good summary of all the research in this area. First, those with preexisting liver conditions, particularly cirrhosis, have a higher risk of liver failure and death due to COVID-19 infection, which is one of the major reasons leading to a higher risk of death. Secondly, the liver is part of the broader multiple organs infected, although it is not the original infected organ. Third, social isolation has been a big change in many people's lifestyles, and some changes like increased consumption of alcohol have caused a higher than usual increase of liver impairment. Lastly, the changed liver function's biochemistry enzymes including AST and ALT might be caused by the overall immune reaction to the infection, using many drugs, and blood clotting problems.

The cirrhosis and liver failure conditions are not within the scope of complementary medicine and TCM practice. But liver damage presented around 20% of all of PCS (post-COVID-19 syndrome) patients with abnormal liver function reading in AST and ALT. It means this condition should be considered seriously, and prior TCM treatment should be provided to prevent hepatitis.

Clinical Characteristics

Characteristics are fatigue/tiredness, anorexia/poor appetite of food, nausea, and indigestion.

Red flag

Red flags are jaundice, bleeding, oedema in the abdomen, and dilated blood vessels visible in the abdomen as the signs of liver failure or cirrhosis, for which medical examination and referral are advised. Only when the patient confirms the diagnosis and the agreed treatment/management plan at home can the TCM practitioners can then provide treatment.

Clinical finding in lab test are as follows:

1. Higher ALT, AST.
2. MRI, CT, ultrasound scanning is commonly recommended.
3. Liver biopsy is not available for most patients under the current circumstances of overstretched medical services.

Syndrome Patterns and Treatment of TCM

Although ancient documents contain rich information on how to treat conditions similar to what happens during PCS, the authors' selection of the syndrome patterns is mostly based on clinical reports in the last 50 years, featuring with treatment observation of hepatitis A and B, chemical hepatitis, and alcohol-led liver damage. The patterns are within the Zang-Fu syndrome pattern system.

Liver Qi Stagnation

Clinical features and signs: Signs are aching in both coastal areas, which is moving around and possibly radiating to the upper abdomen and chest, abdominal distension, poor appetite with belching, hiccupping, mood swings, easily feeling angry, and a light red tongue with less white coating.

Treatment principle in TCM: Dredging *Liver* and promoting *Qi* circulation.

Treatment: Herbal prescription.

Pinyin: Chai Hu Shu Gan Tang.

English name for decoction: Bupleurum Decoction to Spread the Liver.

Role in formula	Name/ Pinyin	Name/Latin	Dose (g)	Function
Chief herb	Chai Hu	Radix Bupleuri	10	Dredges liver *Qi* and promotes general *Qi* movement.
Deputy herb	Bai Shao	Radix Paeoniae Lactiflorae	10–30	Nourishes liver blood and *Yin* to soften the liver.
Assistant herb	Zhi Qiao	Fructus Citri Aurantii	10	Promotes dredging of liver *Qi* and general abdominal *Qi*.
	Chen Pi	Pericarpium Citri Reticulatae	10	Dredges the liver *Qi*, stomach *Qi*, and general *Qi* throughout the body.
	Chuan Xiong	Radix Ligustici Wallichii	10	Releases the blood stasis and eases the pain.
	Xiang Fu	Rhizoma Cyperi Rotundi	10	Supports Chaihu in dredging the stagnated *Qi*.
Guiding herb	Gan Cao	Radix Glycyrrhizae Uralensis	5	Harmonises all the herbs to work well together and regulates the stomach.

Method: The above mentioned herbs are collated as a herbal formula of dry herbs, boiled into a herbal juice, and taken twice daily, or made into be a concentrated herbal powder of which 6 g is taken with warm water twice daily.

Analysis: Chai Hu is the main herb in this formula for dredging *Liver Qi* and promoting general *Qi* movement. Xiang Fu and Zhi Qiao support the main herb to dredge stagnated *Liver Qi*. Chen Pi dispels stagnated *Liver* and *Stomach Qi* to relax the middle burner. Bai Shao nourishes *Liver Blood* and *Yin*. Chuan Xiong dispels blood stasis and eases coastal pain. Gan Cao harmonises all the herbs and regulates *Stomach*. All the herbs in this formula can release *Qi* stagnation in the *Liver*, *Spleen*, and the middle burner. This pattern can be seen as *Liver* inefficiency with some emotional symptoms, including restlessness and stress, during the post-COVID-19 syndrome phase.

Advice: This pattern can be seen as a weaker *Liver* with some emotional symptoms, such as restlessness or stress, during the post-COVID-19 syndrome.

Dampness and Heat accumulated in the Liver and the middle burner

Clinical features: Features are aching at both coastal areas, distension of stomach and abdomen that is radiating to the chest or upper back, nausea, belching, aching and heaviness in the general body, lethargy, feeling sleepy, poor appetite, aversion to greasy food, jaundice in some cases, acne or eczema on the skin, a red tongue with a greasy coating, and a wiry-rolling pulse.

Treatment principle in TCM:

1. Clear *Liver Heat* and releasing *Dampness.*
2. Smooth the *Liver Stagnation* and promoting *Qi* circulation.

Treatment: Herbal prescription.

Pinyin: Huo Xiang Zheng Qi variated with Long Dan Xie Gan Tang.

English name for decoction: Agastache Decoction to Rectify the *Qi* variated with Gentiana Longdancao Decoction to Drain the Liver.

Role in formula	Name/Pinyin	Name/Latin	Dose (g)	Function
Chief herb	Huo Xiang	Herba Agastaches seu Pogostemi	10	Dispels the external and internal dampness.
	Long Dan Cao	Radix Gentianae	10	Releases excessive liver heat in addition to all heat accumulated in the upper and middle burners.
Deputy herb	Hou Po	Cortex Magnoliae Officinalis	10	Dredges the stagnated *Qi* in the liver and the upper and middle burners.
Assistant herb	Zhi Zi	Fructus Gardeniae Jasminoidis	10	Emphasises release of the excessive liver *Qi*.
	Huang Qin	Radix Scutellariae Baicalensis	10	Emphasises release of the excessive *Qi* in both the upper and middle burners.
	Fu Ling	Sclerotium Poriae Cocos	10	Eliminates excessive dampness and fluid.
	Hua Shi	Talcum	10–20	Emphasises elimination of the excessive dampness.

(*Continued*)

(*Continued*)

Role in formula	Name/Pinyin	Name/Latin	Dose (g)	Function
	Ze Xie	Rhizoma Alismatis Orientalis	10	Eliminates excessive dampness and pushes the urine to be released.
	Gan Cao	Radix Glycyrrhizae Uralensis	5	Harmonises all of herbs to work well together and regulates the stomach.
Guiding herb	Chai Hu	Radix Bupleuri	6–10	Dredges stagnated liver *Qi* and leads all the herbs to have an effect on the liver.

Method: The above mentioned herbs are collected as a herbal formula of dry herbs, boiled into herbal juice, and taken twice daily, or made into a concentrated herbal powder of which 6 g is taken with warm water twice daily.

Analysis: Huo Xiang dispels the *External* and *Internal Dampness*, and is also the main herb. Hou Po and Fu Ling release *Excessive Damp* and residual dampness from the coronavirus. Long Dan Cao, Zhi Zi, and Huang Qin emphasise release of excessive *Liver Heat* in addition to all *Heat* accumulated in the upper and middle burners. Hua Shi and Ze Xie eliminate damp-fluid through urination. Chai Hu leads all treatment towards the *Liver* meridian. Gan Cao harmonises all herbs and regulates the *Stomach*. The formula can release excessive *Damp-Heat* from the *Liver*, *Spleen*, and upper-middle burners. This pattern can be seen in patients who are exhibiting some form of lingering coronavirus or abnormal liver function tests with some liver damage, along with dermatological complications or additional symptoms of the *Stomach*.

Advice: This pattern can be seen in patients who still have some corona virus, and have abnormal liver function tests with some liver damage, or have some dermatological complications or some more symptoms in the stomach and digestive system.

Liver Stagnation and Spleen Deficiency

Clinical features and signs: Signs are tiredness, fatigue, aching at both coastal areas and general limbs, distension of stomach and abdomen, loose bowels or diarrhoea, poor appetite or anorexia, mood swings, alight red tongue with teeth marks and less white coating, and a wiry-weaker pulse.

Treatment principle in TCM: Dredging *Liver Qi* and replenishing *Spleen Qi.*

Treatment: Herbal prescription.

Pinyin: Xiao Yao Tang variation or Xiao Yao Tang Plus.

English name for decoction: Bupleurum Rambling Decoction.

Role in formula	Name/ Pinyin	Name/Latin	Dose (g)	Function
Chief herb	Chai Hu	Radix Bupleuri	10	Dredges the liver *Qi* and promotes general *Qi* circulation.
Deputy herb	Dang Gui	Radix Angelicae Sinensis	10	Cultivates *Yin* and blood to soften the liver.
Assistant herb	Chi Shao	Radix Paeoniae Rubrae	10	Nourishes the liver *Yin* and blood.
	Bai Zhu	Rhizoma Atractylodis Macrocephalae	10	Replenishes the spleen *Qi* and general *Qi*.
	Shan Yao	Radix Dioscoreae Oppositae	10	Replenishes the spleen and dries the dampness.
	Fu Ling	Sclerotium Poriae Cocos	10	Replenishes the spleen and pushes for urination.
	Sheng Jiang	Rhizoma Zingiberis Officinalis Recens	10	Warms and strengthens the spleen *Qi* and agitates the general *Qi*.
Guiding Herb	Zhi Gan Cao	Radix Glycyrrhizae Uralensis	5	Harmonises all of herbs to work well together and regulates the stomach.
	Mu Dan Pi	Cortex Moutan Radicis	10	Clears the stagnated liver and blood heat.
	Zhi Zi	Fructus Gardeniae Jasminoidis	10	Clears the stagnated the liver and heart heat.

Method: The above mentioned herbs are collated as a herbal formula of dry herbs, boiled into herbal juice, and taken twice daily, or made into a concentrated herbal powder of which 6 g is taken with warm water twice daily.

Analysis: Chai Hu dredges the *Liver Qi* and promotes general *Qi* circulation as the main herb. Dang Gui softens the *Liver* and cultivates *Blood*, with Bai Shao nourishing *Liver Yin* and *Blood*. Bai Zhu, Shan Yao, and Fu Ling replenish *Spleen Qi* and encourage general *Qi Deficiency*. Sheng Jiang agitates *Qi* and *Yang* in the middle burner. Zhi Gan Cao harmonises all the herbs and supports the *Stomach*. Excess *Heat* accumulated in the *Liver* can be mitigated by adding Zhi Zi and Mu Dan Pi into the formula, further consolidating the formula of Xiao Yao Tang Plus. This pattern is commonly seen in the post-COVID-19 syndrome with liver damage, in which the patients exhibit both excess and deficiency in the *Liver* and *Spleen*, either with or without abnormal liver functions.

Advice: This pattern can commonly be seen in the post-COVID-19 syndrome with liver damage, wherein the patients exhibit both excess and deficiency in the *Liver* and *Spleen*, either with or without abnormal liver function.

Liver and Kidney Yin Deficiency

Clinical features and signs: Signs are slight or indistinct aching at the coastal areas, continuous existence and worse with exertion, dizziness and unclear vision, dry unsmooth eyes, dryness of eyes and mouth, empty heat in both palms, a red tongue with less coating or without coating, and a wiry-fine pulse.

Treatment principle in TCM:

1. Nourishing *Yin* and comforting *Liver*.
2. Cultivating *Blood* and promoting circulation.

Treatment: Herbal prescription.

Pinyin: Yi Guan Jian variation.

English name for decoction: The Liver Reinforcing Decoction.

Role in formula	Name/ Pinyin	Name/Latin	Dose (g)	Function
Chief herb	Sheng Di Huang	Radix Rehmanniae Glutinosae	10-30	Nourishes liver *Yin* and blood, cultivates kidney *Yin* and essence.
Deputy herb	Bei Sha Shen	Radix Glehniae Littoralis	10	Nourishes liver and lung *Yin* and blood.
Assistant herb	Mai Men Dong	Tuber Ophiopogonis Japonici	10	Nourishes liver and general *Yin* on the upper and middle burners.
	Dang Gui	Radix Angelicae Sinensis	10	Cultivates liver blood and *Yin* to soften the liver.
	Gou Qi Zi	Fructus Lycii	10	Nourishes the kidney and liver *Yin*.
Guiding herb	Chuan Lian Zi	Fructus Meliae Toosendan	10	Dredges the stagnated liver *Qi* and clears the liver heat, leads all of herbs into the liver.

Method: The above mentioned herbs are collected as a herbal formula of dry herbs, boiled into herbal juice, and taken twice daily, or made into a concentrated herbal powder of which 6 g is taken with warm water twice daily.

Analysis: Sheng Di Huang as the main herb nourishes *Liver Yin* and clears *Empty Heat*. Bei Sha Shen and Mai Men Dong emphasise the nourishment of *Liver Yin*. Dang Gui softens *Liver Yin* and cultivates *Liver Blood*. Chuan Lian Zi eliminates the *Liver Heat*. Gou Qi Zi nourishes *Kidney Yin*. The herbal formula nourishes the *Liver* and *Kidney Yin* and releases *Liver Heat*.

Advice: This pattern can be seen in liver weakness or in cases of minor liver failure presenting as *Empty Heat* and *Deficiency*; other combined symptoms may include both digestive and psychological disorders.

Liver and Kidney Yang Deficiency with Fluid Retention

Clinical features and signs: Signs are aching and distension at both coastal areas, distension of the stomach and abdomen, swollen abdomen and legs, aversion to cold, cold limbs and palms, pale and puffy face, anorexia, tiredness, fatigue, diarrhoea, lethargy, sleepiness, depression or lower spirit, a pale and swollen tongue with white-slippery coating, and a rolling-fine pulse.

Treatment principle in TCM:

1. Warming *Liver* and strengthening *Kidney Yang*.
2. Releasing excessive fluid and dredging three burners.

Treatment: Herbal prescription.

Pinyin: Ji Sheng Shen Qi variated with Wu Ling San.

English name for decoction: Life Saver Kidney *Qi* Decoction variated with Five-Ingredient Formula with Poria.

Role in formula	Name/ Pinyin	Name/Latin	Dose (g)	Function
Chief herb	Rou Gui/ Gui Zhi	Cortex or Ramulus Cinnamomi Cassiae	5–10	Warms and strengthens the kidney and liver yang *Qi*.
Deputy herb	Gan Jiang	Rhizoma Zingiberis Officinalis	10	Supports warming of yang *Qi* in the middle and lower burners.
	Shu Di Huang	Radix Rhemanniae Glutinosae Praeparata	10–30	Strengthens kidney and liver *Yin* and *Qi*.
	Shan Zhu Yu	Fructus Corni Officinalis	10	Promotes nourishing of the kidney *Yin* and essence.
	Shan Yao	Radix Dioscoreae Oppositae	10	Replenishes the kidney and spleen *Qi* and releases excessive dampness.
	Fu Ling	Sclerotium Poriae Cocos	10	Replenishes the spleen and kidney *Qi* and releases excessive dampness.
	Ze Xie	Rhizoma Alismatis Orientalis	10	Eliminates excessive dampness and pushes the urine out.

(*Continued*)

Role in formula	Name/ Pinyin	Name/Latin	Dose (g)	Function
	Che Qian Zi	Semen Plantaginis	10	Emphasises to release excessive dampness and fluid.
	Zhu Ling	Sclerotium Polypori Umbellati	10–30	Emphasises release of excessive dampness and fluid.
	Bai Zhu	Rhizoma Atractylodis Macrocephalae	10–30	Replenishes the spleen and general *Qi*, dries the dampness.
	Zhi Gan Cao	Radix Glycyrrhizae Uralensis	5	Harmonises all of herbs to work well together and regulates the stomach.
Guiding herb	Chuan Niu Xi	Radix Cyathulae Officinalis	10–15	Leads all the herbs to affect the lower burners and removes the blood stasis.

Method: The above mentioned herbs are collected as a herbal formula of dry herbs, boiled into herbal juice, and taken twice daily, or made into a concentrated herbal powder of which 6 g is taken with warm water twice daily.

Analysis: Rou Gui replaces Fu Zi as the main herb to warm and strengthen *Kidney* and *Liver Yang Qi*. We can also use Gui Zhi for replacement of Fu Zi to warm and agitate *Yang Qi*. Shu Di Huang, Shan Zhu Yu, and Shan Yao are three reinforcing herbs to promote *Liver* and *Kidney Yang Qi*. Fu Ling, Ze Xie, and Mu Dan Pi as the three reducing herbs eliminate excessive fluid. Chuan Niu Xi leads the formula down to the middle and lower burners. Che Qian Zi emphasises the elimination of fluid through urination; if excessive dampness and fluid accumulate, Wu Ling San is added. Zhu Ling, Ze Xie, and Fu Ling release fluid. Bai Zhu reinforces the *Spleen* and dries *Dampness*. Gui Zhi agitates *Yang Qi* in the middle burner. This formula is designed for warming and strengthening the *Liver* and *Kidney Yang Qi* and releasing accumulated *Dampness* and fluid. This pattern can be seen with *Liver* function failure or fibrosis causing fluid accumulation in the abdomen and legs, which presents in the severe stages. If patients are still given treatment from the mainstream healthcare system, we can manage herbs, focusing more on the *Qi* and *Yang* replenishment to complement allopathic medicine.

Advice: This pattern can be seen in liver function failure or fibrosis causing fluid accumulation in the abdomen and legs, which presents in the severe stages. If patients are still given treatment from the mainstream healthcare system, we can manage herbs by focusing on the *Qi* and yang replenishment to complement allopathic medicine.

Liver Blood Stasis

Clinical features and signs: Signs are significant or sharp aching or pain at the coastal areas, stomach and abdominal distension, headache, stress, depression, restlessness, a dark complexion and tongue with stasis marks at the sides with less coating, and a deep-wiry pulse. All the symptoms are worse at night.

Treatment principle in TCM:

1. Activating *Blood* and removing *Blood Stasis*.
2. Promoting *Blood* circulation to relieve pain.

Treatment: Herbal prescription and acupuncture.

Pinyin: Xue Fu Zhu Yu Tang variation.

English name for decoction: Drive Out Stasis in the Mansion of Blood Decoction variation.

Role in formula	Name/ Pinyin	Name/Latin	Dose (g)	Function
Chief herb	Dang Gui	Radix Angelicae Sinensis	10	Replenishes and nourishes *Yin* and blood.
	Sheng Di Huang	Radix Rehmanniae Glutinosae	10–30	Nourishes kidney and general *Yin*.
Deputy herb	Tao Ren	Semen Pruni Persicae	10	Invigorates blood circulation, eases pain, and softens solid stasis.

(*Continued*)

Role in formula	Name/Pinyin	Name/Latin	Dose (g)	Function
	Hong Hua	Flos Carthami Tinctorii	10	Invigorates blood circulation, eases pain, and softens solid stasis.
Assistant herb	Zhi Qiao	Fructus Citri Aurantiio	10	Removes general stagnated *Qi* and softens the solid stasis.
	Chi Shao	Radix Paeoesniae Rubraeo	10	Invigorates the blood stasis and removes stagnated *Qi* in the blood.
	Chai Hu	Radix Bupleuri	10	Dredges the stagnated *Qi*.
	Chuan Xiong	Radix Ligustici Wallichii	10	Invigorates the blood stasis, eases the pain, and removes stagnated *Qi* in the blood.
	Chuan Niu Xi	Radix Cyathulae Officinaliso	10–15	Releases stasis blood.
	Gan Cao	Radix Glycyrrhizae Uralensis	5	Harmonises all of herbs to work well together and regulates the stomach.
Guiding herb	Jie Geng	Radix Platycodi Grandiflori	6–10	Jie Geng leads all the herbs to the lung meridian and removes the lung *Qi*'s circulation.

Method: The above mentioned herbs are collated as a herbal formula of dry herbs, boiled into herbal juice, and taken twice daily, or made into a concentrated herbal powder of which 6 g is taken with warm water twice daily.

Analysis: Sheng Di Huang, Dang Gui, Chi Shao, and Chuan Xiong form the full composition of Si Wu Tang for *Nourishing Blood*. Tao Ren and Hong Hua move blood circulation, ease pain, and soften solid stasis. Chuan Ni Xi removes the *Blood Stasis* in the middle and lower burners. Jie Geng removes the *Blood Stasis* in the upper burner and promotes the *Qi* circulation. Gan Cao harmonises all the herbs and calms the *Stomach*. The formula can remove *Blood Stasis* from the *Liver* and whole body. This pattern can be seen in the patients with significant pain and solid lumps in the liver or liver function failure and fibrosis damage.

Advice: This pattern can be seen in the patients with remarkable pain and solid lumps in the liver or liver function failure and fibrosis damage.

Acupuncture point selection and rationale

Main points: Baihui DU20, Zhongwan REN15.

Assistant points: Waiguan (SJ5), Zulinqi (GB41), Hegu (LI4), Taichong (LIV3); Xiawan (REN10), Qihai (REN6), Guanyuan (REN4); Ququan (LI8), Xingjian (LIV2), Yanglingquan (GB34), Qiuxu (GB40); Yingu (KI10), Taixi (KI3), Zhaohai (KI6); Zusanli (ST36), Yinlingquan (SP9), Sanyinjiao (SP6).

Analysis: DU20 governs the general and *Vital Qi*. REN15 emphasises and regulates *Qi Stagnation* or insufficiency in the middle burner as the main points. SJ5 and GB41 are the cross points and dredge the stagnated *Qi* through the meridians. LI4 and LIV3 are the formation of the four gates and clear accumulated *Heat*. REN10, REN6, and REN4 *Nourish Yin* in general along with the *Conceptive Vessel*. LIV8 and LIV2 are both the He-sea point and *Ying-Spring* point of the liver meridian and nourish Liver *Yin* and blood. GB34 and GB40 are *He-sea* and Yuan-original points of the *Gallbladder* meridian and remove stagnated *Liver Qi*. KID10, KID6, and KID3 reinforce *Kidney Qi* and *Yin*. ST36, SP9, and SP6 reinforce the *Spleen*. All these points can be selected to treat *Liver Inefficiency*, liver failure, and fibrosis according to individual case presentation.

Case Study

Ms. P. Smith, a 58-year-old female officer, visits the TCM clinic for aching coastal areas, accompanied by depression and tiredness with a higher Alanine Aminotransferase (ALT) in the liver function test for 3 months, indicating possible challenge of multiple pathologies, including infection. A positive PCR was confirmed in August 2020, with fever, cough, nausea, and diarrhoea for a period of 2 weeks. During the infectious and illness phase, she stayed at home resting and sleeping for most of the time. However, she continued to be afflicted with the feeling of lethargy, fatigue, nausea, and diarrhoea following the 2-week period. Her ALT levels remained high, with a confirmed elevation to 145, which is one item of the liver function in the blood test, and a slight enlargement on her liver. However, the PCR became negative. It was confirmed at the consultation that this patient had suffered from hepatitis C for a period of 10 years, although it had been controlled well until 2 years ago. Liver function is triggered by coronavirus, which contributed to her feeling unwell after the infectious period of COVID-19. She also had a light red tongue with white coating and a wiry-fine pulse.

Clinical features and signs: Signs were aching local to the right coastal area, compressed pain in the stomach, nausea, no appetite, distension of the abdomen, loose bowels with a frequency of 3–4 times daily, restlessness, nervousness, feeling weepy, and disturbed sleep.

WM diagnosis:

1. Post-COVID-19 syndrome.
2. Recurrent hepatitis/liver functional failure.

Differentiation syndromes of TCM:

1. *Liver Qi Stagnation.*
2. *Spleen Qi Deficiency.*

Treatment: Herbal prescription and acupuncture.

Pinyin: Xiao Yao Tang Plus.

English name for decoction: Augmented Rambling Decoction Plus.

Herbal powders (g):

Dang Gui	Radix Angelicae Sinensis 10 g
Chi Shao	Radix Paeoniae Rubrae 10 g
Chai Hu	Radix Bupleuri 10 g
Bai Zhu	Rhizoma Atractylodis Macrocephalae 10 g
Shan Yao	Radix Dioscoreae Oppositae 10 g
Bo He	Herba Menthae Haplocalycis 5 g

Chuan Xiong	Radix Ligustici Wallichii 10 g
Gan Jiang	Rhizoma Zingiberis Officinalis 10 g
Mu Dan	Pi Cortex Moutan Radicis 10 g
Zhi Zi	Fructus Gardeniae Jasminoidis 10 g
Zhi Gan Cao	Radix Glycyrrhizae Uralensis 5 g

Method: The above mentioned herbal prescription is made into herbal powder of which 6 g is taken with warm water twice daily for a month. The patient is given regular acupuncture once a week as well. He/She feels relaxed, the coastal and stomach pain are much lessened, and the ALT is decreased, after which we change the herbs to a pill form.

Herbal prescription adjustment

The above mentioned prescription herbs are changed to a pill form:

- Jia Wei Xiao Yao Wan (Augmented Rambling Pills).
- Bu Zhong Yi Qi Wan (Tonify the Middle and Augment the *Qi* Pills).

Results: She is still taking these pills and does acupuncture once every 2 weeks, or irregularly when she needs to maintain her liver function at a normal level and to ensure that all other symptoms are under control.

Method: The above mentioned herbal prescription is changed to a herbal powder of which 6 g with is taken warm water twice daily for a month.

Analysis: She continued taking the herbal pills and also receiving acupuncture treatment once every 2 weeks, or whenever when she needs support to maintain and stabilise her liver function to a normal level, including keeping her symptoms under control.

Acupuncture point selection and rationale

Acupuncture: Moxibustion Shenque (REN8); Baihui (DU20), Yintang (Ext), Jiuwei (REN15), Zhongwan (REN12), Qihai (REN6), Tianshu (ST25), Zusanli (ST36), Yinlingquan (SP9), Sanyinjiao (SP6);

Yanglingquan (GB34), Zulinqi (GB41), Waiguan (SJ5), Hegu (LI4), Taichong (LIV3).

Treatment result and analysis: After treatment, she feels relaxed, the coastal and stomach pain has significantly improved and the elevated liver function of the ALT has decreased, which prompted the change to the herbal tablet prescription, along with the decision to realign to an acupuncture maintenance treatment to maintain stability of symptoms for the patient.

References

CDC. (2021). What to know about liver disease and COVID-19. Centers for Disease Control and Prevention, USA. Available at: https://www.cdc.gov/coronavirus/2019-ncov/need-extra-precautions/liver-disease.html (Accessed 18 February 2022).

Cichoż-Lach, H. and Michalak, A. (2021). Liver injury in the era of COVID-19. *World Journal of Gastroenterology*, 27(5), 377–390. https://doi.org/10.3748/wjg.v27.i5.377.

Du, M., Yang, S., Liu, M., and Liu, J. (2022). COVID-19 and liver dysfunction: Epidemiology, association and potential mechanisms. *Clinics and Research in Hepatology and Gastroenterology*, 46(2), 101793. https://doi.org/10.1016/j.clinre.2021.101793.

Marjot, T., Webb, G. J., Barritt, A. S., *et al.* (2021). COVID-19 and liver disease: Mechanistic and clinical perspectives. *Nature Reviews Gastroenterology & Hepatology*, 18, 348–364. https://doi.org/10.1038/s41575-021-00426-4.

Sonzogni, A., Previtali, G., Seghezzi, M., *et al.* (2020). Liver histopathology in severe COVID 19 respiratory failure is suggestive of vascular alterations. *Liver International*, 40(9), 2110–2116. https://doi.org/10.1111/liv.14601.

Tsutsumi, T., Saito, M., Nagai, H., Yamamoto, S., Ikeuchi, K., *et al.* (2021). Association of coagulopathy with liver dysfunction in patients with COVID-19. *Hepatology Research*, 51(2), 227–232. https://doi.org/10.1111/hepr.13577.

Chapter 7

Kidney System Damage

Nephropathy in COVID-19 and Post-COVID-19 Syndrome

As a close part of the multi-system inflammatory condition of COVID-19, the kidney is also a commonly affected organ due to the structurally dominating blood vessels within it. It has been discussed in Chapter 5 that blood vessels are the second most likely tissues to be infected by the SARS-CoV-2 virus. The damage in kidney due to COVID-19 infection thus is inevitable.

Early discussions (Carratalá *et al.*, 2020) from observations in Spain indicate that patients with kidney disease had a higher risk of morbidity and mortality when COVID-19 occurred. There was also a suggestion that some patients of COVID-19 developed vascular lesions in their kidney as part of the vascular system impairment. These impairments will cause problems in the near future when they recover from acute COVID-19.

Dennis *et al.* (2021) in the UK followed 201 individuals 141 days after COVID-19 infection. The finding revealed that 4% of patients have kidney impairment among the patients as one of the organs impaired in the multiple-organs impairment of 29% of all of participants. This is an early source confirming that kidney damage among the PCS population is not rare.

Sperati (2020) suggested that up to 30% of patients hospitalised with COVID-19 in China and New York developed moderate and severe kidney injury. This is indicated by high levels of protein in the urine test and other blood tests, suggesting kidney problems. He did not provide information about how many of the problems were preexisting and how many were newly discovered. Four possible ways that kidney impairment developed during COVID-19 were proposed: Coronavirus attacks the kidney cells via ACE_2 receptor, deprivation of oxygen leads to kidney malfunction, cytokine storm kills kidney cells, and blood clotting chokes the kidney tissues. As above, speculation with regard to the mechanism of kidney impairment remains the hypothesis.

Zhang *et al.* (2021) carried out a 4-month follow-up observation after hospital discharge on 143 patients with new-onset kidney disease during the COVID-19 pandemic. After 4 months, 91% (130 of 143) of patients recovered from kidney disease, and 9% (13 of 143) of patients failed to recover. Two elements are related to the non-recovery: the age of the patient being 10 years older than those who recovered and a higher serum creatinine level when they were discharged.

According to Bowe *et al.* (2021), the largest survey so far which was carried out on American veterans (1,726,683; 89,276 COVID-19 survivors vs 1,637,467 control group) revealed a higher risk of kidney damage 30 days after COVID-19 infection, measured by higher Acute Kidney Injury (AKI), eGFR decline ≥30%, ESKD (End Stage of Kidney Disease means receipt of chronic outpatient dialysis or kidney transplant), and major adverse kidney events (MAKE, a combined eGFR decline of ≥50%, ESKD, or all-cause mortality). The total risk has increased 1.46 per thousand from the non-COVID-19 population to COVID-19 survivors (30 days after infection). However, more worryingly, among all reported PCS, 30% of them showed kidney function damage, and the damage was silent, symptomless. People do not report the symptoms of kidney damage but bear the damage.

Generally speaking, due to the relatively short period of observation, most cases of newly added kidney impairments are classified as Acute Kidney Injury (AKI); although the name is linked to physical damage of the body structure, it has little connection to any physical injury. The name of the condition is best for describing impairment in the kidney due to the long-lasting effect of COVID-19. As time goes on, a better picture of both acute and chronic impairment of the kidney could be drawn. However, chronic diagnosis is limited at this stage.

Among AKI sufferers, some of them need dialysis regularly, along with staying in the hospital, which limits the patients' access to TCM treatment. However, most of them are treated as out-patients, and TCM treatment could provide a value to existing medical/drug treatment.

Clinical Features

Many patients do not show typical symptoms of AKI, although most patients do. The common symptoms of AKI are as follows: Tiredness, nausea, diarrhoea, dehydration, reduced amount of urine, confusion, and drowsiness.

Diagnosis:

1. Blood test: eGFR decline ≥30%. Creatinine level-based index.
2. Urine test: Protein, blood cells in urine, sugar, and waste products.
3. Ultrasound scan of kidney, or CT/MRI scan of kidney.

Syndrome Patterns and Treatment by TCM

Kidney Qi Deficiency

Clinical features and signs: Signs are tiredness, frequency in urination, decreased hearing, weak and sore in the back, uterus prolapse, habitual miscarriage, breathlessness, minor swelling (oedema) in the lower legs, ankle, or feet during exertion, pale complexion, a pale tongue with thin white coating, and a fine-weak pulse.

Treatment principle in TCM: Replenishing *Kidney Qi* agitates the original and *Vitality Qi.*

Treatment: Herbal prescription.

Pinyin: Jin Kui/Gui Shen Qi Tang.

English name for decoction: Kidney *Qi* Decoction from the Golden Cabinet.

Role in formula	Name/Pinyin	Name/Latin	Dose (g)	Function
Chief herb	Shu Di Huang	Radix Rhemanniae Glutinosae Praeparata	10–30	Nourishes the kidney *Yin* and complements the kidney essence.
Deputy herb	Shan Zhu Yu	Fructus Corni Officinalis	10	Promotes nourishing of the kidney *Yin* and holds the kidney essence.

(*Continued*)

(*Continued*)

Role in formula	Name/Pinyin	Name/Latin	Dose (g)	Function
Assistant herb	Shan Yao	Radix Dioscoreae Oppositae	10	Replenishes the spleen and dries the dampness.
	Fu Ling	Sclerotium Poria Cocos	10	Releases excessive dampness and replenishes the spleen; supports Shan Yao to replenish the spleen.
	Mu Dan Pi	Cortex Moutan Radicis	10	Eliminates the liver fire and general fire in the lower burner.
	Ze Xie	Rhizoma Alismatis Orientalis	10	Eliminates the kidney fire and general fire in the lower burner.
	Xiang Fu	Rhizoma Cyperi Rotundi	10	Warms the kidney yang. This is a replacement for Fu Zi in the original formula.
Guiding herb	Gui Zhi	Ramulus Cinnamomi Cassiae	6–10	Warms the kidney yang and agitates general yang *Qi* in the low burner.

Method: The above-mentioned herbs are collected as herbal formula of dry herbs, boiled into herbal juice, and taken = twice daily, or made into a concentrated herbal powder of which 6 g is taken with warm water twice daily.

Analysis: Shu Di Huang and Shan Zhu Yu replenish *Kidney Qi* for strengthening *Pre-Heaven Qi*. Shan Yao replenishes *Spleen Qi,* thus promoting the *Post-Heaven Qi* and consolidating the *Vital Qi* and original *Qi*. Fu Ling and Ze Xie eliminate accumulated fluid. Mu Dan Pi releases the

Empty Heat. Xiang Fu and Gui Zhi replace the Fu Zi and Rou Gui, which are barred in Europe, and promote the general *Qi* and warm them for agitating all the organic (original) *Qi.*

Advice: This pattern can be seen with *Kidney Inefficiency* and a gentle stage of kidney failure during post-COVID-19 syndrome.

Kidney Yang Deficiency and Fluid accumulation

Clinical figures and signs: Signs are anorexia and nausea; dizziness; headache; blood in urine; frequent urination; muscle cramps; aversion to cold; cold and soreness in the lower back; breathlessness; lethargy; impotence or erectile dysfunction in men; no sexual drive in female; poor spirit; swollen legs, ankles, and feet; and a pale or pale-plump tongue with white-slippery coating.

Treatment principle in TCM: Warming and strengthening *Kidney Yang*; releasing accumulated fluid.

Treatment: Herbal prescription.

Pinyin: You Gui Yin variation with Zhen Wu Tang.

English name for decoction: Restore the Right Kidney Drink variation True Warrior Decoction.

Role in formula	Name/ Pinyin	Name/Latin	Dose (g)	Function
Chief herb	Shu Di Huang	Radix Rhemanniae Glutinosae Praeparata	10–30	Nourishes the kidney yin as the foundation to promote the kidney yang; complements the kidney essence.
	Rou Gui	Cortex Cinnamomi Cassiae	5–10	Warms and agitates the kidney yang.
Deputy herb	Shan Zhu Yu	Fructus Corni Officinalis	10	Supports nourishing of the kidney yin to promote building of the kidney yang.
	Sheng Jiang	Rhizoma Zingiberis Officinalis Recens	10	Supports warming and agitating of the kidney yang.

(*Continued*)

(*Continued*)

Role in formula	Name/ Pinyin	Name/Latin	Dose (g)	Function
Assistant herb	Shan Yao	Radix Dioscoreae Oppositae	10	Replenishes the spleen *Qi* and middle burner and releases excessive dampness.
	Du Zhong	Cortex Eucommiae Ulmoidis	10	Warms and replenishes the kidney yang and strengthens the muscles, tendons, and bones.
	Gou Qi Zi	Cortex Cinnamomi Cassiae	10	Nourishes the kidney and liver yin and blood as the foundation to build the kidney yang.
	Bai Zhu	Rhizoma Atractylodis Macrocephalae	10–30	Replenishes the spleen and releases excessive dampness.
	Bai Shao	Radix Paeoniae Lactiflorae	10	Nourishes the kidney and liver yin and blood.
	Fu Ling	Sclerotium Poria Cocos	10	Releases the excessive dampness and replenishes the spleen.
Guiding herb	Zhi Qiao	Cao Radix Glycyrrhizae Uralensis	10	Agitates and removes general *Qi* in the middle and lower burners and and avoids all tonic herbs to cause stagnation.

Method: The above-mentioned herbs are collected as herbal formula of dry herbs, boiled into herbal juice, and taken twice daily, or made into a concentrated herbal powder of which 6 g is taken with warm water twice daily.

Analysis: Shu Di Huang, Shan Zhu Yu, and Shan Yao replenish Kidney *Qi*. Du Zhong strengthens *Kidney Yang*. Gou Qi Zi nourishes *Kidney Yin*. Rou Gui agitates *Yang Qi*. Bai Zhu, Sheng Jiang, and Fu Ling release accumulated fluid. Bai Zhu reinforces *Spleen Qi* for promoting *Kidney Qi*. Zhi Gan Cao harmonises the *Stomach*, promoting the acceptance of all the herbs. All these herbal prescriptions can strengthen *Kidney Yang* and release accumulated fluid and can be used for kidney failure with fluid tension.

Advice: This pattern can be seen with someone tolerating an extended duration of disease history or a severe state of post-COVID-19 syndrome, and a weaker general constitution, so he/she needs a strong enough treatment to reinforce the *Qi* and warm up the yang.

Kidney Yin Deficiency

Clinical features and signs: Signs are tiredness, dizziness, tinnitus, aching back with ejaculation, premature ejaculation, hot flashes during the night with sweating, poor sleep, constipation, a red tongue with less coating or without coating, and a fine-rapid pulse.

Treatment principle in TCM: Nourishing *Kidney Yin*; releasing *Empty Heat.*

Treatment: Herbal prescription.

Pinyin: Zhi Bai Di Huang Wan or Zuo Gui Wan.

English name for decoction: Anemarrhena, Phellodendron, and Rehmannia Decoction or Restore the Left Kidney Decoction.

Role in formula	Name/Pinyin	Name/Latin	Dose (g)	Function
Chief herb	Sheng Di Huang	Radix Rehmanniae Glutinosae	10–30	Nourishes the kidney yin and clears the empty heat.
	Huang Bai	Cortex Phellodendri	10	Releases the empty heat and dries the dampness.
Deputy herb	Mu Dan Pi	Cortex Moutan Radicis	10	Clears the heat in the blood and kidney and lower burner.
	Zhi Mu	Radix Anemarrhenae Asphodeloidis	10	Emphasises nourishing of the kidney yin and clears the empty heat.
Assistant herb	Zhan Zhu Yu	Fructus Corni Officinalis	10	Nourishes the kidney yin and essence.
	Shan Yao	Radix Dioscoreae Oppositae	10	Replenishes the spleen *Qi* and dries the dampness.
	Fu Ling	Sclerotium Poria Cocos	10	Dries the dampness and replenishes the spleen.
	Ze Xie	Rhizoma Alismatis Orientalis	10	Dredges the stagnated *Qi* and accumulated dampness.

Method: The above-mentioned herbs are collected as herbal formula of dry herbs, boiled into herbal juice, and taken twice daily, or made into a concentrated herbal powder of which 6 g is taken with warm water twice daily.

Analysis: Overall, the *Kidney Qi* and *Yin* are replenished by Sheng Di Huang, Shan Zhu Yu, and Shan Yao. Huang Bai and Zhi Mu support Mu Dan Pi to release *Empty Heat.* Fu Ling and Ze Xie assist to reduce excessive *Dampness.* All of formulae nourish *Kidney Yin*, rather than reinforcing *Kidney Qi*. This pattern can be seen in *Kidney Inefficiency* or in a gentle stage of kidney failure accompanied by *Empty Heat.*

Advice: This pattern can also be seen in the patients with an enduring diseased history in addition to a weaker constitution, although some upright *Qi* is still prevailing inside the body, so he/she manifests a deficiency pattern with *Empty Heat* during post-COVID-19 syndrome.

Damp-Heat in the Bladder

Clinical features and signs: Signs are recurrent or persistent soreness, distension or burning sensation in the lower abdomen, frequency or *urgency* of urination, fever, backache, blood in the urine, nausea, sickness, lose or sluggish bowel movements, unclear urination, a red or light red tongue with greasy or greasy-yellow coating, and a rolling-rapid pulse.

Treatment principle in TCM: Release the excessive damp-heat; Clear the lower burner.

Treatment: Herbal prescription.

Pinyin: Ba Zheng San variation.

English name for decoction: Eight-Herb Decoction for Rectification variation.

Role in formula	Name/ Pinyin	Name/Latin	Dose (g)	Function
Chief herb	Che Qian Zi	Semen Plantaginis	10	Reduces the excessive accumulated damp-heat in the lower burner.
Deputy herb	Qu Mai	Herba Dianthi	10	Emphasises reduction of the accumulated damp-heat in the lower burner.
Assistant herb	Bian Xu	Herba Polygoni Avicularis	10	Assists in reducing excessive accumulated damp-heat in the lower burner.
	Hua Shi	Talcum	10	Eliminates excessive dampness and promotes urine elimination.
	Zhi Zi	Fructus Gardeniae Jasminoidis	10	Releases the excessive heat in the bladder and lower burner.
	Tong Cao	Medulla Tetrapanacis Papyriferi	10	Eliminates excessive dampness and promotes urine elimination.
	Dan Huang	Radix et Rhizoma Rhei	10	Purges the bowel movement to treat constipation.
Guiding herb	Gan Cao	Radix Glycyrrhizae Uralensis	5	Harmonises the stomach to receive all herbs and promote effectiveness.

Method: The above-mentioned herbs are collected as a herbal formula of dry herbs, boiled into herbal juice, and taken twice daily, or made into a concentrated herbal powder of which 6 g is taken with warm water twice daily.

Analysis: Che Qian Zi, Ju Mai, and Bian Xu reduce excessive accumulated *Damp-Heat* in the lower burner. Hua Shi and Tong Cao (replacing Mu Tong which is barred from use in Europe) dredge the elimination passage to release *Damp-Heat.* Zhi Zi accentuates *Heat Clearing.* Da Huang stimulates the intestinal passage for movement. Bai Zhu and Gan Cao harmonise the middle burner and consolidate the three burners. This pattern can be seen in patients with recurrent attacks of bladder inflammation including *Kidney Inefficiency* or kidney failure as a result of post-COVID-19 syndrome.

Advice: This pattern can be seen in patients with recurrent bladder inflammation, or those suffering from the interstitial cystitis as a chronic state in the post-syndrome of COVID-19, so herbal treatment is still needed to release the pathogenic factors.

Acupuncture

Main points: Baihui (DU20), Yintang (Ext).

Group 1: Juiwei (REN15), Zhongwan (REN12), Qihai (REN6), Guanyuan (REN4), Yingu (KI10), Fuliu (KI7), Zhaohai (KI6), Taixi (KI3), Tianshu (ST25), Zusanli (ST36).

Group 2: Yaoyangguan (DU3), Mingmen (DU4), Dazhui (DU14), Shenshu (BL23), Pishu (BL20), Ganshu (BL18), Dachangshu (BL25), Yinlingquan (SP9), Sanyinjiao (SP6), Waiguan (SJ5), Zulinqi (GB41), or Hegu (LI4), Taichong (LIV3), Fengchi (GB20).

Analysis: Baihui governs general *Qi* and can dredge stagnated *Qi* in the whole body. Yintang with cold-inducing needle technology can release *Empty Heat* and clear the front head as the main points.

Group 1: Jiuwei, Zhongwan, Qihai, and Guanyuan are located along the conception vessel, capable of reinforcing *Vitality Qi* and cultivating general *Yin-Essence.* Yingu, Fuliu, Zhaohai, and Taixi as the *He-sea* point, *Jing-River* point, *Shu-Stream*, and *Yuan-Original* points of the *Kidney* meridian are able to regulate as well as reinforce kidney disorder with various needle technologies. Tianshu and Zusanli call attention to strengthen the middle and lower burners.

Group 2: Yaoyangguan and Mingmen strongly reinforce *Original* and *Kidney Qi* and *Essence.* Dazhui excites general *Yang Qi* along with regulating any disorder at the upper burner. Sheshu, Pishu, or Ganshu is selected according to the presentation of clinical symptoms. Dachangshu is the back shu point of the *Large Intestine* and can regulate the intestines and resolve constipation. Waiguan and Zulinqi are selected to remove stagnated *Kidney* or *Liver Qi.* Hegu and taichong are selected to clear *Excessive Heat.* Fengchi is given to eliminate headache or dizziness caused by *Excessive Wind* at the top of the head.

Case Study

Ms. R. Kail, a 58-year-old Pakistani housewife, had been feeling tired, fatigue, and recurrent dizziness for nearly a year after she suffered from COVID-19 in April 2020. She passed on the virus to one of the grandchildren in the family, whom manifested a fever, cough, nausea, and general aching within a couple of weeks. She has not felt well since, feeling lethargic, fatigued, anorexia with no appetite all the time, having poor sleep, and dizziness, which resulted in her admission to the hospital for further examination. Chronic nephropathy was confirmed with a creatinine level of 315 ml/min, urea 20, resulting in the offer of regular dialysis. A previous surgery to resect the left kidney due to cancer 5 years ago gave rise to worry in her family and therefore they decided to seek TCM treatment and postpone doing dialysis.

Clinical features and signs: Signs are recurrent dizziness, tiredness, fatigue, headache, anorexia, no appetite with nausea, loose bowels or sluggish bowels, aversion to cold, a light red-dark tongue with less white coating, and a deep-fine pulse.

Examination: BP 198/104 P 89/min.

Last kidney function report:

- Creatinine 315 ml/min.
- Urea 20 ACR.
- Hb 7.8.

Diagnosis:

1. Post-COVID-19 syndrome.
2. Kidney failure/Chronic nephropathy.
3. Hypertension.
4. Anaemia.

Differentiation syndromes of TCM:

1. Both *Kidney* and *Spleen Qi* and *Yin Deficiency*.
2. *Liver Qi Stagnation* and *Internal Wind* rising inside.

Treatment: Herbal prescription and acupuncture.

Acupuncture

Main points: Baihui (DU20), Yintang (Ext); Jiuwei (REN15), Zhongwan (REN12), Qihai (REN6), Guanyuan (REN4); Yingu (KI10), Fuliu (KI7), Zhaohai (KI6), Taixi (KI3); Yinlingquan (SP9), Sanyinjiao (SP6), Tianshu (ST25), Zusanli (ST36); Waiguan (SJ5), Zulinqi (GB41).

Herbal prescription

Herbal powders (g):

Shu Di Huang	Radix Rehmanniae Glutinosae 20 g
Dang Gui	Radix Angelicae Sinensis 10 g
Chi Shao	Radix Paeoniae Rubrae 10 g
Chuan Xiong	Radix Ligustici Wallichii 10 g
Dang Shen	Radix Codonopsis Pilosulae 10 g
Bai Zhu	Rhizoma Atractylodis Macrocephalae 10 g
Fu Ling	Sclerotium Poriae Cocos 10 g
Huang Qi	Radix Astragali Membranacei 10 g
Shi Jue Ming	Concha Haliotidis 15 g
Shan Zha	Fructus Crataegi 10 g
Shen Qu	Massa Medica Fermentata 10 g
Bai Dou Kou	Fructus Amomi Cardamomi 10 g
Yu Zhu	Rhizoma Polygonati Odorati 10 g

Gou Teng	Ramulus cum Uncis Uncariae 10 g
Zhi Gan Cao	Radix Glycyrrhizae Uralensis 5 g

The above herbs amount to 160 g, out of which the patient was advised to take 6 g with warm water twice daily. The patient visited the clinic every 2 weeks and continued taking herbal powders. She was given a blood transfusion occasionally by the NHS (2022) and does not do dialysis.

References

Bowe, B., Xie, Y., Xu, E., and Al-Aly, Z. (2021). Kidney outcomes in long COVID. *Journal of the American Society of Nephrology*, 32(11), 2851–2862. doi:10.1681/ASN.2021060734.

Carratalá, P. V., Górriz-Zambrano, C., Ariño, M. C., Caro, L. J. L., Gorriz, J. L., *et al.* (2020). COVID-19 and cardiovascular and kidney disease: Where are we? Where are we going? *SEMERGEN*, 46(Suppl 1), 78–87. Spanish. doi:10.1016/j.semerg.2020.05.005. Epub 2020 May 11.

Dennis, A., Wamil, M., Alberts, J., Oben, J., Cuthbertson, D. J., *et al.* (2021). Multiorgan impairment in low-risk individuals with post-COVID-19 syndrome: A prospective, community-based study. *BMJ Open*, 11(3), e048391. doi:10.1136/bmjopen-2020-048391.

NHS (National Health Service). (2022). Acute kidney injury. NHS. Available at: https://www.nhs.uk/conditions/acute-kidney-injury/.

Sperati, J. (2020). Coronavirus: Kidney damage caused by COVID-19. Johns Hopkins Medicine. Available at: https://www.hopkinsmedicine.org/health/conditions-and-diseases/coronavirus/coronavirus-kidney-damage-caused-by-covid19 (Accessed 18 February 2022).

Zhang, N. H., Cheng, Y. C., Luo, R., *et al.* (2021). Recovery of new-onset kidney disease in COVID-19 patients discharged from hospital. *BMC Infectious Diseases*, 21, 397. https://doi.org/10.1186/s12879-021-06105-8.

Chapter 8

Brain and Neurological Disorders

The nervous system is partially involved in COVID-19 infection through several pathways which could be the reduced oxygen supply, vessel infection and clotting, and long-term fight–flight reaction. In the PCS stage, the damages are clearly detectable and they continue to cause problems in sufferers.

According to Origier (2020), based on early reports of COVID-19 related neurological damage, hypotheses of how such damage might take place were proposed. Among them are hypoxemia due to the reduced oxygen supply, viral invasion into the brain, and psychological factors. And, these lead to chronic neuro-inflammation, demyelination, and degenerative changes. Early speculation is still valuable when looking at the situation of the post-COVID-19 population.

Lu's research team in China found that, in this follow-up stage, neurological symptoms were presented in 55% of COVID-19 patients. In the scanned images of their brain, these patients indicated a significant increase of grey matter volume (GMV) in the olfactory cortices, hippocampi, insula, left Rolandic operculum, left Heschl's gyrus, and right cingulate gyrus and a general decline of MD, AD, and RD accompanied by an increase of FA in white matter, especially AD in the right CR, EC, and SFF, and MD in SFF. Their studies revealed a possible disruption to microstructural and functional brain integrity in the recovery stages of COVID-19. They also suggest that the changes are not individually related to one peripheral nerve which might allow for the virus to enter the CNS.

Caress *et al.* (2020) reviewed 37 published cases of Guillain-Barré syndrome (GBS) associated with COVID-19 to summarise this information as an emerging theme in COVID-19 neuropathy. The mean time between the onset of COVID-19 symptoms and GBS symptoms was 11 days. The clinical presentation and severity of these GBS cases were similar to those with non-COVID-19 GBS. The EDx pattern was considered demyelinating in approximately half of the cases. CSF demonstrated albuminocytologic dissociation in 76% of the cases. Serum antiganglioside antibodies were absent in 15 of 17 patients tested. Most patients were treated with a single course of intravenous immunoglobulin, and improvement was noted within 8 weeks in most cases. GBS-associated COVID-19 appears to have been an uncommon condition with similar clinical and EDx patterns to GBS before the pandemic. The Uncini *et al.* (2020) review put more effort into the GBS clinical manifestation, reporting that the most common clinical features were limb weakness (76.2%), hyporeflexia (80.9%), sensory disturbances (66.7%), and facial palsy (38.1%).

Spectrum of Symptoms in Nervous System Impairment

According to Khatoon *et al.* (2021), COVID-19 causes multiple forms of damage when infection happens, not limited to the respiratory system but in the nervous system as well. A broad spectrum of neurological conditions were reported in acute COVID-19 sufferers, which included encephalopathy, impaired consciousness, confusion, agitation, seizure, ataxia, headache, anosmia, ageusia, and degenerative neuropathy. The evidence suggests that the SARS-CoV-2 virus enters the brain via the olfactory nerve or the peripheral nerve, with a possible route through the blood vessels. Most of the damage reported turns out to be extensive overtime, and repair/recovery will be very slow, moving into a chronic stage.

It was speculated that due to the neuro-invasive nature of SARS-CoV-2, and the chronic neuro-inflammation, some of the damage to neurons could be non-reversible and that can lead to degenerative illness in the long term (Norouzi *et al.*, 2021), including Alzheimer's disease (AD).

To verify the damage in the central nervous system (CNS), Virhammat *et al.* (2021) carried out a test on proven biomarkers indicating CNS impairments in 19 patients who showed neurological symptoms during COVID-19. Analysis of cerebrospinal fluid (CSF), for measurement of biomarkers of CNS injury (neurofilament light chain [NFL] protein, glial fibrillary acidic protein [GFAp], and total tau), was performed and compared to neurological features and disease severity. Pleocytosis is detected in two patients, increased immunoglobulin was found in four patients, and increased NFL protein, total TAU, and GFAp were seen CSF in 63%, 37%, and 16% of patients, respectively. However, interestingly, neuronal autoantibodies had not been detected. The abnormality of biomarkers could not lead to a clear cause of the CNS damage, but can exclude autoimmune problems.

Headache

Headache is a common symptom in the patients with post-COVID-19 syndrome (PCS) which could be a result of the brain neurological disorders, or part of fibromyalgia, ME, or some other causes. Most PCS patients did not report headache as the primary symptom, which is more likely to be dull or tension related; however, some did suffer from severe headache as a new illness, or triggered a new episode of headache severe enough to cause serious distraction to their life. In such situations, the headache still follows the common patterns of tension-type headache, migraine, and trigeminal pain. At this stage, no controlled clinical study has been conducted to reveal how the incident of headache compares to non-COVID-19 sufferers. Besides, there no specific pathology has been discovered to reveal if the headaches in PCS patients are different from those not related to COVID-19.

If the headache is a violent one accompanied by vomiting, vision change, and a stiff neck, then medical examination is needed to exclude stroke. There is no specific biomarker or image investigation for diagnosing this type of headache, and one mainly relies on medical history and excluding other conditions.

TCM diagnosis

Key TCM questions/examination for diagnosis

Nature of the pain

Sharp pain indicates *Excess* pattern; dull aching suggests *Deficiency*; burning pain results from *Heat; Cold pain* is caused by cold; distending pain is from *Qi Stagnation;* and fixed sharp pain indicates *Blood Stasis.* Pulsation with a banging/beating feeling accompanied by pain is due to

Liver Yang Rising/hyperactive *Liver Yang*. Most headaches are intermittent, suggesting excess patterns, while some are constant, lasting for more than a day, suggesting deficiency pattern.

The severity of a headache is now commonly measured by Visual Analog Scale (VAS) of pain, with 0 meaning no pain, while 10 is the worst imaginable pain which leads to full occupation of the mind, and nothing else can be noticed while one is in pain. If the pain is changing, then VAS should be asked in three levels, the worst, the average, and the best time, particularly when the patient does not feel much of the pain during the visit to or treatment in the clinic.

Location of the pain

Pain in the forehead is a problem of *Yang Ming* channels, *Stomach* Channel, and *Large Intestine* Channel; when only on one lateral side, it is possible for it to be migraine, and the *Shao Yang* channels, *Gallbladder* Channel, or *San Jiao* Channels are affected; pain at the back of the head is of *Tai Yang* (*Urinary Bladder* Channel, BL/UB, and *Small Intestine* Channel); and when the headache is on the top, then it is the *Liver* Channel and *DU* Channel.

The trigger factors are very important for syndrome pattern differentiation. When triggered by cold environment/wind blowing, it is related to *Cold/Cold-Dampness* invasion or *Yang Deficiency*; if the headache is mostly experienced after some heavy work, it is more likely to be *Qi* and/or *Blood Deficiency*; and if emotions trigger the headache, it is *Liver Qi Stagnation.*

Treatment of headache with acupuncture is widely considered to be both effective and cost effective; in addition, it is recommended in the national guidelines. The best example is the UK NICE guidelines on headache which recommend acupuncture for tension-type headache and migraines (NICE, 2012). The authors believe that the recommendation is well supported by clinical evidence and applies to headache in PCS. Although TCM herbs are not mentioned, their clinical evidence and the clinical cases observed by the authors also support their use in treatment of PCS.

Common patterns on headache

These patterns are classified for use in herbal medicine, according to the special clinical symptoms and observed signs of the tongue and pulse of the individual.

External pathogenic invasion — Headache with external damp-wind

Clinical features and signs: Headache presenting on the front or back of the head with catarrh, with blocked nose, is always a tension and heavy headache. If there is aversion to cold without sweat and sudden occurrence, with wheezing and distension of the chest, it indicates wind-damp with cold. A sore throat, minor sweating, and choky cough indicate wind-damp with heat. Another sign is a light red tongue with less white coating, and a floating-wiry pulse.

Treatment principle in TCM: *Dispel Wind* and release *Damp.*

Treatment: Herbal prescription.

Pinyin: Huo Xiang Zheng Qi San variation.

English name for decoction: Agastache Powder to Rectify the *Qi*.

Role in formula	Name/ Pinyin	Name/Latin	Dose (g)	Function
Chief herb	Huo Xiang	Herba Agastaches seu Pogostemi	12	Dispels the external wind and dampness from the exterior and the upper burner.
Deputy herb	Zi Su Ye	Folium Perillae Frutescentis	5	Promotes and dispels the external wind and dampness from the exterior and the upper burner.
Assistant herb	Da Fu Pi	Pericarpium Arecae Catechu	5	Eliminates excessive dampness and promotes easy discharge of the urine.
	Fu Ling	Sclerotium Poria Cocos	5	Eliminates the dampness and replenishes the spleen.
	Bai Zhu	Rhizoma Atractylodis Macrocephalae	10	Replenishes the spleen and strengthens the middle burner; releases excessive dampness.
	Ban Xia	Rhizoma Pinelliae Ternatae	10	Dries the dampness and expels the phlegm to ease cough.
	Chen Pi	Pericarpium Citri Ret	10	Dries the dampness and replenishes the spleen.
	Hou Po	Cortex Magnoliae Officinalis	10	Expels the accumulated dampness and eliminates the stagnated *Qi*.
	Sheng Jiang	Rhizoma Zingiberis Officinalis Recens	10	Warms and excites the stomach to encourage and dispel the external Wind-damp-cold.
	Da Zao	Fructus Zizyphi Jujubae	10	Harmonises the stomach and spleen.
	Gan Cao	Radix Glycyrrhizae Uralensis	5	Harmonises the stomach to receive all herbs and influence congruence.
Guiding herb	Bai Zhi	Radix Angelicae Dahuricae	5	Dispels the external wind and leads the formula to ascend and drive to the exterior.

If accompanied by *Cold*, Gui Zhi, Niu Bang Zi, or Gan Jiang can be added; however, if accompanied by heat, Yin Hua, Lian Qiao, or Lu Gen can be added. When aching in the back is more prevalent, Qian Huo or Fang Feng can be added. When there is blocked nose presenting, Bo He or Jing Jie can be added.

Method: The above mentioned herbs are collated as a herbal formula of dry herbs, boiled into herbal juice, and taken twice daily, or made into a concentrated herbal powder, with 6 g taken in warm water, twice daily.

Analysis: Huo Xiang and Zi Su Ye dispel *External Wind* and *Dampness.* Bai Zhi dispels *External Wind* and leads all herbs in the prescription to affect the top of the body. Fu Ling and Da Fu Pi dredge the fluid passage to release excessive *Dampness*. Bai Zhu, Ban Xia, and Chen Pi dry the *Damp* and reinforce *Spleen Qi*. Hou Po and Sheng Jiang regulate and spread the external and internal *Qi* throughout the body. Da Zhao and Gan Cao harmonise the *Stomach* and adjust all the herbs, combining them and ensuring that they work together.

Acupuncture

Main points: Fengchi (GB20), Touwei (ST8), Tongtian (BL7).

Assistant points: Hegu (LI4), Sanyangluo (SJ8).

Variation: Shangxing (DU23), Yangbai (GB14), use for frontal headache; Baihui (DU20), Qianding (DU21), use for top of head headache; Tianzhu (BL10), Houding (DU19), use for posterior headache; Shuaigu (GB8), Taiyang (Ext).

All these points are given with reducing or balanced handling method.

Analysis: Tongtian releases the pathogenic *Wind-Damp* from the larger *Yang* meridian. Fengchi harmonises the lesser *Yang*. Touwei dispels the bright *Yang* in all three points and is able to clear all pathogenic factors from the three *Yang* meridians. Hegu manages all the problems on the face to help ease the headache. Sanyanluo dredges *Stagnated Qi* in general. These varied points will be selected according to the specific body location or the affected meridian and the location of the expressing headache.

Advice: This pattern can be seen in the patients suffering from a cold, flu, or recurrent virus which lasts 1–2 days, so the pathogenic factors (邪气) are not very strong, and a good general *Upright Qi* (正气) exists in the body. The herbs should be effective in releasing the pathogenic factors or virus.

Liver Qi Stagnation and Liver Yang flare-up

Clinical features and signs: The headache expresses on the top of the head or either the left or right temporal areas; sharp pain or throbbing pain, stress, loss of temper, depression, nervousness, worries, easily angry; restless and difficult sleep; aching of both coastal areas, bitter taste, red or sore eyes, or unclear vision; and red tongue with a thin yellow coating.

Treatment principle in TCM: *Dredge Liver Qi* and dispel general *Stagnated Qi*; Clear and calm down the *Liver Heat.*

Treatment: Herbal prescription.

Pinyin: Chai Hu Shu Gan Decoction variation.

English name for decoction: Bupleurum Decoction to Spread the Liver variation.

Role in formula	Name/ Pinyin	Name/Latin	Dose (g)	Function
Chief herb	Chai Hu	Radix Bupleuri	10	Dredges the stagnated liver *Qi* to release the stress.
Deputy herb	Chen Pi	Pericarpium Citri Reticulatae	10	Harmonises the stomach and releases the stagnated *Qi*; reinforces the spleen.
Assistant herb	Chi Shao	Radix Paeoniae Rubrae	10	Softens the liver and nourishes its blood to ease the headache.

(Continued)

(*Continued*)

Role in formula	Name/ Pinyin	Name/Latin	Dose (g)	Function
	Chuan Xiong	Rhizoma Cyperi Rotundi	10	Releases the stasis blood to ease the headache.
	Xiang Fu	Rhizoma Cyperi Rotundi	10	Supports to eliminate the stagnated liver *Qi* and general *Qi*.
	Gan Cao	Radix Glycyrrhizae Uralensis	5	Harmonises the stomach to receive all herbs and influences collaboration.
Guiding herb	Zhi Qiao	Fructus Citri Aurantii	10	Pushes the stagnated *Qi* and dredges the liver.

If the headache is severe there is a possibility that it may cause hypertension or stroke, Tian Ma Gou Teng Yin can be selected for calming down *Liver Yang* and releasing the excessive *Internal Wind.* When excessive *Heat* is strong, Chuan Lian Zi or Huang Qin should be added to release excessive *Liver Heat.* If Liver *Heat* is accompanied by *Dampness,* Long Dan Xie Gan Tang is selected to clear *Heat* and dispel *Dampness.* If poor sleep is presenting, Ye Jiao Teng, San Zao Ren and Fu Shen are added for nourishing the *Liver* and calming down the spirit.

Method: The above mentioned herbs are collected as a herbal formula of dry herbs, boiled into herbal juice, and taken twice daily, or made into a concentrated herbal powder, with 6 g taken in warm water, twice daily.

Analysis: Chai Hu dredges the *Stagnated Liver Qi.* Chi Shao softens the liver and nourishes *Liver Blood.* Chuan Xiong removes *Liver Blood Stasis* and restrains the headache. Zhi Qiao and Xiang Fu support Chai Hu to dredge the *Stagnated Qi.* Chen Pi releases the *Stagnated Qi* and reinforces the *Spleen.* Gan Cao harmonises all herbs and comforts the *Stomach.*

Acupuncture

Main points: Xuanlu (GB5), Heyan (GB4).

Assistant points: Taichong (LIV3), Taixi (KI3).

Variation: Guanchong is punctured to bleed to release accumulated heat; Neiting (ST44) used to release the excessive *Heat* in the *Bright Yang* meridian.

Analysis: If the headache is caused by *Liver Qi Stagnation* and flares upwards, occurring at the temporal side, use Xuanlu and Heyan in the *Gallbladder* meridian to release *Heat* and *Wind*, along with no restraint in the local pain. Taichong clears *Liver Heat.* Taixi nourishes *Kidney Yin* and pushes *Yang* down.

Advice: This pattern can be seen with stress attacks, migraine, or trigeminal neuralgia seizures, or some manifestations of psychiatric disorders; if the headache is getting stronger, it may be a precursor of hypertension or a stroke, or post-stroke TIA (transient ischaemic attacks). This is the commonest pattern in the brain and neurological damage of post-COVID-19 syndrome.

Liver Blood and Kidney Yin Deficiency

Clinical features and signs: An empty headache, headache with dizziness, dull aching, or faint headache; depression, ignoring aching at coastal areas, back, and legs, fatigue, poor spirit and memory, tinnitus, lack of sleep, unclear vision, red or light red tongue without coating or less coating; wiry-fine, or deep-fine pulse.

Treatment principle in TCM: *Nourish Liver* and *Kidney Yin*; Clear the *Empty Heat.*

Treatment: Herbal prescription.

Pinyin: Liu Wei Di Huang or Zhi Bai Di Huang Tang variation.

English name for decoction: Six-Ingredient Decoction with Rehmannia or Anemarrhena, Phellodendron, and Rehmannia Decoction variation.

Role in formula	Name/ Pinyin	Name/Latin	Dose (g)	Function
Chief herb	Sheng Di Huang	Radix Rehmanniae Glutinosae	10–30	Nourishes the kidney *Yin* and clears the empty heat.
	Huang Bai	Cortex Phellodendri	10	Releases the empty heat and dries the dampness.
Deputy herb	Mu Dan Pi	Cortex Moutan Radicis	10	Clears the heat in the blood, kidney, and the lower burner.
	Zhi Mu	Radix Anemarrhenae Asphodeloidis	10	Accentuates and nourishes the kidney *Yin* and clears the empty heat.
Assistant herb	Zhan Zhu Yu	Fructus Corni Officinalis	10	Nourishes the kidney *Yin* and essence.
	Shan Yao	Radix Dioscoreae Oppositae	10	Replenishes the spleen *Qi* and dries the dampness.
	Fu Ling	Sclerotium Poria Cocos	10	Dries the dampness and replenishes the spleen.
	Ze Xie	Rhizoma Alismatis Orientalis	10	Dredges the stagnated *Qi* and accumulated dampness.

If the headache is significant, Chuan Xiong and Bai Zhi are added. If hot flashes or Empty Heat symptoms are prevalent, Zhi Bai Di Huang should be used. When a headache presents with unclear vision, Qi Ju Di Huang should be used. If poor sleep is affecting the patient, Suan Zao Ren and Bai Zi Ren are added. When psychiatric symptoms are expressed, He Huan Pi and Mei Gui Hua are added.

Method: The above mentioned herbs are collected as a herbal formula of dry herbs, boiled into herbal juice, and taken twice daily, or made into a concentrated herbal powder, with 6 g taken in warm water, twice daily.

Analysis: Sheng Di Huang, Shan Zhu Yu, and Shan Yao are the three reinforcing herbs to nourish the *Liver* and *Kidney Yin*. Mu Dan Pi, Ze Xie, and Fu Ling are the three reducing herbs to clear *Empty Heat* and *Dampness*, creating the full composition of Liu Wei Di Huang Tang and performing the key effect of nourishing the *Liver* and *Kidney Yin*. Zhi Mu and Huang Bai are added to promote clearing of *Empty Heat* as components of Zhi Bai Di Huang Tang. Ju Hua and Gou Qi Zi are added to increase and nourish *Liver Yin* for clearing the eyes. Chuan Xiong and Bai Zhi can remove *Liver Blood Stasis* to restrain the headache. He Huan Pi and Mei Gui Hua can remove *Liver Qi Stagnation,* relax the spirit, and calm down the mind.

Acupuncture

Main points: Shangxing (DU23), Xuehai (SP10).

Assistant points: Qihai (REN6), Guanyuan (REN4).

Variation: Ganshu (BL18), Pishu (BL20), Shenshu (BL23), if more deficiency symptoms are manifested.

Analysis: Shangxing dredges the *Governing Vessel* (Du) for harmony of all meridians to restrain the headache. Xuehai nourishes *Liver Blood.* Qihai and Zhongji nourish *Original Yin* and *Essence* to cultivate the root. These three shu-points along the *Bladder* meridian are used to replenish and *Nourish Blood, Yin*, and *Qi* together.

Advice: This pattern can be seen in the chronic and long-term presentation of COVID-19 syndrome. Headaches occur persistently or intermittently, always manifesting in a dull pain or gentle pain, as well as being accompanied by both insomnia and psychological disorders.

Liver Qi Stagnation and Spleen Qi Deficiency

Clinical features and signs: The headache suffered is strong with changeability: sharp, throbbing, or dull; indicated seizure at the temporal aspect, or unilateral of the head; whole or part of head, fixed or moveable headache; accompanied by mood swings, anxiety, depression, or loosing ones' temper easily; tiredness, fatigue, lethargy, poor appetite, lose or sluggish bowel movement; in addition to a light red tongue with thin white coating with or without teeth marks, wiry or wiry-weak pulse.

Treatment principle in TCM: Dredge *Liver Qi* and reinforce *Spleen Qi.*

Treatment: Herbal prescription.

Pinyin: Xiao Yao Wan variation.

English name for decoction: Rambling Decoction variation.

Role in formula	Name/ Pinyin	Name/Latin	Dose (g)	Function
Chief herb	Chai Hu	Radix Bupleuri	10	Dredges the liver *Qi* and releases the stagnation.
Deputy herb	Dang Gui	Radix Angelicae Sinensis	10	Softens the liver *Yin* and blood to support liver *Qi*'s movement through the body.
	Bai Shao	Radix Paeoniae Lactiflorae	10	Softens the liver *Yin* and blood.
Assistant herb	Bai Zhu	Rhizoma Atractylodis Macrocephalae	10–30	Reinforces the spleen and dries the dampness.
	Fu Ling	Sclerotium Poria Cocos	10	Eliminates the accumulated dampness and reinforces the Spleen *Qi*.
	Sheng Jiang	Rhizoma Zingiberis Officinalis Recens	10	Warms and excites the liver and spleen *Qi*.
Guiding	Bo He	Herba Menthae Haplocalycis	5	Clears the stagnated *Qi* and leads herbs upwards towards the top.
	Zhi Gan Cao	Radix Glycyrrhizae Uralensis	5	Harmonises all herbs and promotes congruence.

If the headache is damaging, Chuan Xiong and Bai Zhi are added. If Internal Heat expresses above the headache with burning and throbbing, loss of temper, or difficulty falling asleep, Mu Dan Pi and Zhi Zi are added as Jia Wei Xiao Yao Wan. When sharp or throbbing pain presents, E Zhu and San Leng, Ru Xiang and Mo Yao can be used.

Method: The above mentioned herbs are collated as a herbal formula of dry herbs, boiled into herbal juice, and taken twice daily, or made into a concentrated herbal powder, with 6 g taken in warm water, twice daily.

Analysis: This is a combined excessive and deficiency pattern, and also the commonest pattern; therefore, the formula is well considered and a mix of both reducing and reinforcing herbs. Chai Hu is designed as the main herb to *Dredge Liver Qi* and promote general *Qi* circulation in the whole body. Dang Gui and Bai Shao soften *Liver Yin* and nourish *Liver Blood* as the main herbs for calming down the mind. Bai Zhu and Fu Ling reinforce *Spleen Qi* and are suitable for patients with chronic and longer illness durations. Sheng Jiang excites *Qi* and *Yang* supports the Chai hu effect. Bo He dredges the *Stagnated Qi* at the orifice of the head and face and promotes ascension of the formula. Zhi Gan Cao harmonises all herbs and comforts the *Stomach.* Mu Dan Pi and Zhi Zi clear excessive *Liver Heat*. E Zhu and San Leng, or Ru Xiang and Mo Yao are stronger herbs that restrain a severe headache and other kinds of severe pain.

Acupuncture

Main points: Taiyang (Ext), Fengchi (GB20).

Assistant points: Waiguan (SJ6), Zulinqi (GB41), Hegu (LI4), Taichong (LIV3).

Variation: Sanyinjiao (SP6), Zusanli (ST36), if tiredness is more prevalent than other symptoms and manifested as more deficiency.

Analysis: *Tai Yang* releases the stagnated *Liver Qi* and eases headache at the temporal regions of the head. Fengchi dispels excessive Wind from the *Liver* and *Gallbladder* meridians. Waiguan and Zulinqi as one pair of the 8 points of the Cross vessels are selected to eliminate the excessive stagnated *Qi* from the liver meridian and the general body. Hegu and Taichong as the combination of the four gate points can clear excessive *Liver Heat,* calm the mind, and promote good sleep. Sanyinjiao is the meeting point of the three *Yin* meridians on the legs to nourish the *Yin* in all three meridians. Zusanli replenishes the *Stomach Qi* to build up the *Spleen* and general *Qi* in the body.

Advice: This pattern is commonly seen in the clinic as every kind of headache in the post-COVID-19 syndrome and is related to brain and neurological damage. For example, chronic dull headache appears after chronic blood thrombosis and post-stroke, with unstable blood pressure; this includes severe headache attacks, like migraine, trigeminal neuralgia, and headache caused by psychiatric disorders.

Phlegm and Dampness accumulated within

Clinical features and signs: Woozy headache with confusion, distension of chest and stomach, nausea and vomiting phlegm, sluggish reaction, heavy or aching feeling in general, lethargy, and tiredness; plump and light red tongue with teeth marks and greasy coating, deep-rolling, or deep-wiry pulse.

Treatment principle in TCM: Strengthen *Spleen* meridian and dispel accumulated *Phlegm*; encourage rebellion *Liver Qi* to descend and restrain the pain.

Treatment: Herbal prescription.

Pinyin: Ban Xia Bai Zhu Tian Ma Tang variation.

English name for decoction: Pinellia, Atractylodes Macrocephala, and Gastrodia Decoction variation.

Role in formula	Name/Pinyin	Name/Latin	Dose (g)	Function
Chief herb	Ban Xia	Rhizoma Pinelliae Ternatae	10–15	Releases accumulated phlegm and dries the dampness.
Deputy herb	Chen Pi	Pericarpium Citri Reticulatae	10	Releases accumulated phlegm and dampness, and replenishes the spleen.
Assistant herb	Bai Zhu	Rhizoma Atractylodis Macrocephalae	10–30	Replenishes the spleen and dries the accumulated dampness.
	Gou Teng	Rhizoma Gastrodiae Elatae, which is replaced by Tian Ma	10	Eliminates the external or internal wind, calms the mind to ease headache or dizziness.
	Fu Ling	Sclerotium Poria Cocos	10	Releases excessive dampness and reinforces the spleen.

(*Continued*)

Role in formula	Name/ Pinyin	Name/Latin	Dose (g)	Function
	Man Jing Zi	Fructus Viticis	10	Removes blood stasis to release the headache, and leads to the ascending of herbs towards the head.
	Sheng Jiang	Rhizoma Zingiberis Officinalis Recens	10	Warms and excites the yang *Qi* in the stomach, releases the external wind.
	Da Zao	Fructus Zizyphi Jujubae	4	Harmonises the stomach.
Guiding herb	Gan Cao	Radix Glycyrrhizae Uralensis	5	Harmonises the stomach and promotes cohesiveness of herbs.

If the headache is enduring, Chuan Xiong and Bai Zhi are added. When the headache is severe, E Zhu and San Leng are added. When there is a persistent headache and dizziness, Tian Ma Gou Teng Yin is replaced. When there is wooziness and confusion indicating *Phlegm* accumulation, Zhu Ru, Zhi Shi, and Huang Qin are added. For a fixed headache, Wang Bu Liu Xin or San Qi is added.

Method: The above mentioned herbs are collated as a herbal formula of dry herbs, boiled into herbal juice, and taken twice daily, or made into a concentrated herbal powder, with 6 g taken in warm water, twice daily.

Analysis: Ban Xia and Chen Pi are the main herbs to release the accumulation of *Phlegm.* Fu Ling releases and drains the excessive *Phlegm Fluid.* Tian Ma is a plant at a stage of imminent extinction and is banned from use in the West; therefore, Gou Teng is a replacement to dispel accumulation of *Phlegm* and dredge stagnated *Liver Qi* to restrain the headache. Man Jing Zi removes *Liver Qi* and leads the ascension of herbs to the head and is a superior herb for easing headache. Sheng Jiang excites general Yang Qi; Da Zao and Gan Cao comfort the *Stomach* and harmonise all the herbs. Chuan Xiong and Bai Zhi eliminate *Blood Stasis* to ease headache. E Zhu and San Leng release *Blood Stasis* to decrease intense headache. Tian Ma Gou Teng Yin is another formula that can descend the reversed liver *Qi* and remove the liver stagnation, and is also specific to *Liver Wind* flaring upwards. Zhu Ru, Zhi Shi, and Huang Qin respond to release accumulated *Phlegm* and clear the confusion in the mind. Wang Bu Liu Xing and special San Qi eliminate *Blood Stasis* to restrain the headache.

Acupuncture

Main points: Baihui (DU20), Yintang (Ext).

Assistant points: Zhongwan (REN12), Fenglong (ST40).

Variation: Neiguan (P6) eases nausea and vomiting; Tianshu (ST25) and Yinlingquan (SP9) restrain a loose bowel or diarrhoea.

Analysis: Baihui (DU20) with Yintang clears and releases the bursting at the top of the head. When *Excess Heat* is accumulated within, Yintang can be used clear excessive heat to ease the headache. Zhongwan (REN 12) with Fenglong (ST40) dispels excessive *Damp Phlegm* and strengthens the *Spleen* and *Stomach.* Neiguan (PC6) calms down the mind and restrains nausea. Tianshu (ST25) with Yinlingquan (SP9) tonifies *Spleen Qi* and Yang to speed up *Damp Fluid* elimination.

Advice: This pattern can be seen in patients with headaches caused by blood stasis or clots occurring in the brain or neurological system while they are infected by coronavirus, or post-stroke and some mental disorders during post-COVID-19 syndrome.

Blood Stasis

Clinical features and signs: Signs are sharp headache, like being punctured by a needle at the fixed position, or severe headache; chronic persistent headache not completely released; headache with probable external injury or operation; lumps found in the brain or other places in the body; a purple tongue or light red tongue with blood stasis marks and thin white coating; a deep-fine, fine-choppy pulse.

Treatment principle in TCM: Unblock stuffy orifice; Activate *Blood* to remove *Blood Stasis.*

Treatment: Herbal prescription.

Pinyin: Tong Qiao Huo Xue Tang.

English name for decoction: Open the Portals and Quicken the Blood Decoction.

Role in formula	Name/Pinyin	Name/Latin	Dose (g)	Function
Chief herb	Chi Shao	Radix Paeoniae Rubrae	3	Activates the blood stasis and restrains the headache.
Deputy herb	Chuan Xiong	Radix Ligustici Wallichii	3	Promotes and activates blood stasis to restrain the headache.
Assistant herb	Tao Ren	Semen Pruni Persicae	9	Promotes and activates blood stasis and moistens the large intestine.
	Hong Hua	Flos Carthami Tinctorii	9	Promotes and activates the blood stasis and warms the meridians.
	Sheng Jiang	Rhizoma Zingiberis Officinalis Recens	9	Warms and excites the yang *Qi* to support the blood circulation.
	Da Cong	Bulbus Allii Fistulosi	3	Drives and opens the orifices and leads to upwards ascension of the herbs.
	Da Zao	Fructus Zizyphi Jujubae	3	Harmonises the stomach and moistens the large intestines.
Guiding herb	San Qi, which is replaced by She Xiang	Radix Pseudoginseng	3	Strengthens and activates the blood stasis and restrains the headache; promotes circulation of herbs.

She Xiang 0.15 (banned in the West as an animal material) is replaced by San Qi.

When headache manifests in the temporal region, Chai Hu, Yu Jin, or Xiang Fu can be added. For headache in the posterior of the head, Qiang

Huo and Man Jing Zi can be added. For a frontal headache, use Ge Gen and Gui Zhi. If headache occurs at the top of the head, Chuan Ni Xi could be added.

Method: The above mentioned herbs are collected as a herbal formula of dry herbs, boiled into herbal juice, and taken twice daily, or made into a concentrated herbal powder, with 6 g taken in warm water twice daily.

Analysis: Chi Shao and Chuan Xiong are the main herbs to activate the *Blood Stasis* and restrain the headache. Tao Ren and Hong Hua promote the release of *Blood Stasis* and restrain the headache. Shen Jiang and Da Cong (spring onion) excite *Yang Qi* and evacuate the *Stagnated Qi*. Da Zao comforts the *Stomach.* She Xiang is an important herb in this prescription and superior for dredging the stuffy orifices and removing *Blood Stasis*, and therefore releasing the intense headache. We use San Qi to replace She Xiang in the West and it is able to remove deep stasis in the blood vessels, meridians, and viscera, and is useful to restrain the headache.

Acupuncture

Main points: Ashi points, painful areas palpated.

Assistant points: Hegu (LI4), Sanyinjiao (SP6).

Variation: Zanzhu (BL2) for headache located over the eyebrow; Taiyang (Ext) for temporal headache; Qimai (SJ18) for posterior headache; Sishencong (Ext) for headache presenting at the top of the head.

Analysis: Headache caused by Blood Stasis always manifests as a fixed position of pain, and therefore, finding the point of intense pain is key to releasing the pain in general. The sensitive point is punctured after pressing with a finger. Afterwards, the needle is removed with a reducing handle technique, or deliberately pierced to bleed, allowing pathogenic *Heat* to be removed. Hegu drives *Qi* and Blood flow. Sanyinjiao is reduced to dispel three burners and ease pain.

Advice: This pattern can be seen in patients with a long duration of chronic disease or with a severe headache attack, like migraine, trigeminal neuralgia; or with general aching or pain; or headache with paralysis, numbness, or abnormal limb activity, like post-stroke. Recurrent headache is caused by blood clot production or blood stasis during post-COVID-19 syndrome.

Case Study

Ms. Y. Liu, 25, master's student, has had recurrent headaches for a half year. Since she was infected with COVID-19 last Aug, she has reoccurring tension headaches, 2–3 times per week, worse before menstruation. Although she had a negative PCR, she suffers from headache attacks, with frequency of attacks increasing since she returned to normal study and started carrying out research. When the headache appears, she takes Nurofen, Paracetamol, or another painkiller, which provides temporary relief from the headache. Therefore, she seeks acupuncture and TCM to help with the treatment.

Clinical features: She has recurrent tension headache, 2–3 times per week; lasting a few of hours or 1–2 days depending on the frequency of taking painkillers. Due to more regular headache attacks, she feels anxious, nervous, and restless with disturbed sleep. The headache can appear frontally, temporally, or on the top of the head. Tension is felt in the neck and upper back. She has regular menstruation, although suffering from dysmenorrhea, which has been worse the last 2–3 circles. She has loose bowels and is easily tired. Her tongue is light red with white coating, and she has wiry-fine pulse.

Diagnosis:

1. Post-COVID-19 syndrome, tension headache.
2. Chronic neck pain.
3. Psychiatric disorders, stress.

Differentiation syndromes of TCM:

1. Liver *Qi* Stagnation with Excessive Heat flaring upwards.
2. Spleen *Qi* Deficiency.

Treatment principle in TCM: Dredge *Stagnated Liver Qi* and general *Qi*; clear excessive *Liver Heat*; replenish *Spleen Qi* and build up general *Vitality Qi*.

Acupuncture: Baihui (DU20), Shangxing (DU23), Taiyang (Ext), Fengchi (GB20); Waiguan (SJ5), Zulinqi (GB41), Yanglingquan (GB34), Sanyinjiao (SP6), Yinlingquan (SP9).

Herbal prescription

Pinyin: Jia Wei Xiao Yao variation.

Herbal powders (g):

Chai Hu	Radix Bupleuri 10 g
Dang Gui	Radix Angelicae Sinensis 10 g
Chuan Xiong	Radix Ligustici Wallichii 10 g
Ge Gen	Radix Puerariae 10 g
Bai Shao	Radix Paeoniae Lactiflorae 10 g
Qiang Huo	Rhizoma et Radix Notopterygii 10 g
Bai Zhu	Rhizoma Atractylodis Macrocephalae 10 g
Fu Ling	Sclerotium Poriae Cocos 10 g
Bo He	Herba Menthae Haplocalycis 10 g
Gan Jiang	Rhizoma Zingiberis Officinalis 10 g
Yan Hu Suo	Rhizoma Corydalis 10 g
E Zhu	Rhizoma Curcumae Ezhu 10 g
Zhi Gan Cao	Radix Glycyrrhizae Uralensis 5 g

Method: The above-mentioned herbs are mixed as a concentrated herbal powder, with 6 g taken in warm water, twice daily. She has acupuncture treatment once a week and continues taking herbal powder regularly. After a month, she feels more relaxed in the neck and clear in the mind. So, she continues body acupuncture once every 2 weeks and a herbal prescription of Jia Wei Xiao Yao Wan and Qiang Hua Sheng Shi Wan, 6 g, twice a day, until the headache attack stops.

Dizziness

Dizziness is very common in acute COVID-19 and could reflect the state of dehydration, inflammation in the upper respiratory tract, and general unease of movement. It is not considered to be very specific in terms of clinical judgement, and there are no specific biomarkers for its diagnosis.

In prolonged illness, dizziness is often presented as a feeling of unstable body position or in ability to keep the body steady while standing or walking. It is usually described as "light-headedness". The cause of this light-headed sensation is thought to be lack of blood supply to the brain due to hypotension (lower blood pressure, LBP) or hypoglycaemia (lower blood sugar) or a combination of both. When patients stand up quickly, some of them might also experience a feeling of loss of vision partially (visual field disappears or becomes black) which is described by many as black-out where they recover in a minute or so. However, as this light dizziness is not life threatening, it is rarely investigated seriously in pathology and diagnosis, and is considered to be a non-specific symptom, with no treatment specified for this. In PCS, this is always a suggestion of some deficiency in TCM syndrome pattern differentiation.

A severe form of dizziness is vertigo, a sensation where the whole body, or otherwise the whole outside world, is moving fast, swirling or spinning. This leads to very bad whole-body reaction characterised by tension in all muscles, nausea, vomiting, cold hands and feet, and fast heart rate. Vertigo has been an important clinical subject and neurological and internal ear problems are the main source. Examples of causes include Meniere's disease and Labyrinthitis of the inner ear, transient ischemic attack (TIA) or stroke, and brain tumours (original or immigrated). However, many other problems could also cause vertigo, for example, cervical spondylosis.

Diagnosis

Case history is crucial for further diagnostic examinations

- For illness involving the inner ear along with present hearing impairment, tinnitus, or deafness, and therefore, investigation, the examination should be focused on the structure of inner ear, and CT/MRI scan and Meniere's test should be employed.
- When brain damage is suspected, EEG, CT/MRI, and other neurological tests should be the main methods used.
- Cervical spondylosis is mainly diagnosed by X-ray of the neck or CT.

Common patterns of TCM and treatment

Liver Fire and Yang flare-up

Clinical features and signs: Signs are dizziness with tinnitus, headache, and tension, anger and aggravation, irritability, restlessness, distension of chest and both of coastal areas, insomnia with dreams, red face and bitter taste, a red tongue with yellow or greasy coating, and a wiry-rapid or wiry-fine-rapid pulse.

Treatment principle in TCM: Clears and descends the liver *Fire* or *Yang*; nourishes *Liver Blood* and *Kidney Yin.*

Treatment: Herbal prescription.

Pinyin: Tian Ma Gou Teng Yin variation.

English name for decoction: Gastrodia and Uncaria Decoction variation.

Role in formula	Name/ Pinyin	Name/Latin	Dose (g)	Function
Chief herb	Gou Teng	Rhizoma Gastrodiae Elatae,	10–30	Clears the liver heat and causes descension of liver yang *Qi.*
Deputy herb	Shi Jue Ming	Concha Haliotidis	10–30	Supports descension of the liver yang *Qi.*
Assistant herb	Huang Qin	Radix Scutellariae Baicalensis	10	Clears the excessive liver heat.
	Zhi Zi	Fructus Gardeniae Jasminoidis	10	Promotes and clears the excessive liver heat.
	Yi Mu Cao	Herba Leonuri Heterophylli	10	Activates the blood stasis and drives the circulation.
	Fu Shen	Sclerotium Poriae Cocos Paradicis	10	Calms the mind and eases dizziness.
	Ye Jiao Teng	Caulis Polygoni Multiflori	10	Calms the mind and promotes good sleep.
	Du Zhong	Cortex Eucommiae Ulmoidis	10	Replenishes the kidney and strengthens the essence.
	Sang Ji Sheng	Ramulus Loranthi	10	Strengthens the kidney and releases the external wind to ease the dizziness.
Guiding herb	Chuan Niu Xi	Radix Cyathulae Officinalis	10–15	Activates the blood stasis and leads all herbs into the relevant meridian.

If dizziness is severe with *Excessive Heat,* Long Dan Cao, Mu Dan Pi, and Ju Hua are added. When dizziness is accompanied by *Yin Deficiency,*

Sheng Di Huang, Mai Men Dong, and Bai Shao are added. For shaking hands or trembling limbs, Zhen Zhu Mu, Long Gu, and Mu Li are added. For constipation, Da Huang and Mang Xiao are added.

Method: The above-mentioned herbs are collated as a herbal formula of dry herbs, boiled into herbal juice, and taken twice daily, or made into a concentrated herbal powder, with 6 g taken in warm water, twice daily.

Analysis: Gou Teng is the main herb and clears *Liver Heat* and causes descension. In the UK, Tian Ma is a banned herb, as it is an imminently endangered plant in the west. Therefore, we can use a higher dose of Gou Teng Jue Ming Zi to support and cause descension of *Liver Yang*. Huang Qin and Zhi Zi clear excessive *Liver Heat.* Chuan Niu Xi, Du Zhong, and San Ji Sheng replenish *Kidney Qi* and *Yin*. Fu Shen and Ye Jiao Teng nourish *Blood* and comfort the mind. Yi Mu Cao releases the *Blood Stasis* in the brain. If strong *Heat* exists, Long Dan Cao, Mu Dan Pi, and Ju Hua emphasise and Clear *Heat* as well as unblocking the eyes. When *Yin Deficiency* is present, use Sheng Di Huang, Mai Men Dong, and Bai Shao to double nourish the *Liver* and *Kidney Yin.* If internal *Liver Wind* and *Yang* flare up, Zhen Zhu Mu, Long Gu, and Mu Li are the mineral materials added to promote healing. When constipation appears, Da Huang and Mang Xiao are laxative herbs that can be added. This prescription should restrain dizziness of various severities.

Advice: This pattern can be commonly seen in patients with brain and neurological damage and good constitution, and also in patients with hypertension, post-stroke, blood clots occurring in the brain, and neurological nerves.

Turbid Phlegm accumulated in the head

Clinical features and signs: Signs are dizziness with heaviness and confusion in the brain, bandaged like sensation, blurred vision with a feeling of spinning, nausea and distension of the chest, vomiting and abundant phlegm expelled, a light red tongue with white-greasy coating, and a wiry-slippery pulse.

Treatment principle in TCM: Dry *Dampness* and dispel *Excessive Phlegm*; replenish *Spleen* and comfort *Stomach.*

Treatment: Herbal prescription.

Pinyin: Ban Xia Bai Zhu Tian Ma Tang variation.

English name for decoction: Pinellia, Atractylodes Macrocephala, and Gastrodia Decoction variation.

Role in formula	Name/ Pinyin	Name/Latin	Dose (g)	Function
Chief herb	Ban Xia	Rhizoma Pinelliae Ternatae	10–15	Releases the accumulated phlegm and dries the dampness.
Deputy herb	Chen Pi	Pericarpium Citri Reticulatae	10	Releases the accumulated phlegm and dampness; replenishes the spleen.
Assistant herb	Bai Zhu	Rhizoma Atractylodis Macrocephalae	10–30	Replenishes the spleen and dries the accumulated dampness.
	Gou Teng	Rhizoma Gastrodiae Elatae, which is replaced by Tian Ma	10	Eliminates the external or internal wind, and calms the mind to ease headache or dizziness.
	Fu Ling	Sclerotium Poria Cocos	10	Releases the excessive dampness and reinforces the spleen.
	Man Jing Zi	Fructus Viticis	10	Removes the blood stasis to release the headache, and leads all the herbs in the prescription to affect the head.
	Sheng Jiang	Rhizoma Zingiberis Officinalis Recens	10	Warms and excites the yang *Qi* in the stomach; releases the external wind.
	Da Zao	Fructus Zizyphi Jujubae	4	Harmonises the stomach.
Guiding herb	Gan Cao	Radix Glycyrrhizae Uralensis	5	Harmonises the stomach and leads all herbs to work together well.

If there is dizziness with severe vomiting, Dai Zhe Shi and Zhu Ru are added. If chest or abdominal distension is more prominent, Bai Dou Kou and Sha Ren are added. For heaviness and general aching, Huo Xiang, Pei Lan, and Shi Chang Pu are added. For weak hearing or tinnitus, Cong Bai, Yu Jin, and Shi Chang Pu are added.

Method: The above-mentioned herbs are collated as a herbal formula of dry herbs, boiled into herbal juice, and taken twice daily, or made into a concentrated herbal powder, with 6 g taken in warm water, twice daily.

Analysis: Ban Xia and Chen Pi are the main herbs to release accumulated *Phlegm*. Fu Ling releases the excessive *Phlegm Fluid*. Tian Ma is a plant on the brink of imminent extinction and is banned from use in the West; therefore, Gou Teng is used as a replacement to dispel accumulated *Phlegm* and dredge stagnated *Liver Qi* to restrain dizziness. Man Jing Zi removes *Liver Qi* and leads all herbs to the head and is a superior herb for easing dizziness. Sheng Jiang excites general Yang Qi, and Da Zao and Gan Cao comfort the *Stomach* and harmonise all herbs. Dai Zhe Shi and Zhu Ru comfort the *Stomach* to ease vomiting also dredge stagnated *Liver* and *Spleen Qi* to reduce abdominal distension. Bai Dou Kou and Shah Ren invigorate the *Spleen* to eliminate *Dampness*. Huo Xiang, Pei Lan, and Shi Chang Pu agitate the *Spleen* to dissipate *Dampness*. Cong Bai, Yu Jin, and Shi Chang Pu dredge the *Yang* and open the orifices. This formula will restrain dizziness in excessive *Damp Phlegm* patterns without strong heat.

Advice: This pattern can be seen in patients with dizziness caused by stroke, or cerebrovascular clots, patients with a severe or medium disease, or chronic diseases without a deficient constitution.

Blood Stasis obstructs the orifices

Clinical features and signs: Signs are dizziness with headache accompanied by obliviousness, insomnia, palpitation, spiritlessness, tinnitus and deafness, purple complexion, a purple tongue or light tongue with stasis marks and spots, and a wiry-fine, fine-choppy pulse.

Treatment principle in TCM: Unblock stuffy orifice; Activate *Blood* to remove *Blood Stasis*.

Treatment: Herbal prescription.

Pinyin: Tong Qiao Huo Xue Tang variation.

English name for decoction: Open the Portals and Quicken the Blood Decoction variation.

Role in formula	Name/Pinyin	Name/Latin	Dose (g)	Function
Chief herb	Chi Shao	Radix Paeoniae Rubrae	3	Activates the blood stasis and restrains the headache.
Deputy herb	Chuan Xiong	Radix Ligustici Wallichii	3	Promotes activation of the blood stasis and restrains the headache.
Assistant herb	Tao Ren	Semen Pruni Persicae	9	Emphasises activation of the blood stasis and moistens the large intestine.
	Hong Hua	Flos Carthami Tinctorii	9	Emphasises activation of the blood stasis and warms the meridians.
	Sheng Jiang	Rhizoma Zingiberis Officinalis Recens	9	Warms and excites the yang *Qi* to support the blood circulation.
	Da Cong	Bulbus Allii Fistulosi	3	Pushes open the orifices and leads all herbs to ascend.
	Da Zao	Fructus Zizyphi Jujubae	3	Harmonises the stomach and moistens the intestines.
Guiding herb	San Qi, which is replaced by She Xiang	Radix Pseudoginseng	3	Strengthens activation of the blood stasis and restrains the headache, leading all of herbs into circulation.

She Xiang 0.15, part of the original prescription, is banned in the West as an animal material and can be replaced by San Qi.

If there is more *Qi Deficiency*, Huang Qi with a higher dose 10–30 is added. When there are *Cold* symptoms, Gui Zhi is added. When dizziness is triggered or aggravated by fluctuating weather, Chuan Xiong will be given as double dose. Fang Feng, Bai Zhi, and Jing Jie are also added into the prescription.

Method: The above-mentioned herbs are collated as a herbal formula of dry herbs, boiled into herbal juice, and taken twice daily, or made into a concentrated herbal powder, with 6 g taken in warm water, twice daily.

Analysis: Chi Shao and Chuan Xiong are the main herbs to activate the *Blood Stasis* and restrain dizziness. Tao Ren and Hong Hua promote to release *Blood Stasis* and restrain dizziness. Shen Jiang and Da Cong (spring onion) agitate *Yang Qi* and expel the *Stagnated Qi*. Da Zao comforts the *Stomach*. She Xiang is the important herb in this prescription and superior for dredging a stuffy orifice and removing the *Blood Stasis*; therefore, it can have a good influence in giving relief from severe dizziness. We use San Qi to replace She Xiang effect in the West which can remove deep stasis in the blood vessels, meridians, and viscera, and therefore is a treatment option to restrain dizziness.

Advice: This pattern can be seen in the patients with severe dizziness and stabilized symptoms who commonly suffer from post-stroke or cerebrovascular damage which is becoming a chronic condition.

Acupuncture for dizziness in the excessive patterns

Scalp acupuncture: Vertigo and auditory area.

Body acupuncture:
Main points: Baihui (DU20), Yintang (Ext), Shuiquan (KI5).

Assistant points: Zhongwan (REN12), Guanyuan (REN4); Yinlingquan (SP9), Xingjian (LIV2).

Audial points: Liver, Kidney, Pizhixia, Shenmen.

Analysis: Vertigo and auditory area are stimulated to stimulate brain sensational function. Baihui excites Yangqi and removes *Stagnated Qi* in the brain. Yintang clears the mind to restrain dizziness. Shuiquan descends the reversed liver *Qi* down. Zhongwan and Guanyuan are front-mu points collecting *Yin-Qi* at the Vitality Gate, along with comforting the *Stomach* to ease nausea and vomiting. Yinlingquan is the *He-sea* point of *Spleen* meridian, and harmonises *Spleen Yin.* Xin and Xingjian are *Ying-Spring* points of the *Liver* meridian that lead to descension of *Qi* and restrain dizziness.

Qi and Blood Deficiency

Clinical features and signs: Signs are dizziness and blurred vision, worse with exertion and are triggered by more activity, lethargy, spiritless, pale complexion, palpitation, deprived sleep, a light red or pale tongue with thin white coating, and a fine-weak pulse.

Treatment principle in TCM: Replenish *Qi* and nourish *Blood;* Strengthen *Spleen* and transform *Stomach.*

Treatment: Herbal prescription.

Pinyin: Gui Pi Tang variation.

English name for decoction: Restore the Spleen Decoction variation.

Role in formula	Name/ Pinyin	Name/Latin	Dose (g)	Function
Chief herb	Huang Qi	Radix Astragali Membranacei	10–30	Replenishes the spleen *Qi* and vitality *Qi.*
Deputy herb	Dang Gui	Radix Angelicae Sinensis	10	Nourishes the blood.
Assistant herb	Bai Zhu	Rhizoma Atractylodis Macrocephalae	10–30	Replenishes the spleen and general *Qi*, dries the excessive dampness.
	Dang Shen	Radix Codonopsis Pilosulae	10	Promotes and replenishes the spleen and vitality *Qi.*
	Fu Shen	Sclerotium Poriae Cocos Paradicis	10	Calms the mind down, releases the dampness, and reinforces the Spleen.
	Long Yan Rou	Arillus Euphoriae Longanae	10	Nourishes the *Yin* and blood to tranquilise the mind to promote good sleep.

(*Continued*)

Role in formula	Name/ Pinyin	Name/Latin	Dose (g)	Function
	San Zao Ren	Semen Zizyphi Spinosae	10	Nourishes the liver *Yin* and blood to tranquilise the mind.
	Yuan Zhi	Radix Polygalae Tenuifoliae	10	Tranquilises the mind and nourishes the heart.
	Mu Xiang	Radix Aucklandiae Lappae	6–10	Pushes the *Qi* flow into the meridians and supports the tonic herbs to work cohesively.
Guiding herb	Gan Cao	Radix Glycyrrhizae Uralensis	5	Harmonises the stomach and leads all herbs to perform together.

If there is dizziness with more sweating, a double dose of Huang Qi is given. Fang Feng and Fu Xiao Mai promote defensive *Qi* and ease sweating. When there are signs of accumulated *Dampness* with loose bowels or diarrhoea, Yi Yi Ren, Ze Xie, and Bian Dou are added. When there is aversion to *cold* with faint aching in the abdomen, Gui Zhi and Gan Jiang are added. When *Blood Deficiency* with pale complexion is present, Shu Di Huang, E Jiao, and Zi He Che powders are added. If the middle burner *Qi* descends causing a persistent dizziness, Bu Zhong Yi Qi Tang is replaced.

Method: The above-mentioned herbs are prescribed as a herbal formula in dry herbal or as a concentrated herbal formula to be taken twice daily.

Analysis: Huang Qi replenishes general *Qi* and Dang Gui cultivates *Blood* and the main herbs of this formula, consolidating the middle burner to stimulate the ascending *Qi* and *Blood* towards the head, easing dizziness. Dang Shen, Bai Zhu, and Fu Shen strengthen the *Spleen* and comfort the mind to promote *Spleen Qi* and *Blood.* Long Yan Rou, San Zao Ren, and Yuan Zhi nourish *Blood* and tranquilise the mind to restrain dizziness. Mu Xiang excites the middle burner *Qi* and transform the *Spleen* and *Stomach.* Gan Cao harmonises all herbs and encourages the *Stomach* to receive them. All the variations can emphasise a specific treatment point, and therefore the prescription can be tailored to the individual case.

Advice: This pattern can be seen by patients with chronic diseases, and is weaker in those with a general constitution and severe symptoms are not present; however, there will be a general weaker constitution. Therefore, we should combine reducing and reinforcing treatments together.

Liver and Kidney Yin Deficiency

Clinical features and signs: Signs are persistent chronic dizziness or recurrent seizures, declined vision, dry and gritty eyes, sleep disturbance with oblivious irritability, dry mouth, tinnitus, spiritlessness, soreness, weakness in the back and legs, a red tongue without coating, and a wiry-fine pulse.

Treatment principle in TCM: Nourish *Liver* and *Kidney Yin*; replenish and cultivate *Essence.*

Treatment: Herbal prescription.

Pinyin: Zuo Gui Wan variation.

English name for decoction: Restore the Left Kidney Decoction variation.

Role in formula	Name/ Pinyin	Name/Latin	Dose (g)	Function
Chief herb	Shu Di Huang	Radix Rhemanniae Glutinosae Praeparata	10–30	Nourishes the kidney *Yin* and essence and liver *Yin* and blood.
Deputy herb	Shan Zhu Yu	Fructus Corni Officinalis	10	Nourishes the kidney *Yin.*
Assistant herb	Shan Yao	Radix Dioscoreae Oppositae	10	Replenishes the spleen *Qi* and dries the dampness.
	Gou Qi Zi	Fructus Lycii	10	Nourishes the kidney *Yin* and essence.
	Tu Si Zi	Semen Cuscutae Chinensis	10	Replenishes the kidney *Qi* and nourishes the kidney *Yin.*
	Lu Jiao Shuang	Cornu Cervi Degelatinatum	10	Strengthens the kidney *Qi*, *Yin*, and essence.
	Gui Ban	Plastrum Testudinis	10	Nourishes the kidney *Yin* and essence.
Guiding herb	Chuan Niu Xi	Radix Cyathulae Officinalis	10–15	Activates the blood circulation and drives all herbs to the relevant meridians.

Lu Jiao Shuang *Cornu Cervi Degelatinatum* and Gui Ban *Plastrum Testudinis* are not allowed in the EU, so the following alternatives can be used:

- *Han Lian Cao 15 g,*
- *Nu Zhen Zi 10 g.*

If severe dizziness presents with *Empty Heat,* Zhi Mu, Huang Bai, and Mu Dan Pi can be added. When persistent insomnia occurs, E Jiao, Ji Zi Huang, Suan Zao Ren, and Bai Zi Ren are added. When *Yin Deficiency* presents, Sha Shen, Mai Men Dong, and Yu Zhu are added.

Method: The above-mentioned herbs are collated as a herbal formula in dry herbs or as a concentrated herbal powder, taken twice daily in herbal juices.

Analysis: Shu Di Huang, Shan Zhu Yu, and Shan Yao nourish *Kidney Yin* as three reinforcing herbs. Gou Qi Zi and Tu Si Zi emphasise there enforcement of the *Kidney.* Lu Jiao Shuang replenishes *Kidney Yin* and *Essence.* Chuan Niu Xi strengthens the *Kidney* and leads all *Yang* down to the *Kidney.* Gui Ban nourishes *Yin* and clears *Empty Heat.* Zhi Mu and Huang Bai clear ministerial fire and harmonise the *Heart* and *Kidney* to promote sleep. E Jiao, Ji Zi Huang, Suan Zao Ren, and Bai Zi Ren also nourish the heart and kidney *Yin* and harmonize the heart and kidney yang for tranquilising the heart and the mind. Sha Shen, Mai Men Dong, and Yu Zhu nourish the *Kidney*, *Liver,* and Lungs to restrain dizziness.

Advice: This pattern can be seen in the patients with minor symptoms but lasting longer. In these cases, the brain and neurological system are damaged. The disease occurs in the inner ear or peripheral nervous system.

Acupuncture for dizziness in the deficiency patterns

Scalp acupuncture and auricular acupuncture are the same for excess patterns.

Body acupuncture:
Main points: Baihui (DU20), Fengchi (GB20).

Assistant points: Geshu (BL17), Ganshu (BL18), Pishu (BL20), Shenshu (BL23).

Variation: When palpitation exists, Neiguan (P5) is added; for insomnia, Shenmen (HE7) is added; for tinnitus, Tinggong (SI19) is added.

Analysis: Baihui raises *Yang Qi* and dredges general *Qi Stagnation.* Fengchi releases excessive *Wind.* Ge shu and Gan shu along the governing meridian at the back eliminate the stagnated *Qi*; Pishu and Shenshu replenish the post-heaven and pre-heaven *Qi* to strengthen the general vitality *Qi*. Neiguan calms the mind. Shenmen tranquilises the spirit. Tinggong dredges the audial passage.

Case Study

Ms. J. Stunnifer, 62 years old, a retired teacher, has had recurrent dizziness with tinnitus for a half year. Due to a coronavirus infection, she is still has recurrent dizziness and stubborn tinnitus which disturb her sleep; she is feeling restless, nervous, and annoyed due to palpitations. No treatments are offered by her GP; therefore, she is looking to acupuncture for some help.

Present symptoms: Symptoms were tension in the neck and recurrent dizziness, minor dizziness, stubborn tinnitus causing irritability, restlessness, angers easily, poor sleep on occasion, tiredness, fatigue, alight red tongue with less coating, and a wiry-fine pulse.

Diagnosis:

1. Post-COVID-19 syndrome — Dizziness and tinnitus.
2. Chronic cervical neck pain.

Differentiation syndromes of TCM:

1. *Liver* and *Kidney Yin* Deficiency.
2. *Liver Yang* and *Fire* flare up.

Treatment: Herbal prescription and acupuncture.

Acupuncture

Scalp acupuncture: Vertigo-audial area.

Body acupuncture: Baihui (DU20), Fengchi (GB20); Zhongwan (REN12), Qihai (REN6), Waiguan (SJ5), Zulinqi (GB41).

Herbal prescription

Pinyin: Zhi Bai Di Huang Wan; Qiang Huo Sheng Shi Wan.

Advice: The acupuncture is given once a week for a month, which is then changed to once every 2 weeks. Herbal prescription, 6 g/day, twice a day.

Result: After 2 months of treatment, the dizziness has gone completely; tinnitus changes are intermittent, although much less than previously experienced. There is improvement, therefore, and the treatment of acupuncture and herbs are being continued for the time being.

Atrophy and Muscle Wasting

When the muscles cannot contract to support the physical position or change of tension, most of the conditions are due to problems in the nervous system which controls the movement of the muscle. When a muscle is not used, it starts to lose its nutrition and oxygen supply, and gradually it loses its muscle fibres and become smaller. This is called Withering disease (Wei disease). Such symptoms are called Atrophy, and the modern term for loss of bulk muscle is wasting.

Atrophy could be caused by problems in the central nervous system (CNS) or peripheral nerves. Problems in the peripheral nerves are mostly caused by physical damage to one or more spinal nerves by tumours, physical injuries, and chemical impairments during diabetes. So, peripheral neuropathy is not relevant to PCS in general. Problems caused by CNS impairments could be the main concern in PCS, excluding tumours. In this chapter, paralysis/atrophy is listed in the next section. Also, serious motor nerve impairment conditions like Amyotrophic Lateral Sclerosis, ALS, are excluded from this discussion.

There is a long tradition in TCM for treating atrophy/paralysis caused by stroke or stroke sequela, which is centred on muscular incapacity of movement. After more than 40 years of clinical experience, acupuncture and herbal treatment were standardised by the Acupuncture Society of the National Administration of TCM China. The authors have been using such protocols for treating patients who have lost the ability to move, and very good clinical results have been observed; therefore, the same protocols are used in treating PCS conditions presenting muscular impairment, whether it shows damage in one muscle or hemiplegia (half body) as the principles are the same.

WM diagnosis

CT/MRI is performed to identify if it is a tumour, a stroke, or CIA.

Nerve conduction tests, PECT, or fMRI could be further used to identify the damaged pathway of the nerves.

In terms of PCS, most of the conditions are suspected to be TIA. There is no evidence yet to suggest that COVID-19 can cause brain tumours. So, when a tumour is diagnosed, it is not within PCS.

Diagnosis with TCM perspective

The levels of muscular strength should be recorded for monitoring the progression:

Level 0: No visible muscle contraction with the best effort.
Level 1: Muscle contraction is visible, but not causing physical movement of the body part connected to it.
Level 2: Muscle contraction can lead to horizontal movement of the body part, but not against the weight or resistance (not able to lift).
Level 3: Muscle contraction is able move the body part up or against resistance.
Level 4: Muscle can make all-round movement, although slow and weaker.
Level 5: Normal movement achieved.

When a muscle shrinks, it is necessary to measure the size of the muscle, the circumference of the limb, and movement is a good way to evaluate the muscle state.

If an infrared camera or thermo-camera is available, the image should be taken before and after every treatment/visit.

Rigidity is a big issue in treatment. When a muscle is not controlled by the nerve system, it can gain contraction without control, which shows high tension in the muscle but not relaxation. This suggests prolonged damage at a deeper level.

TCM acupuncture treatment

For paralysis as the main symptom which is caused by damage in the brain and neurological systems, acupuncture is the best therapy, so multiple acupuncture technologies should be the first choice to create a suitable and strong enough treatment for individual cases as the key technology to release paralysis.

TCM acupuncture

Main points: Baihui (DU20), Fengchi (GB20).

Assistant points:

- Paralysis: Quchi (LI11), Hegu (LI4); Xuehai (SP10), Sanyinjiao (SP6).

Original-yuan point/Shu-stream point and He-sea point on relevant meridian such as:

- Lung: Taiyuan (LU9), Chize (LU6).
- Spleen: Taibai (SP2), Yinlingquan (SP9).
- Liver: Taichong (LIV3), Ququan (LIV8).
- Kidney: Taixi (KI2), Yingu (KI10).

Remaining points for building up *Qi* and *Yin* to treat chronic state:

- Mu-points: Jiuwei (REN15), Zhongwan (REN12), Qihai (REN6), Zhongji (REN4).
- Back-points: Ganshu (BL18), Geshu (BL17), Pishu (BL20), Shenshu (BL23).

Scalp acupuncture:

- The foot motor sensory area for paralysis or loss of balance.
- The motor area at the relevant local part for paralysis or difficult movement.
- The sensory area for numbness, or pain occurrence at relevant part.
- The secondary and tertiary speech areas for slurring or difficult speech.
- The chorea-trembling controlled area for loss of balance or shaking and trembling of limbs.

Scalp acupuncture can be used alone, or with electric support, combined with body acupuncture or other technology.

Electric acupuncture: The electricity is connected to the end of the needles when they are put into the selected points. Both the positive and negative ends from the electric acupuncture machine are always connected on the points of the same meridian.

Rarefaction wave: It provides stronger stimulation to the points via the needles, so it causes contraction of muscles and increment of the tension in muscle and ligament, so it is good to treat paralysis or muscular tendons.

Dense wave: It may induce an inhibitory effect on the sensory nerve and motor nerve, so it is used for sedation and pain relief, relaxation of muscles, and vessel spasm.

Rarefaction-dense wave: This uses two waves, each wave lasting one and a half seconds, and is good for pain relief and paralysis.

Intermittent wave: It may increase the excitability of muscular tissue and has a fine simulative and contractive effect on the striated muscle. This it is commonly used for muscular weakness, atrophy, and paralysis.

Analysis: In scalp acupuncture, the points are selected according to the relevant anatomic areas in the brain, and the selected points are guided by the combination of medical science and TCM theories, corresponding to the local paralysis or impaired function.

Baihui dissipates the *Stagnated Qi* of the upper head and general body. Fengchi eliminates the excessive *Wind* from the top of the head. Quchi and Hegu as points along *Bright Yang* meridian of the hand are selected to dredge the stagnated *Qi* and *Blood* at the arms, according to the treatment principle of TCM: "treating points are selected for limbs paralysis from *Bright Yang* meridian only". Xuehai and Sanyinjiao from the *Larger Yin* meridian are selected to dredge the stagnated *Qi* and *Blood* at the legs. Then, the shu-stream points and the *He-sea* points are selected from each meridian to dredge their *Qi Stagnation* and *Blood* obstruction according to the affected meridian on an individual case. They will assist the main points to create a robust treatment level.

Whether electricity is used or not, according to the severity of the paralysis, a higher level of treatment should be given. In electric acupuncture treatment stimulation, needles are put into the body to maximise the treatment level. Multiple acupuncture technologies can be used for gentle or minor limb weakness and numbness as pre-clinical conditions, and for paralysis, hemiplegia or paraplegia, as post-syndrome of stroke or other organic diseases which have damaged the brain or neurological system.

Common patterns of TCM and herbal medicine treatment

Residual Damp-phlegm-heat accumulate through three burners

Clinical features and signs: Weakness, numbness, or paralysis of the limbs with minor local swelling, heavy feeling in general, distension of the chest and abdomen, confusion of the mind, poor appetite, hot flashes, warm palms, red-plump tongue with yellow-greasy thick coating, and rapid-fine soft pulse.

Treatment principle in TCM: Clear excessive *Heat* and eliminate *Dampness*; dredge the meridians and *Blood* vessels.

Treatment: Herbal prescription.

Pinyin: Gan Lu Xiao Du Dan variated with Qiang Huo Sheng Shi Tang.

English name for decoction: Sweet Dew Special Decoction to Eliminate Toxin variated.

Role in formula	Name/ Pinyin	Name/Latin	Dose (g)	Function
Chief herb	Hua Shi	Talcum	10–30	Eliminates excessive dampness and heat from the three burners.
Deputy herb	Huang Qin	Radix Scutellariae Baicalensis	10	Promotes elimination of the excessive dampness and heat.
	Yin Chen	Herba Artemisiae Capillaris	10	Promotes elimination of the excessive dampness and heat.
Assistant Herbs	Shi Chang Po	Rhizoma Acori Graminei	10	Dredges the stagnated *Qi* in the chest and pushes the *Qi* flow into the meridians.
	Tong Cao	Semen Pruni Persicae	10	Releases the excessive dampness in the meridian and promotes elimination of urine.
	Huo Xiang	Herba Agastaches seu Pogostemi	10	Eliminates the dampness in the exterior and interior.
	Bai Dou Kou	Fructus Amomi Cardamomi	10	Dredges the stagnated *Qi* in the stomach and general *Qi*.
	Qiang Huo	Rhizoma et Radix Notopterygii	10	Releases the excessive dampness in the muscles and joints, and in the meridians.
Guiding herb	Chuan Xiong	Radix Ligustici Wallichii	10	Activates the blood circulation and promotes the movement of the deep obstructions to surface.

Method: The above-mentioned herbs are collated as a formula and boiled into herbal juice with dry herbal medicine, or made into a concentrated herbal powder, taken twice daily.

Analysis: Hua Shi eliminates excessive *Dampness* and *Heat* from three burners. Huang Qin dries *Dampness* and releases *Heat* from the upper burner. Shi Chang Pu opens the chest and dredges accumulated *Qi* from the chest. Yin Chen and Huo Xiang dispel *Damp* and heat from the upper and middle burners. Tong Cao which replaced Mu Tong expels excessive *Dampness* and urine. Qiang Huo and Chuan Xiong resolve obstruction and stagnated meridians to release *Blood Stasis*. All these formulas can release excessive *Damp-Heat* to dredge the meridian for treating paralysis.

Advice: This pattern can be seen in patients suffering from weakness, numbness, or paralysis as part of post-COVID-19 syndrome. Some symptoms are still recurrent occurrences with coronavirus as ordinary viral pathogens have not been eliminated.

Qi and Fluid Deficiencies in the Lung with Empty Heat

Clinical features and signs: After a fever, the limbs appear flaccid, with fatigue, lethargy, aching in general, irritability, dry mouth, arid skin, dry throat and choky cough with less phlegm, constipation, red tongue with dry-yellow coating, and fine-rapid pulse.

Treatment principle in TCM: *Clear Heat* and nourish *Lung*; cultivate meridians and vessels.

Treatment: Herbal prescription.

Pinyin: Qing Zao Jiu Fei Tang variation.

English name for decoction: Eliminate Dryness and Rescue the Lung Decoction variation.

Role in formula	Name/ Pinyin	Name/Latin	Dose (g)	Function
Chief herb	Sang Ye	Folium Mori Albae	10	Ventilates the lung and clears excessive heat in the lung meridian.
	Shi Gao	Gypsum Fibrosum	30	Clears excessive heat in the lung and chest.
Deputy herb	Mai Men Dong	Tuber Ophiopogonis Japonici	10	Nourishes the lung *Yin* and fluid.
	Huo Ma Ren	Semen Cannabis Sativae	10–30	Nourishes the lung *Yin* and intestinal *Yin*.
Assistant herb	Ren Shen	Radix Ginseng	10	Reinforces the spleen *Qi* and blends with Gancao, a sweet flavour, to produce more fluid.
	Xing Ren	Semen Pruni Armeniacae	10	Releases lingering phlegm and eases cough.
	Pi Ba Ye	Folium Eriobotryae Japonicae	6–10	Ventilates the lungs and eases the cough.
Guiding herb	Gan Cao	Radix Glycyrrhizae Uralensis	5	Harmonises the stomach and promotes cohesive working of the herbs.

Method: The above-mentioned herbs are made into a dry herbal prescription or concentrated herbal powders, and taken twice daily as a drink in water.

Analysis: Ren Shen, Mai Men Dong, and Gan Cao promote lung fluid richness with their sweet flavour and moist nature to reinforce *Qi* and nourish *Yin* in the middle burner. Shi Gao, Sang Ye, Huo Ma Ren, and Xing Ren clear *Heat*, nourish *Yin,* and ventilate the *Lung.* Pi Ba Ye moistens the *Lung* and promotes fluid. All these herbs are mixed to clear *Heat*, nourish *Yin*, and release the *Stagnated Qi* and *Blood Stasis* in the meridians.

Advice: This pattern can be seen in patients with weakness, numbness, or gentle paralysis in a shorter disease time, indicating both pathogenic factors and the upright *Qi* not being resilient.

Spleen Qi Deficiencies with Blood Stasis

Clinical features and signs: Signs are flaccid limbs and general body weakness which is worse during the daytime, paralysis of face or limbs, fatigue and pale complexion, shortage of breath, lethargy and spiritlessness, loose bowels and poor appetite, a pale or light red tongue with stasis spots and marks, and a deep-fine or deep-weak pulse.

Treatment principle in TCM: Replenish *Spleen* and *Vitality Qi*; activate *Blood* to remove *Blood Stasis.*

Treatment: Herbal prescription.

Pinyin: Shen Ling Bai Zhu San variated with Bu Yang Huan Wu Tang.

English name for decoction: Ginseng, Poria, and Atractylodis Macrocephalae Powder variated with Tonified Yang to Restore Five-Tenth Decoction.

Role in formula	Name/ Pinyin	Name/Latin	Dose (g)	Function
Chief herb	Huang Qi	Radix Astragali Membranacei	10–30	Reinforces the spleen and general *Qi*.
Deputy herb	Shan Yao	Radix Dioscoreae Oppositae	10	Promotes to reinforce the spleen *Qi* and dries the dampness.

(*Continued*)

Role in formula	Name/ Pinyin	Name/Latin	Dose (g)	Function
Assistant herb	Fu Ling	Sclerotium Poria Cocos	10	Releases the accumulated dampness.
	Sha Ren	Fructus Amomi	10	Dredges the stagnated stomach and harmonises general *Qi*.
	Yi Yi Ren	Semen Coicis Lachryma-Jobi	10–30	Eliminates the accumulated dampness and promotes diuresis.
	Dang Gui	Radix Angelicae Sinensis	10	Nourishes the blood and *Yin* in the meridians.
	Chi Shao	Radix Paeoniae Rubrae	10	Nourishes the blood and activates blood stasis in the meridians.
	Chuan Xiong	Radix Ligustici Wallichii	10	Activates the blood stasis and eases the pain.
	Tao Ren	Semen Pruni Persicae	10	Activates the blood stasis and nourishes the intestines.
	Hong Hua	Flos Carthami Tinctorii	10	Activates the blood stasis and promotes the circulation.
Guiding herb	Gan Cao	Radix Glycyrrhizae Uralensis	5	Harmonises the stomach and leads all herbs to work cohesively.

Method: The above-mentioned herbs are mixed as a dry herbal or concentrated herbal prescription and taken trice daily.

Analysis: Huang Qi is the main herb that reinforces the *Spleen* and general *Qi*. Shan Yao and Fu Ling promote increase of *Qi* and release *Dampness*. Sha Ren and Yi Yi Ren harmonise the *Stomach* and dispel *Dampness* and fluid accumulation in the meridians. Dang Gui, Chi Shao, and Chuan Xiong nourish *Blood* and release the *Blood Stasis* in the meridians and blood vessels. Tao Ren and Hong Hua support and release *Blood Stasis* in the meridians and collaterals. Gan Cao comforts the *Stomach* and causes the herbs to work cohesively.

Advice: This is the commonest pattern with paralysis in the post-COVID-19 syndrome. Either facial palsy or post-stroke can be treated with this method; it can be used for a case with shorter disease duration or a chronic type with longer duration of suffering.

Liver and Kidney Qi and Yin Deficiencies

Clinical features and signs: Signs are weakness of leg(s) with slower movement, flaccid leg(s) and foot/feet, sore and weak at the back and knee(s), unable to stand for longer periods of time accompanied by dizziness, tinnitus, premature or nocturnal emission, irregular menstruation, possible collapse of leg(s) with complete paralysis and muscular a trophy of leg(s), a red tongue with less coating, and a deep-thread pulse.

Treatment principle in TCM: Replenish *Liver* and *Kidney*; nourish *Yin* and clear *Heat.*

Treatment: Herbal prescription.

Pinyin: Hu Qian Wan variation.

English name for decoction: Hidden Tiger Decoction variation.

Role in formula	Name/ Pinyin	Name/Latin	Dose (g)	Function
Chief herb	Sang Ji Sheng	Ramulus Loranthi	10	Replenish the kidney *Qi* to strengthen ligaments, tendons, myofascia, and muscles; promote active joints.
Deputy herb	Suo Yang	Herba Cynomorii Songarici	10	Promotes strengthening of ligaments, muscles, and joints.
Assistant herb	Dang Gui	Radix Angelicae Sinensis	10	Nourishes *Yin* and blood.
	Bai Shao	Radix Paeoniae Lactiflorae	10	Nourishes *Yin* and blood.
	Huang Bai	Cortex Phellodendri	10	Clears the empty heat in the lower burner.
	Shu Di Huang	Radix Rhemanniae Glutinosae Praeparata	10–30	Nourishes the kidney and general *Yin.*
	Zhi Mu	Radix Anemarrhenae Asphodeloidis	10	Nourishes the kidney *Yin* and general *Yin.*
	Gui Ban	Plastrum Testudinis	10	Emphasises nourishing the kidney and general *Yin.*
Guiding herb	Gan Jiang	Rhizoma Zingiberis Officinalis	10	Warms and excites the spleen, kidney, and vitality *Qi.*

If pale complexion or palpitation is manifested, Huang Qi, Dang Shen, and Ji Xue Teng are added; if aversion to the cold, impotence, or longer urination is manifested Zi He Che and bone marrow are increased.

Method: The above-mentioned herbs are mixed as a dry herbal or concentrated herbal prescription and taken trice daily.

Analysis: Sang Ji Sheng, which is replacing Hu Gu (tiger bone), and Suo Yang strengthen ligaments, myofascia, and muscles, and promote active joints. We can use bone marrow from pork or cow to replace Hu Gu as the main herbal material. Dang Gui and Bai Shao soften the *Liver*, nourish the *Blood*, and cultivate tendons. Huang Bai, Zhi Mu, Shu Di Huang, and Gui Ban nourish *Yin*, reinforce the *Kidney*, and clear *Heat*.

Advice: This pattern can be seen in patients with chronic paralysis as part of the post-COVID-19 syndrome. If the patient is suffering from these syndromes for a longer duration, then *Qi* and *Yin* deficiency will be predominant leading to pathogenic dampness and heat accumulation.

Case Study

Mr. L. Jarman, 69 years old, is a retired technician. He suffered from coronavirus a month ago along with his wife. They took herbs to heal and relax. Jarman suddenly experienced a headache, with dizziness; in a day, he felt weakness in the left arm and leg; he visited the accident and emergence services and was diagnosed with TIA (Transient Ischemic attack). He had an MRI scan, and was then discharged and advised to fully rest without any treatment. He visited the clinic again complaining of tiredness, weakness of the left arm and leg, intermittent dizziness and recurrent headache at the right temporal region and front head, restlessness, nervous and disturbed sleep, light red tongue with less coating, and wiry pulse. He had minor elevated blood pressure (160/98) with slower pulse (56/min).

Diagnosis:

1. Post-COVID-19 syndrome.
2. TIA (minor stroke).

Differentiation syndromes of TCM:

1. *Liver Wind-Heat* flare up.
2. *Spleen Qi Deficiency* with *Blood Stasis*.

Treatment principle in TCM: Tranquilise *Liver* and Clear *Heat,* replenish *Spleen Qi*, and activate *Blood Stasis* to promote circulation.

Acupuncture

Scalp acupuncture: The foot motor sensory area and the motor area at the top and middle part.

Body acupuncture: Baihui (DU20), Fengchi (GB20); Yinlingquan (SP9), Taibai (SP3), Sanyinjiao (SP6); Quchi (LI11), Hegu (LI4), Waiguan (SJ5), Zulinqi (GB41).

When he visited the clinic the following week, all symptoms had decreased, and the same treatment was provided every 2 weeks, in addition to a recommendation for regular Taiji exercise. He has been maintaining a healthy condition.

Facial Palsy/Bell's Palsy (Facial Paralysis)

Peripheral facial palsy is a condition where muscles on one side of the face suddenly lose the ability to move; this is not accompanied by pain. This results in abnormal facial expression, facial imbalance of the two side, and the inability to hold one's breath. It is also called facial paralysis, and is the result of impairment of the facial nerve (the 7th cranial nerve) which controls the muscles in the face. Most of the cases (three quarters) are idiopathic and are named Bell's palsy (BP), which means the cause is not clear. A quarter of the cases can be clearly identified/diagnosed as due to cancer/tumour, viral infection in the CNS, autoimmune damage in CNS, Ramsay-Hunt-Syndrome, and Lyme Neuroborreliosis (Zimmermann *et al*., 2019). Regarding BP, speculations on the role of the herpes simplex and herpes zoster viruses were supported by research but could not be firmly ratified by results. The hypothesis is that the herpes virus hides inside the body but is unable to cause damage when the immune system is working normally. When the immune system is struggling against other infections, the weakness provides the virus a chance to attack a peripheral nerve, which can be in the form of Bell's palsy or Shingles. When the immune function returns to normal, the virus is then cleared. Some patients of BP recover within 9 months of onset; however, 80–90% did not. Non-recovery is possibly due to the damage of the nerve–muscle connection.

With regard to COVID-19 and PCS, the case of BP has been observed more often in medical practice than before the COVID-19 period.

A higher occurrence of facial palsy during the COVID-19 outbreak was observed compared to the same period of the year before the pandemic, with an increase of 21%. This study provides evidence of the correlation between BP and COVID-19. However, the report could not provide a long-term follow-up to confirm if it is the same trend in the post-COVID-19 stage.

The condition was recorded in TCM very early as Facial Paralysis or wry face. A very rich experience has been accumulated by using acupuncture and herbal medicine. Great success rates were reported when the non-recovery cases were treated. Acupuncture alone can achieve very good results; however, considering the root of the condition is more about the weakened defensive system, herbal medicine should always be used in conjunction with acupuncture, particularly for those with disease lingering into a chronic stage.

Diagnosis

Clinical features and signs: Signs are sudden occurrence of numbness, weakness, deviation of mouth, and even paralysis on one side of the face. Pain is not often reported. Dripping saliva, eye tearing, and flat face without wrinkle could be observed. The damage in the facial muscle is limited to the face only. If the muscles in the limbs are also involved, it is not a facial palsy and needs thorough medical examination for diagnosis. History and physical examination are the main clinical diagnosis procedures. CT/MRI and CFS are applied to exclude/establish causes.

Acupuncture

Acupuncture is the best treatment method for facial palsy.

Body acupuncture:
Main points: Taiyang (EXT), Dicang (ST4), Jiache (ST6).

Assistant points: Yangbai (GB14), Sibai (ST2), Hegu (LI4), Neiting (ST44).

- Eyebrow drooping, Zanzhu (BL2) is added.
- Flat nasolabial fold, Yingxiang (LI 20) is added.
- Pain at the mastoid behind ear, Yifeng (SJ17) is added.
- Deviation of the face and mouth Renzhong (DU26) is added.
- Deviation of mentolabial sulcus, Chengjiang (RN24) is added.
- Tongue numbness, loose taste, Lianquan (RN23) is added.

Electric acupuncture: Dicang (ST4), Jiache (ST6), Yangbai (GB14), and Hegu (LI4) can connect with electricity using minor waves to encourage the patient to feel comfortable, and minor muscle throbs can be treated with a fit dose of electricity.

Syndrome patterns and treatment of TCM herbal treatment

External Wind-Cold based on Spleen Qi Deficiency

Clinical features and signs: Signs are sudden occurrence of facial numbness, weakness, paralysis on the one side, eyebrow drops down, unclosed eye, deviated mouth with breathing out at the corner of the mouth on the affected side, tiredness, fatigue, and aversion to wind without sweating. Facial palsy occurs after coronavirus infection or a long time after being vaccinated, or even after excessive expending of energy. Other signs are a light red or pale tongue with less, thin white coating and a floating and weak pulse.

Treatment principle in TCM: Dispel the external *Wind-Cold*; replenish *Spleen* and general *Qi*.

Treatment: Herbal prescription.

Pinyin: Bu Zhong Yi Qi Tang variation.

English name for decoction: Tonify the Middle and Augment the *Qi* Decoction variation.

Role in formula	Name/ Pinyin	Name/Latin	Dose (g)	Function
Chief herb	Huang Qi	Radix Astragali Membranacei	10–30	Reinforces the spleen and strengthens the weak muscle.
Deputy herb	Ren Shen	Radix Ginseng	10	Promotes reinforcement of the spleen *Qi* and general vitality *Qi*.
Assistant herb	Bai Zhu	Rhizoma Atractylodis Macrocephalae	10–30	Reinforces the spleen *Qi* and strengthens muscles.
	Chen Pi	Pericarpium Citri Reticulatae	10	Excites the spleen *Qi* and dredges the stagnated *Qi* in the Meridians.
	Dang Gui	Radix Angelicae Sinensis	10	Nourishes liver *Yin* and blood to cultivate muscles.
	Sheng Ma	Rhizoma Cimicifugae	6–10	Ascends herbs to the face and pushes *Qi*.
	Chai Hu	Radix Bupleuri	6–10	Dredges the liver *Qi* and promotes general *Qi* movement.
Guiding herb	Zhi Gan Cao	Radix Glycyrrhizae Uralensis	5	Harmonises the stomach and promotes cohesiveness of herbs.

If Bell's palsy has just started and is gradually developing with catarrhal, Fang Feng and Jing Jie are added. If there is some facial muscle spasm, Wei Ling Xian Qiang Huo and Bai Sao are added.

Method: The above-mentioned prescription can be made into a herbal decoction or concentrated herbal powder which is given in case of a sudden occurrence, severe appearance of the problem, and when the patient wants to quickly control the problem.

Analysis: Huang Qi as the main herb reinforces the *Spleen* and leads the *Spleen* energy up to strengthen the weak muscle. Ren Shan and Bai Zhu support the main herb in reinforcing the Spleen *Qi*. Chen Pi and Chai

Hu release the stagnated *Qi* and relax the muscle spasm. When a spasm exists, Bai Shao can be increased to 30 g to relax the muscle spasm. Dang Gui nourishes *Yin* and Blood to fill the facial muscle. Sheng Ma eliminates excessive wind in the blood. Fang Feng, Qiang Huo, etc., are added to have a stronger effect to eliminate the external wind. Zhi Gan Cao harmonises the *Stomach* and promotes herbs to work together. This prescription will give robust support to facial muscles and control its palsy.

Advice: This pattern is seen as a typical pattern of the Bell's palsy after an infection of COVID-19. When the *Vitality Qi* and *Spleen Qi* are weaker from the struggle against coronavirus, a facial palsy is caused due to external wind invasion. Therefore, strengthening general *Qi* can heal not only Bell's palsy but also post-COVID-19 syndrome.

External Wind-Heat based on Liver Qi Stagnation

Clinical features and signs: Signs are sudden occurrence of facial numbness, weakness, paralysis on one side; eyebrow drops down, unclosed eye, deviated mouth with breathing out from the corner of the mouth at the affected side; nervousness, panic attacks, restlessness, headache, redness in the affected eye; sore throat or ear sore, possible insomnia after coronavirus or vaccination. This facial palsy can occur during or after a coronavirus infection, when a patient is very nervous during his/her infection, or when infection extends for a long time, increasing the stress response. Patients might have red tongue with less yellow or thin white coating and wiry pulse.

Treatment principle in TCM: Eliminate external Wind-Heat; dredge Liver Stagnation to promote general *Qi* circulation.

Treatment: Herbal prescription.

Pinyin: Jia Wei Xiao Yao Tang variation.

English name for decoction: Augmented Rambling Decoction variation.

Role in formula	Name/ Pinyin	Name/Latin	Dose (g)	Function
Chief herb	Chai Hu	Radix Bupleuri	10	Dredges the liver *Qi* and releases the stress to promote *Qi* flow in the meridians through the body.
Deputy herb	Dang Gui	Radix Angelicae Sinensis	10	Softens the liver and cultivates the liver *Yin* and blood.
Assistant herb	Chi Shao	Radix Paeoniae Rubrae	10	Activates the blood stasis and softens the liver to help the *Qi* and blood circulation.
	Fu Ling	Sclerotium Poria Cocos	10	Replenishes the spleen and dries the accumulated dampness.
	Bai Zhu	Rhizoma Atractylodis Macrocephalae	10	Replenishes the spleen and strengthens the muscles.
	Gan Jiang	Rhizoma Zingiberis Officinalis	10	Warms and excites the spleen *Qi* and general *Qi*.
	Bo He	Herba Menthae Haplocalycis	5	Promotes herbs to ascend and release the external wind.
	Mu Dan Pi	Cortex Moutan Radicis	10	Clears the excessive heat in the middle burns and general heat in the blood.
	Zhi Zi	Fructus Gardeniae Jasminoidis	10	Clears the excessive heat in the liver and heart to promote relaxation.
	Gan Cao	Radix Glycyrrhizae Uralensis	5	Harmonises the stomach and promotes cohesiveness of herbs.

Method: The above-mentioned prescription can be made into an herbal decoction or concentrated herbal powder and given in the cases of a sudden occurrence, severe appearance of the problem and also when the patient wants to quickly control the problem.

Analysis: Chai Hu dredges the stagnated *Liver Qi* and eliminates the external *Wind* as the main herb. Dang Gui and Chi Shao soften the *Liver Yin* and *Blood* to nourish the fascia. Fu Ling and Bai Zhu reinforce the *Spleen Qi* to strengthen muscle recovery. Gan Jiang promotes the main herb to release the stagnated *Qi* and promotes ascension of the herbs.

Bo He clears the *Heat* at the head or face and unblocks the closed eye. Mu Dan Pi and Zhi Zi release the excessive Heat. Gan Cao is a harmonising herb that promotes and regulates the *Stomach* to a good condition. All the herbs are combined to release stress and support healing of inadequate muscles.

Advice: This pattern is seen in patients suffering from a facial palsy triggered by stress or due to psychiatric symptoms after he/she is healing from a COVID-19 infection.

Case Study

Mr. T. Zhao, 28 years old, Ph.D. student, was infected with COVID-19 and suffered a minor fever and cough during a stressful time of study commitments. He rested for a couple of weeks and felt better, therefore returning to his research. However, he felt and noticed a deviated right face in a morning after waking up. He was unable to completely close his right eye and mouth, causing tearing and discharge from the month when talking or smiling. Due to the inconvenience of seeing a doctor during the lockdown, he sought support from and made an appointment at a TCM clinic. He also provided proof of a negative PCR examination.

Clinical features and signs: Signs were paralysis and deviation of the right side of the face with no wrinkles on the forehead; he was unable to close the right eye, causing tearing, and unable to close the right side of the mouth, causing discharge when speaking. He has aversion to cold, stress, nervousness, restlessness, and poor sleep before consultation. No fever, cough, or sore throat was present. He had a light red tongue with less white coating, and a floating-wiry pulse.

Diagnosis:

1. Bell palsy after COVID-19 as part of the post-COVID-19 syndrome.
2. Stress.

Differentiation syndromes of TCM:

1. External *Wind-Cold* invasion.
2. *Liver Qi Stagnation* and *Spleen Qi Deficiency.*

Treatment principle in TCM:

1. Eliminate external *Wind-Cold.*
2. Dredge *Liver Qi* and strengthen *Spleen Qi.*

Treatment: Herbal prescription and acupuncture.

Acupuncture

Main points: Baihui (DU20), Taiyang (Ext); Dicang (ST4), Jiache (ST6), Sibai (ST2), Yingxiang (LI20), Fengchi (GB20), Hegu (LI4), Taichong (LIV3), Zusanli (ST36), Sanyinjiao (SP6).

Herbal prescription

Pinyin: Xiao Yao Wan Plus Bu Zhong Yi Qi Wan.

Result: The above mentioned herbs were taken 5 g each, twice daily, for a week, after which his deviated face gradually returned into its normal shape in 2 weeks. He took another PCR exam with a negative result.

References

Caress, J. B., Castoro, R. J., Simmons, Z., Scelsa, S. N., Lewis, R. A., *et al.* (2020). COVID-19-associated Guillain-Barré syndrome: The early pandemic experience. *Muscle & Nerve*, 62(4), 485–491. doi:10.1002/mus.27024.

Codeluppi, L., Venturelli, F., Rossi, J., *et al.* (2021). Facial palsy during the COVID-19 pandemic. *Brain Behavior*, 11, e01939. https://doi.org/10.1002/brb3.1939.

Khatoon, F., Prasad, K., and Kumar, V. (2021). COVID-19 associated nervous system manifestations. *Sleep Medicine*, 91, 231–236, https://doi.org/10.1016/j.sleep.2021.07.005.

Lu, Y., Li, X., Geng, D., Mei, N., Wu, P., Huang, C., Jia, T, Zhao., Wang, D., Xiao, A. (2020). Cerebral micro-structural changes in COVID-19 Patients — An MRI-based 3-month follow-up study. *eClinicalMedicine*, (*Lancet*), 25, 100484. https://doi.org/10.1016/j.eclinm.2020.100484.

NICE. (2012). Headaches in over 12s: Diagnosis and management. National Institute for Health and Care Excellence. Available at: https://www.nice.org.uk/guidance/cg150/ifp/chapter/treatments-for-tensiontype-headache, (Accessed on 1 March 2022).

Norouzi, M., Miar, P., Norouzi, S., *et al.* (2021). Nervous system involvement in COVID-19: A review of the current knowledge. *Molecular Neurobiology*, 58, 3561–3574. https://doi.org/10.1007/s12035-021-02347-4.

Ogier, M., Andéol, G., Sagui, E., and Dal Bo, G. (2020). How to detect and track chronic neurologic sequelae of COVID-19? Use of auditory brainstem responses and neuroimaging for long-term patient follow-up. *Brain, Behavior, and Immunity — Health*, 5, 100081. doi:10.1016/j.bbih.2020.100081.

Uncini, A., Vallat, J. M., and Jacobs, B. C. (2020). Guillain-Barré syndrome in SARS-CoV-2 infection: An instant systematic review of the first six months of pandemic. *Journal of Neurology, Neurosurgery and Psychiatry*, 91(10), 1105–1110. doi:10.1136/jnnp-2020-324491.

Virhammar, J., Nääs, A., Fällmar, D., Cunningham, J. L., Klang, A., *et al.* (2021). Biomarkers for central nervous system injury in cerebrospinal fluid are elevated in COVID-19 and associated with neurological symptoms and disease severity. *European Journal of Neurology*, 28(10), 3324–3331. https://doi.org/10.1111/ene.14703.

Zimmermann, J., Jesse, S., Kassubek, J., *et al.* (2019). Differential diagnosis of peripheral facial nerve palsy: A retrospective clinical, MRI and CSF-based study. *Journal of Neurology*, 266, 2488–2494. https://doi.org/10.1007/s00415-019-09387-w.

Chapter 9

Psychological Disorders

From most sources available on post-COVID-19 syndrome (PCS), anxiety disorders, including anxiety, post-traumatic stress disorder (PTSD), feeling and being overstressed, and frustration, accompanied by emotional outcry are very common, affecting about 36% of all patients (Domigo *et al.*, 2021; Michelen, 2020; Taquet *et al.*, 2021; Whitaker *et al.*, 2021). There is huge difference between the people infected with COVID-19 and the people not infected. The problem can also extend into depression.

From previous pandemic experience, it is true that any pandemic will lead to a huge blow to the sufferer's mental and psychological health. The impact could be from the infection itself, from the overreaction of the people in their environment and the wider society, the shock of being placed in special wards, and observing many other patients in the ICU, in addition to death. Some previous studies suggested that when facing a new/unknown disease without proven treatment, people panic because of the uncertainty they are dealing with. The lack of authentic/validated information and the oversupply of wrong information also have a psychological impact on the population.

New cases of psychological problems are observed, and it is also important to know that many previously healed or well-managed psychological conditions are relapsing, due to either the impact of the shock received or the interruption of the care/treatment they were provided (Vadivel *et al.*, 2021; Pereira-Sanchez *et al.*, 2020). From another point of view, the healthcare workers/home carers who are in charge of COVID-19 patients were subject to very high demands and unguided decision-making, coupled with the shortage of staff due to isolation requirements, all contributing to a society of anxiety. They might have also reflected this back to the sufferers.

TCM has been a very promising alternative in treatment and management of psychological conditions, from situational anxiety (Tang *et al.*, 2021) to general anxiety disorder (GAD) (Yang *et al.*, 2021) and post-traumatic stress disorder (PTSD) (Hu, 2021). The advantage is that acupuncture, TCM herbs, Qigong, Taiji, and Daoyin (self-stimulation of channels) are applied integrating with and complementary to each other, providing a holistic and all-round behavioural change based on the mind–body–action strategy to help the patients in the short and long term.

Anxiety

Anxiety disorders refer to a group of clinical conditions featuring a free flow of disturbing ideas, fused with worry, fear, and unsettled feelings. Some patients feel anxiety purely in the mind, while many have both subjective and objective feelings, which could be described as butterflies in stomach. In the worst scenario, a panic attack could happen in an overwhelming loss of control of bodily feeling and movement. The most commonly mentioned anxiety disorders include general anxiety disorder (GAD), post-traumatic stress disorder (PTSD), panic attack, and phobia disorder. In the context of post-COVID-19 syndrome, anxiety is mostly discussed as a symptom or is maybe extended to GAD, because the diagnosis of anxiety disorder requires a 6-month period of consistent presenting of the symptoms, which might require more time.

Besides the constant feeling of worry, being distracted easily due to other worrying aspects, and feeling blank-minded, being clueless on what to do and irritability/frustration are other common feelings. Furthermore, fatigue is experienced by most of the patients. Physically, tension builds up and leads to general aching and hypertonicity. Sleep becomes disturbed and includes dreams with themes of worrying. The quality of life (QoL) is significantly reduced and the efficiency of working is lowered. Its manifestations overlap with many clinical complaints of “Brain Fog”, which relates to lack of freshness/alertness of the mind. However, that feeling can be improved by drinking tea/coffee, although anxiety disorders do not response to tea/coffee.

In this discussion, anxiety disorders are discussed as a whole for the convenience of diagnosis and treatment in TCM.

Diagnosis

According to the world's most-used diagnostic tool in mental health, DSM-5 (America Psychiatric Society, 2016), the diagnosis for GAD relies on history taking and exclusion of other illnesses which can cause such disorders.

The key symptom is the excessive anxiety and worry about most activities, self, or closely related persons, lasting 6 months or more. Worrying is difficult to control and overcome. Excessive or free-floating worry means a worry is unwarranted compared to the possible risk when a decision is made about whether something poses any threat. Mostly, the worry is generated due to a personal way of thinking.

The main symptom is accompanied by at least three other symptoms from the list of six as follows:

(i) Edginess or restlessness.
(ii) Feeling tired or fatigued easily.
(iii) Poor concentration or the feeling of blankness frequently.
(iv) Irritability (even not observable to others).
(v) Increased muscle aches or soreness due to tension.
(vi) Difficulty sleeping (due to trouble falling asleep or staying asleep, restlessness at night, or unsatisfying sleep).

PTSD clearly features most of the anxiety manifestations, plus a unique experience of "flashback" of the trauma scenery, violence, bloodiness, screaming, etc., that the patient was involved in, witnessed, or suffered from. The flashback is a vivid playback of the image and sound, like watching a short film of the traumatic event. When a flashback happens, the body is triggered into a "fight–flight–freeze" response, with increased heartbeat, tremors, coldness, and many other symptoms. It could happen in sleep or be triggered by any reminder of the bad experience.

A panic attack is an episode of sudden loss of control of self and being overpowered or gripped by the fear/horror the patient perceives. It is always related to the phobia of something. The panic attack is characterised by sudden loss of strength, faintness, confusion, sweating, and tremors. The episode could last from half an hour to a few days in the worst cases. It is easily linked to some environment (closed spaces like in a lift), a person posing a threat, or a challenging situation (asked to speak in a public meeting).

In TCM, anxiety was named *Jing Ji* (frightened and heart beating wildly), and the treatment was always suggested as a combination of acupuncture, herbal medicine, and body–mind exercise.

Syndrome pattern and treatment in TCM

Heart Qi Deficiency with Qi Stagnation

Clinical features and signs: Signs are worrying a lot, panic attacks with sweating of palms, palpitation, breathlessness, recurrent dull aching in the central chest, fatigue and lethargy which are worse on exertion and better at rest, pale face or lips, pale or light red tongue with less white coating, and wiry-fine pulse, weaker at left cun (heart) position.

Treatment principle in TCM: Reinforce *Heart Qi* and promote general circulation.

Acupuncture: Jianshi (P5), Shenmen (HE7), Xinshu (BL15), Zusanli (ST36); For severe panic attacks: Daling (P7) is added; for intense sweating, Gaohuang Shu (BL43).

Analysis: Juque (CV14) accompanies Xinshu as a pair of Mu (募) — Shu (腧) points reregulate the heart *Qi*. Shanzhong (REN17) promotes *Heart* and general *Qi* circulation. Jianshi (P5) and Shenmen (HE7) strengthen *Qi* flowing in the *Pericardium* and *Heart* meridians. Zusanli reinforces general *Vitality Qi.* Daling assists Jianshi to dredge stagnated *Heart Qi*. Gaohuang also assists *Heart Qi* to be stronger and fills the whole meridian to ease sweating, due to sweat flowing out at the tip of *Heart* meridian.

Treatment: Herbal prescription.

Pinyin: Sheng Mai Yin and Gui Zhi Long-Mu Decoctions.

English name for decoction: Generate the Pulse Decoction varied with Cinnamon Twig Decoction Plus Dragon Bone and Oyster Shell Decoction.

	Name/Pinyin	Name/Latin	Dose (g)	Function
Chief herb	Ren Shen	Radix Ginseng	10	Replenishes the heart *Qi* and general *Qi*.
Deputy herb	Mai Men Dong	Tuber Ophiopogonis Japonici	10	Nourishes the heart *Yin* and general *Yin*.
Assistant herb	Wu Wei Zi	Fructus Schisandrae Chinensis	10	Nourishes the heart and liver *Yin*, and general *Yin*.
	Gui Zhi	Ramulus Cinnamomi Cassiae	5–10	Excites the heart *Qi* and general *Qi*.
	Chi Shao	Radix Paeoniae Rubrae	10	Activates the blood stasis and softens the liver to promote relaxation.
	Long Gu	Os Draconis	15	Calms the mind down and tranquilises the spirit to restrain anxiety.
	Mu Li	Concha Ostreae	15	Calms the mind down and tranquilises the spirit to restrain anxiety.
Guiding herb	Gan Cao	Radix Glycyrrhizae Uralensis	5	Harmonises the stomach and promotes cohesiveness of all herbs.

Method: The above-mentioned herbal prescription is the main formula where the herbs are mixed as a decoction to create a variation, according to specific individualised symptoms, and then boiled or made into concentrated herbal powders to be consumed with warm water, twice daily.

Analysis: Ren Shen reinforces the *Heart Qi* and general *Q*i. Mai Men Dong nourishes the *Heart Yin.* Wu Wei Zi has a sour taste and is to be mixed with Gan Cao with sweet taste to co-nourish the *Heart Yin*. Gui Zhi warms and reinforces *Qi-Yang* for moving *Qi* and *Blood* circulation in the *Heart* and in general. Chi Shao nourishes *Yin* and dredges stagnated *Heart Stasis.* Long Gu and Mu Li tranquilise the spirit and calm the mind down.

All the above prescriptions can reinforce *Qi* as a main effect, and can also nourish *Yin* and dredge stagnated *Qi* and *Blood*, so they can ease and release anxiety and many kinds of psychiatric disorders.

Advice: This pattern can be seen with anxiety as an initial or gentle stage during an infection or suspected infection of COVID-19, and is a part of post-COVID-19 syndrome.

Heart Blood Deficiency or Heart Yin Deficiency with Empty Fire flare-up

Clinical features and signs: Signs are palpitation, panic attacks with breathlessness, sore or pressure aches in the chest, poor sleep with many dreams which is worse with contemplation (overthinking), dizziness, pale face, easily annoyed, upset, tinnitus, dry mouth, red-slim tongue without coating, and fine-rapid pulses.

Treatment principle in TCM: Nourish *Heart Blood* and promote general circulation; clear *Empty Heat.*

Acupuncture

Main points: Tongli (HE5), Shentang (BL44).

Assistant points: Geshu (BL17), Pishu (BL20), Yinlingquan (SP9), Xuehai (SP10); If extremely annoyed, Laogong (P8) is added; For tinnitus, Zhongzhu (SJ3) is added; When heart is more empty, Taixi (KI3) is added.

Analysis: Tongli as a Collateral-Luo point of the *Heart* meridian accompanies Shentang to nourish *Heart Yin* and *Blood* to tranquilise the spirit and calm the mind as the main points. Xuehai is a collection of *Blood* and accompanies Yinlingquan, which nourishes *Heart Blood.* Geshu dredges stagnated *Heart Qi.* Pishu reinforces the *Post-Heaven Qi* to maintain blood production. Laogong as the stream point of the pericardium meridian promotes blood flow to activate the mind. Zhongzhu as the Spring-Shu point of three burner meridian dredges all *Stagnated Qi* and *Stasis*

Blood to eliminate tinnitus. If *Empty Heart* heat flares up, Taixi is the paring point of the *Kidney* and is used to clear *Heart Heat.*

Treatment: Herbal prescription.

Pinyin: Si Wu and An Shen Bu Xin Decoctions.

English name for decoction: Four-Substance Decoction variated to Calm the Mind and Reinforce the Heart Decoction.

Role in formula	Name/ Pinyin	Name/Latin	Dose (g)	Function
Chief herb	Shu Di Huang	Radix Paeoniae Lactiflorae	10–30	Nourishes the heart *Yin* and blood to cultivate the mind.
Deputy herb	Bai Shao	Radix Paeoniae Lactiflorae	10	Nourishes the heart *Yin* and liver blood to support relaxation.
Assistant herb	Chuan Xiong	Radix Ligustici Wallichii	10	Activates the blood stasis and eases pain or angina.
	Dang Gui	Radix Angelicae Sinensis	10	Nourishes the heart *Yin* and liver blood.
	Yuan Zhi	Radix Polygalae Tenuifoliae	10	Tranquilises the spirit and calms the mind down.
	Huang Qin	Radix Scutellariae Baicalensis	10	Clears accumulated heat in the chest and heart.
	Bai Zhu	Rhizoma Atractylodis Macrocephalae	10–30	Replenishes the spleen and general *Qi*, releases the dampness.
	Suan Zao Ren	Semen Zizyphi Spinosae	10	Nourishes the liver *Yin* and blood to promote the heart *Yin.*
	Gan Cao	Radix Glycyrrhizae Uralensis	5	Harmonises the stomach and promotes cohesiveness of herbs.

Method: The above-mentioned herbal prescription is the main formula where the herbs are mixed as a decoction, which can be variated according to specific individual symptoms, and then boiled or made into concentrated herbal powders to be consumed with warm water, taken twice daily.

Analysis: Si Wu Tang decoction, which means four-herb mixture made with Shu Di Huang, Dang Gui, Chi Shao, and Chuan Xiong as the main herbs, can nourish the *Heart Yin* and Blood, chill the *Empty Heat*, and eliminate stagnant *Blood* in the *Heart* meridian. Yuanzhi nourishes *Heart Yin* and *Blood,* and Suan Zao Ren nourishes *Heart* and *Liver Yin,* both of which can tranquilise the spirit and calm the mind down. Huang Qin clears *Excessive Heat* in the upper burner. Bai Zhu reinforces *Spleen Qi* at the middle burner to strengthen the *Post-Heaven Qi.* Gan Cao harmonises herbs to support cohesiveness or settle the *Stomach.*

Advice: This pattern can be seen in sufferers with chronic, extended disease, often seen in the post-COVID-19 syndrome. This is always accompanied by both depression and insomnia; in some cases, this pattern can involve a real heart attack — angina.

Heart Fire-Phlegm flare-up

This is an excess pattern in patients, manifesting extra symptoms, although there is no appearance of deficiency symptoms.

Clinical features and signs: The signs are panic attacks in the day and night with apparent sweating, breathlessness, and occasional palpitation. The panic attacks can last a few minutes, hours, or a while according to its severity. The patients might also feel nervous or restless, with a fogginess in the mind and a general feeling of heaviness. Severe cases can appear such as obsessive-compulsive disorder (OCD), which means the sufferer has negative intrusive thoughts or images and is engaging in compulsive or repetitive behaviour. Depression or insomnia always accompanies it. The patient can also have a red or light red tongue with white-greasy coating and wiry-rolling pulses.

Treatment principle in TCM: Dispel *Excessive Damp-Phlegm* and dredge *Stagnated Qi*; clear excessive *Heat* and still the mind.

Acupuncture

Main points: Lingdao (HE4), Ximen (P4).

Assistant points: Chize (LU5), Fenglong (ST40), Feishu (BL13); For Insomnia, add Lidui (ST45); For constipation, add Dachangshu (BL25).

Analysis: Lingdao (HE4) is the River-Jing point of the *Heart* meridian and Ximen (P4) is Space-Xi point of the *Pericardium* meridian used to tranquilise the spirit and calm the mind. Chize (LU5) and Feishu (BL13) eliminate *Stagnated Lung Qi*; Chize (LU5) eliminates the stagnated lung *Qi*, while Feishu (BL13) as a back shu point promotes it. Fenglong harmonises *Damp-Phlegm* and dredges *Stagnated Qi* to clear *Fire-Phlegm.*

Treatment: Herbal prescription.

Pinyin: Wen Dan Decoction and Chang Pu Yu Jin Decoction variation.

English name for decoction: Warm Gallbladder Decoction varied with Modified Acorus and Curcuma Decoction.

Role in formula	Name/ Pinyin	Name/Latin	Dose (g)	Function
Chief herb	Ban Xia	Rhizoma Pinelliae Ternatae	10–15	Eliminate the damp-phlegm and dredge the stagnated *Qi* in the chest.
Deputy herb	Chen Pi	Pericarpium Citri Reticulatae	10	Promotes drying of the damp-phlegm, ventilates the lung, and dredges stagnated *Qi* in the chest.
Assistant herb	Zhi Shi	Fructus Immaturus Citri Aurantii	10	Dredges the stagnated *Qi* in the chest and general body.
	Fu Shen	Sclerotium Poriae Cocos Paradicis	10	Dries the dampness and calms the mind down.
	Zhu Ru	Caulis Bambusae in Taeniis	10	Releases the excessive dampness and phlegm from the chest.
	Gan Jiang	Rhizoma Zingiberis Officinalis	10	Agitates the general *Qi* and the *Qi* gathering in the chest.
	Shi Chuang Pu	Rhizoma Acori Graminei	10	Ventilates the stagnated *Qi* in the chest and expels the damp-phlegm.
	Yu Jin	Tuber Curcumae	10	Dredges the stagnated *Qi* and regulates the mood.
Guiding herb	Zhi Gan Cao	Radix Glycyrrhizae Uralensis	5	Harmonises the stomach and promotes cohesiveness of herbs.

Method: The above-mentioned herbal prescription is the main formula where the herbs are mixed as a decoction, which can be variated according to specific individual symptoms, and then boiled into a preparation or made into concentrated herbal powders to be consumed with warm water, taken twice daily.

Analysis: Ban Xia and Chen Pi harmonise *Damp-Phlegm* and dredge the stagnated *Qi* in the chest. Fu Shen releases excessive *Dampness* and calms the mind. Zhi Shi and Zhu Ru dispel stagnated *Qi* and release *Damp-Phlegm.* Shi Chang Pu and Yu Jin eliminate stagnated *Qi* in the chest and tranquilise the mind. Gan Jiang warms the *Stomach.* Zhi Gan Cao harmonises all of herbs, causing them to work cohesively.

Advice: This pattern can be seen for anxiety of medium or severe cases. A typical case can accompany COVID-19 or post-COVID-19 syndrome. It can become a chronic and refractory case.

Heart Blood Stasis

Clinical features and signs: The signs are palpitation or panic attacks lasting for an extended time and gradually getting worse, wheezing and breathlessness accompanying a panic attack, recurrent dull ache or pain in the chest which is worse with exertion, light-dark tongue or light red tongue with purple stasis marks at tip or sides, and choppy-fine pulse with irregular missing beats.

Treatment principle in TCM: Remove the *Blood Stasis* and push the *Heart* and general Blood; circulation; tranquilise the spirit and calm the mind down.

Acupuncture

Main points: Quze (P3), Shaohai (HE3).

Assistant points: Qihai (REN6), Xuehai (SP10).

If accompanied by frequent palpitation and panic attacks, add Neiguan (P6) and Gongsun (SP4); For depression, add Waiguan (SJ5) and Zulinqi (GB41); For insomnia, add Hegu (LI4) and Taichong (LIV3).

Analysis: Quze (P3) is the Sea-He point of the pericardium meridian and Shaohai (HE3) is the Sea-He point of the *Heart* meridian which reinforce

Heart Qi and tranquilise the spirit. Qihai excites the governing vessel and *Vitality Gate*. Xuehai promotes blood support to the *Heart* and *Pericardium* meridians. These points can strengthen these meridians to calm the mind down to ease panic attacks.

Treatment: Herbal prescription.

Pinyin: Guanxin II Formula and Chai Hu Long Mu Decoction.

English name for decoction: Recipe #2 for Coronary Heart Disease variated with Bupleurum Plus Dragon Bone and Oyster Shell Decoction.

Role in formula	Name/ Pinyin	Name/Latin	Dose (g)	Function
Chief herb	Chi Shao	Radix Paeoniae Rubrae	10	Activates the blood to remove blood stasis.
Deputy herb	Chuan Xiong	Radix Ligustici Wallichii	10	Promotes activation of the blood stasis.
Assistant herb	Dan Shen	Radix Codonopsis Pilosulae	10	Activates the blood stasis and dredges the Stagnated *Qi* in the blood.
	Hong Hua	Flos Carthami Tinctorii	10	Activates the blood stasis.
	Chai Hu	Radix Bupleuri	10	Dredges the stagnated liver *Qi*, relaxes anxiety, and eases the depression.
	Huang Qin	Radix Scutellariae Baicalensis	10	Clears the stagnated heat in the chest.
	Ban Xia	Rhizoma Pinelliae Ternatae	10	Disperses the phlegm and impels the lung *Qi*.
	Long Gu	Os Draconis	15	Calms the mind down to restrain panic attacks.
	Mu Li	Concha Ostreae	15	Calms the mind down to restrain panic attacks.
Guiding herb	Jiang Xiang	Lignum Dalbergiae Odoriferae	2–3	Dispels the blood stasis and dredges the stagnated *Qi*, leads herbs effectively towards the chest.

Method: The above-mentioned herbal prescription is the main formula where the herbs are mixed into a decoction, which can be variated according to specific individual symptoms, and then boiled or made into concentrated herbal powders to be consumed with warm water, taken twice daily.

Analysis: Chi Shao and Chuan Xiong activate *Blood* to remove *Blood Stasis*, and the main herbs Dan Shen and Hong Hua emphasise the effect. Jiang Xiang dispels *Blood Stasis* and dredges *Stagnated Qi.* Chai Hu unblocks *Qi* and *Blood Stasis.* Huang Qin releases excessive *Heat* accumulation in the chest. Ban Xia disperses the *Phlegm* and impedes *Lung Qi.* Long Gu and Mu Li calm the mind to still panic attacks.

Advice: This pattern can be seen in patients with post-COVID-19 syndrome with an extended history of suffering, a chronic condition, and a refractory case.

Case Study

Ms. P. Flower, 73, divorced, a retired teacher, was worried for many years about daily life, about her son, daughters, and grandchildren. Since she became infected with COVID-19, she was gradually getting worse. Having healed from COVID-19, the panic attacks became more frequent over the last 2 months, appearing more than 10 times a day. Worry and fear occurred and presented with sweating, palpitation, breathlessness, and insomnia, in addition to not being able to stay home alone. Recently, she became worried about her granddaughter suffering from and dying of cancer; however, the girl suffers from a common disease. The patient was given antidepressants which did not control her symptoms. Therefore, she was referred to a psychiatric consultant. She was diagnosed with anxiety and OCD (Obsessive compulsive disorder). She visited the clinic for acupuncture treatment. She had a light red tongue with white-greasy coating, and wiry-rolling pulse.

Diagnosis:

1. Anxiety/OCD (obsessive compulsive disorder).
2. Post-COVID-19 syndrome.

Differentiation syndromes of TCM:

1. Accumulated *Damp-Phlegm* in the chest.
2. *Qi Stagnation* of *Heart* and *Liver*.

Treatment: Herbal prescription and acupuncture.

Acupuncture

Main points: Baihui (DU20), Shenting (DU24), Touwei (ST8); Daling (P7), Quze (P3), Gongsun (SP4), Taichong (LIV3); Shanzhong (REN17), Zhongwan (REN15), Qihai (REN6), Guanyuan (REN4).

Herbal prescription

Pinyin: Wen Dan Tang plus Chai Hu Shu Gan San.

Result: She felt relaxed 10 min after the needles were inserted. She continued treatment twice a week, and regularly took herbal pills. The frequency of panic attacks gradually decreased daily and she was able to stay at home alone, but she wished to continue receiving acupuncture and herbal treatment.

Depression

Depression is another common mental health disorder involved in the post-COVID-19 stage. Clinically, this is the most common symptom, the diagnosis for which requires 6 months to establish with many patients who consider their condition of depression to be new not having reached the milestone to be diagnosed yet. However, there are numerous reports of relapse of previously diagnosed cases or existing cases getting worse due to the pandemic, and not limited to COVID-19 sufferers.

Depression as a symptom refers to a lasting episode of unhappiness with hopelessness, losing interest in the things one used to enjoy, and sometimes becoming very tearful. It is very commonly described as feeling blue or melancholic. If feeling blue is short term and obviously event related, it will eventually go away. The depression is not related to a particular event or life experience.

When depression becomes an illness or mental disorder, in a mild range, feelings of guilt, helplessness, weight loss or gain, fatigue, and poor concentration and sleeping difficulties are developed, and most patients will not actively seek help. In the middle range, the patients stay away from groups or social activities, becoming disconnected or dejected. In social situations, they speak less and are reluctant to initialise conversation. In the worst case (major depressive disorder, MDD), thoughts of suicide, hallucinations, and delusions could also take place.

Depression as a mental disorder has long been considered to be purely psychological. But in the last 50 years, researchers have tended to agree that the change in the central nervous system (CNS), particularly the brain cortex, is the pathology of it, although no visible destruction of any important part of brain is recorded. The changes in the brain mainly affect the frontal lobe and hippocampus in reduced response to stimuli due to the impaired neurons and the reduced production of neurotransmitters. The cause is prolonged and excessive stress which takes the route of the hypothalamic–pituitary–adrenal axis (HPA axis) to cause a neurotoxic response causing direct atrophy in neurons or an immune response of inflammatory reaction (Dafsari & Jessen, 2020). The damage is considered to be reversible if the stress is cleared in time.

Antidepressants have clearly proved the biomechanism of increased neurotransmitters in the brain to release the abnormal mood produced by depression. However, antidepressants do not work for all patients, and psychological therapies, mostly CBT, are strongly recommended.

Depression is called Yu Zheng (sorrow illness or blocked illness) in TCM and has had recorded treatment strategies for 2,000 years. It was broadly agreed to be an emotional imbalance and should be treated with comprehensive approaches, from acupuncture and herbal medicine to emotional interventions. Modern clinical studies focus on failure of the *Liver* to regulate the emotion, along with a *Weak Yang* being unable to lift the spirit in the *Heart*.

Diagnosis

According to NICE (2022), depression as a mental disorder is only considered when at least one of the two "core" symptoms has been present most days, most of the time, for at least 2 weeks:

- Disturbed sleep (decreased or increased compared to usual).
- Decreased or increased appetite and/or weight.
- Fatigue/loss of energy.
- Agitation or slowing of movements.
- Poor concentration or indecisiveness.

- Feelings of worthlessness or excessive or inappropriate guilt.
- Suicidal thoughts or acts.

The severity could vary significantly and MDD is a major contributor of suicide worldwide. So, mental health regulations restrict practice with patients of MDD. The criteria for diagnosing MDD could be found in DSM-5 (America Psychiatric Society, 2016). Complementary medicine practitioners are advised to seek clarification from relevant authorities in treating MDD. If suicide is imminent, it is important to treat the situation as a "red flag" and signpost to seek professional help.

Syndrome pattern and treatment of TCM

Accordingly, the *Liver* governs emotions, which is the foundational theory of TCM, so *Liver Qi Stagnation* should be the main reason and causation of low mood and negative thoughts. The *Liver* also governs *Qi* movement in the general body; therefore, *Liver Qi*, a wood meridian, has the potential capability to influence other organs; for example, Liver *Qi* stagnation as an excessive pathogenic factor can enlarge its stagnation to the stomach to cause an excessive pattern; it can also overact the spleen as an earth meridian to produce a deficiency pattern. *Spleen Qi Obstruction* can disturb fluid metabolism causing accumulation of dampness in *Phlegm* in the chest as a lump, known as "Plum nuclear gas" (梅核气). *Stagnated Liver Qi* can become *Heat* and flare up, exhibiting symptoms. Separate explanations and details of these patterns are listed as follows.

Liver Qi Stagnation with Stomach Qi accumulation

Clinical features and signs: Signs are low emotion, annoyance, silence, nervousness, weeping easily, loss of confidence; declined appetite, bloated abdomen, distension, constipation, difficult sleeping, light red tongue with thin white coating, and wiry pulse.

Treatment principle in TCM: Dredge *Stagnated Liver Qi*; regulate Stomach Qi and descend.

Acupuncture

Main points: Baihui (DU20), Shenting (DU24).

Assistant points: Touwei (ST8), Waiguan (SJ5), Zulinqi (GB41); Hegu (LI4), Taichong (LIV3).

When accompanied by headache, use Yintang (Ext); For constipation, add Yanglingquan (GB34), Sanyinjiao (SP6).

Analysis: Baihui and Shenting agitate and unblock the governing vessel and drive *Qi* and move it. Shenting assists Touwei as the emotion area in scalp acupuncture and stimulates the mood centre of the brain. Waiguan and Zulinqi assist Baihui and encourage general *Qi* movement. Hegu and Taichong are used to push Stagnated *Qi*, remove and clear excessive *Liver Heat* to promote better sleep.

Treatment: Herbal prescription.

Pinyin: Chai Hu Shu Gan Decoction.

English name for decoction: Bupleurum Decoction to Spread the Liver variation.

Role in formula	Name/ Pinyin	Name/Latin	Dose (g)	Function
Chief herb	Chai Hu	Radix Bupleuri	10	Dredges the stagnated liver and general *Qi*.
Deputy herb	Chen Pi	Pericarpium Citri Reticulatae	10	Dredges the stagnated *Qi* in the stomach and the middle burner.
Assistant herb	Xiangfu	Rhizoma Cyperi Rotundi	10	Promotes and dredges the stagnated liver *Qi*.
	Zhi Qiao	Fructus Citri Aurantii	10	Promotes and dredges stagnated stomach and general *Qi*, superior for removing abdominal *Qi*.
	Chuan Xiong	Radix Ligustici Wallichii	10	Activates blood stasis to release headache.
	Chi Shao	Radix Paeoniae Rubrae	10	Activates blood stasis and softens the liver to promote relaxation.
Guiding herb	Zhi Gan Cao	Radix Glycyrrhizae Uralensis	5	Harmonises the stomach and promotes cohesion of herbs.

Method: The above-mentioned herbal prescription is the main formula, although combinations of decoction can be variated according to specific individual symptoms, which is then boiled or made into concentrated herbal powders to be consumed with warm water, taken twice daily.

Analysis: Chai Hu is the main herb, assisted by Xiang Fu, to dredge stagnated *Liver Qi*, and Chen Pi, assisted by Zhi Qiao, regulate *Stagnated Stomach Qi*. Chuan Xiong removes *Stagnated Qi* and Stasis *Blood* to dredge *Liver Qi*, and Chi Shao harmonises *Liver Qi* and nourishes *Liver Yin*, while Zhi Gan Cao regulates all herbs and promotes cohesion in the formula. When *Liver Qi* moves, patients can relax their mind to ease depression.

Advice: This is a typical and a common pattern in patients with depression as part of the post-COVID-19 syndrome. It can also be seen in patient with mild, medium, or severe stage, acute or chronic type, appearing as an excess pattern, without deficiency in the constitution.

Liver Qi Stagnation with accumulated Phlegm in the chest

Clinical features and signs: Signs are low emotion, irritation, negative thought, weeping, restlessness, anguish, feeling obstruction in the throat or chest that one is unable to expel, difficulty swallowing, although ordinarily no difficulty in swallowing food, accompanied by belching, suspicious, oversensitive, light red tongue with white-greasy coating, and wiry or rolling pulse.

Treatment principle in TCM: Dredge *Stagnated Liver Qi*; dissipate *Phlegm* and resolve masses.

Acupuncture

Main points: Shenting (DU24), Shazhong (REN17), Qihai (REN6).

Assistant points: Taichong (LIV3), Chize (LU5), Yuji (LU10) Fenglon (ST40), Hegu (LI4). If accompanied by a sore throat, use Tianding (LI17), Shangyang (LI1). For insomnia, add Lidui (ST45).

Analysis: This pattern is produced by *Liver Qi Stagnation*, causing *Liver Fire* combined with accumulated *Phlegm*. Shenting dredges stagnated *Liver Qi* and agitates general *Qi* circulation. Shanzhong unblocks *Stagnated Qi* in the chest and dissipates *Excessive Phlegm.* Taichong and Hegu are the four gate points and clear accumulated *Liver Fire.* Kouzui and Yuji are Sea-He point and Stream-Ying point of the *Lung* meridian and dredge stagnated *Qi* and dissipate excessive *Phlegm.* Fenglong emphasises dissipation of *Phlegm.*

Treatment: Herbal prescription.

Pinyin: Wen Dan with Ban Xia Hou Po Decoction variation.

English name for decoction: Warm Gallbladder Decoction variated with Pinellia and Magnolia Bark Decoctions.

Role in formula	Name/ Pinyin	Name/Latin	Dose (g)	Function
Chief herb	Ban Xia	Rhizoma Pinelliae Ternatae	10–15	Dissipates phlegm and resolves masses in the throat.
Deputy herb	Hou Po	Cortex Magnoliae Officinalis	10	Dredges the stagnated *Qi* in the upper and middle burners.
Assistant herb	Zi Su	Ramulus Perillae Frutescentis	10	Promotes and dissipates the stagnated *Qi*.
	Chen Pi	Pericarpium Citri Reticulatae	10	Dissipates the stagnated phlegm, promoting relaxation.
	Fu Ling	Sclerotium Poriae Cocos	10	Releases the accumulated dampness and fluid.
	Gan Jiang	Rhizoma Zingiberis Officinalis	10	Agitates and warms the yang *Qi* to release the stagnation.
	Zhi Shi	Fructus Immaturus Citri Aurantii	10	Dredges the stagnated *Qi* in the middle burner and unblocks the obstructive abdominal *Qi*.
	Zhu Ru	Caulis Bambusae in Taeniis	10	Dissipates the accumulated *Qi* and phlegm in the chest.
Guiding herb	Zhi Gan Cao	Radix Glycyrrhizae Uralensis	5	Harmonises the stomach and promotes cohesiveness of herbs.

Method: The above-mentioned herbal prescription is the main formula, which can be combined into decoctions of different variations according to specific individual symptoms, and is then boiled or made into concentrated herbal powders to be consumed with warm water, taken twice daily.

Analysis: Hou Po and Zi Su unblock stagnated *Qi* in the chest. Ban Xia, Chen Pi, and Gan Jiang dissipate Phlegm and resolve masses in the throat. Zhi Shi and Zhu Ru emphasise and dredge *Stagnated Qi* and dispel excessive *Phlegm. Zhi Gan Cao* harmonises herbs and promotes unification.

Advice: This pattern can be seen in patients with depression, accompanied by feelings of obstruction in the chest. This is commonly seen in chronic cases accompanied by a lengthy period of depression after he/she has recovered from COVID-19.

Liver Qi Stagnation with Spleen Qi Deficiency

Clinical features and signs: Signs are prolonged depression, low mood with negative thoughts, lack of interest and confidence, tiredness, fatigue, lethargy, no appetite, hiccups, distension, indigestion, loose bowel, restlessness, nervousness, insomnia, headache, short temper, aching and distension in coastal areas, sudden loss of consciousness for a short period of time, light red tongue with teeth marks with less white coating, and wiry, wiry-fire, or wiry-rapid pulse.

Treatment principle in TCM: Dredge *Liver Qi, reinforce Spleen Qi*; dispel excessive *Liver Heat.*

Acupuncture

Main points: Yintang (Ext), Baihui (DU20).

Assistant points: Neiguan (P6), Gongsun (SP4); Jianshi (P5), Daling (P7); Xingjian (LIV2), Ququan (LIV8); If accompanied by loss of consciousness, add Renzhong (DU26), Zhongchong (P9); For trembling of limbs, add Taichong (LIV3), Yanglingquan (GB34). For hiccups, add Zhongwan (REN12), Zusanli (ST36).

Analysis: For individual depression, Yintang and Baihui excite Yang Qi and dredge *Stagnated Qi* as the main point. Neiguan and Gongsun as a pair of cross points tranquilise the spirit and stimulate the mind. Jianshi and daling encourage the *Heart Qi.* Xinjian and Ququan are the Stream-Ying point and Sea-He point of the *Liver* meridian and strongly stimulate *Liver Qi* to promote a happier and positive mood. These points promote immediate relaxation for patients. Patients have fallen asleep when needles are retained; some patients also cry, releasing negative feeling and relaxing immediately after it. Some patients feel exhausted after his/her *Qi Stagnation* had moved.

Treatment: Herbal prescription.

Pinyin: Xiao Yao San Decoction variation.

English name for decoction: Rambling Decoction variation.

Role in formula	Name/Pinyin	Name/Latin	Dose (g)	Function
Chief herb	Chai Hu	Radix Bupleuri	10	Dredges liver *Qi* and releases the stress and promotes *Qi* flow in the meridians.
Deputy herb	Dang Gui	Radix Angelicae Sinensis	10	Softens the liver and cultivates liver *Yin* and blood.
Assistant herb	Chi Shao	Radix Paeoniae Rubrae	10	Activates blood stasis and softens the liver to help *Qi* and blood circulation.
	Fu Ling	Sclerotium Poria Cocos	10	Replenishes the spleen and dries the accumulated damp.
	Bai Zhu	Rhizoma Atractylodis Macrocephalae	10	Replenishes the spleen and strengthens the muscles.
	Gan Jiang	Rhizoma Zingiberis Officinalis	10	Warms and agitates the spleen *Qi* and general *Qi*.
	Bo He	Herba Menthae Haplocalycis	5	Helps in ascension of herbs, releasing external wind.
	Mu Dan Pi	Cortex Moutan Radicis	10	Clears excessive heat in the middle burner and general heat in the blood.
	Zhi Zi	Fructus Gardeniae Jasminoidis	10	Clears the excessive heat in the liver and heart to promote relaxation.
	Gan Cao	Radix Glycyrrhizae Uralensis	5	Harmonises the stomach and promotes cohesiveness of herbs.

Method: The above-mentioned herbal prescription is the main formula, which can be combined into decoctions of different variations according to specific individual symptoms, and is then boiled or made into concentrated herbal powders to be consumed with warm water, taken twice daily.

Analysis: Chai Hu dredges stagnated *Liver Qi* to motivate the mind, while Dang Gui and Bai Shao nourish *Liver Yin* and blood to harmonise *Liver Qi.* Gan Jiang stimulates *Yang* and *Qi* in the middle burner *for* the *Liver* and *Spleen.* Bo He evacuates the stagnated liver *Qi* to clear the mind. Fu Ling and Bai Zhu nourish the *Spleen* and *Stomach Yin and Qi* to support *Liver Qi* movement. Zhi Gan Cao warms the *Stomach* and unifies the herbs. If there are signs of accumulated heat flaring up, Mu Dan Pi and Zhi Zi are added to dispel excessive *Liver Heat*, calming the mind, promoting peace and tranquillity.

Advice: This pattern can be commonly seen in younger people, like students, intellectuals, officers with stressful jobs, or those who have a preexisting psychological disorder or depression. It is worse after being infected by COVID-19; some people suffer from depression after COVID-19 as a post-COVID-19 syndrome. TCM should provide good support for all of them.

Confusion in Liver Blood and Heart Qi

Clinical features and signs: Signs are wandering mind, absent-mindedness, restlessness, feel ill at ease, suspicious, startling easily, sorrowful, worrying, crying, mood swings, yelling and swearing, unusual behaviours. All these symptoms can be frequent or intermittent as outbursts. Other signs are pale or light red tongue, with less coating, and wiry or wiry-fine pulse.

Treatment principle in TCM: Nourish the Heart and mind; to dredge the Stagnated Liver *Qi.*

Acupuncture

Main points: Yintang (Ext), Shenting (DU24), Baihui (DU20).

Assistant points: Neiguan (P6), Laogong (P8) Shenmen (HE7), Tongli (HE5); Yanglingquan (GB34), Jiaxi (GB43), Xingjian (LIV2), Zhongfeng (LIV4).

Analysis: Yintang, Shentang, and Baihui unblock *Stagnated Qi* and open the *Yang Qi* in the *Yang* meridians at the head to clear the mind. Neiguan and Laogong are the Collateral-Luo point and Stream-Ying point of the *Pericardium* meridian and stimulate *Heart Qi* as a *Yang* meridian. Shenmen and Tongli are Collateral-Luo point and Spring-Shu point of *Heart* meridian and nourish *Heart Yin* and *Blood* as a *Yin* meridian. Yanglingquan and Jiaxi are Sea-He point and Stream-Ying point of *Gallbladder* meridian and agitate stagnated *Liver Qi* as a *Yang* meridian. Xingjian and Zhongfeng are Stream-Ying point and River-Jing point of *Liver* meridian and nourish *Liver Yin* and *Blood.* All points work together to open the mind and inspire the spirit which can ease confusion.

Special acupuncture technologies

Scalp-acupuncture: Chorea-tremor control area; Dizziness and auditory area; Mania control area; Spirit-emotion area.

Auri-acupuncture: Heart, under sebum, Brain, Liver, Endocrine, Shenmen.

Treatment: Herbal prescription.

Pinyin: Gan Mai Da Zao Decoction variation.

English name for decoction: Liquorice, Wheat, and Jujube Decoction variation.

Role in formula	Name/ Pinyin	Name/Latin	Dose (g)	Function
Chief herb	Fu Xiao Mai	Semen Tritici Aestivi Levis	10–15	Nourishes the heart *Yin* and tranquilises the mind.
Deputy herb	Gan Cao	Radix Glycyrrhizae Uralensis	10	Harmonises the middle burner and promotes relaxation.
Assistant herb	Da Zao	Fructus Zizyphi Jujubae	10	Replenishes both heart and general *Qi*, and nourishes the brain.

If accompanied by bad confusion, add Zhen Zhu Mu, Guo Teng. For shaking, add Sheng Di Huang, Dang Gui. For insomnia, add Suan Zao Ren, Bai Zi Ren, and Fu Shen.

Method: The above-mentioned herbal prescription is the main formula and can be combined with decoctions of different variations according to specific individual symptoms, and is then boiled or made into concentrated herbal powders to be consumed with warm water, taken twice daily.

Analysis: Gan Cao harmonises, Xiao Mai reinforces *Qi*, and Da Zao nourishes *Blood*. These three simple herbs can inspire the mind and release confusion. Zhen Zhu Mu and Gou Teng can tranquilise the spirit and calm the mind, and are able to dispel *Excessive Wind*, to accentuate clarity and ease shaking of limbs. Sheng Di Huang and Dang Gui nourish *Liver Blood* and *Yin* to nourish *Liver Yin*. Suan Zao Ren and Fu Shen calm and clear the mind.

Advice: This pattern is seen as a severe attack of mental disorder and suffering over an extended period with depression or the sudden appearance of depression, as a result of existing or preexisting psychological disorders, which are triggered or aggravated by COVID-19. However, this pattern can also happen as part of the primary post-COVID-19 syndrome. For a severe case, the patient may be admitted to a psychological health hospital for intensive treatment. They can be treated by acupuncture or herbs before or after.

Case Study

Mrs. Linsey, 42 years old, a clerk by profession, has demonstrated depression, anxiety, restlessness, nervousness, and palpitation since her husband was suspected to have suffered from a mild state of COVID-19. She is burdened with constant worry, is always annoyed, and weeps that her husband may die of COVID-19 if the infection is too severe. She worries that she and her children are also infected. The daily anxiety has caused insomnia, tiredness, and loss of appetite. When she enquired about treatment for her husband's COVID-19 infection, her husband reported she is the one in most need of treatment.

Observation indicates a light red tongue with a thin white coating, highlighting that she may have pandemic dampness and can be considered to have suffered from COVID-19, in addition to a psychiatric disorder as the main health problem.

Diagnosis:

1. Psychological disorders occur during COVID-19.
2. Depression and anxiety attack.

Differentiation syndromes of TCM:

1. *Liver Qi Stagnation.*
2. *Dampness engaging* at *Spleen* and *Heart.*

Treatment: Herbal prescription.

Pinyin: Chai Hu Shu Gan Decoction variation.

Herbal powders (g):

Chai Hu	Radix Bupleuri 10 g
Jiang Nan Xia	Rhizoma Pinelliae Ternatae 15 g
Chen Pi	Pericarpium Citri Reticulatae 10 g
Fu Ling	Sclerotium Poriae Cocos 10 g
Xiang Fu	Rhizoma Cyperi Rotundi 10 g
Zhi Qiao	Fructus Citri Aurantii 10 g
Huang Qin	Radix Scutellariae Baicalensis 10 g
Chi Shao	Radix Paeoniae Rubrae 10 g
Shi Chang Pu	Rhizoma Acori Graminei 10 g
Yu Jin	Tuber Curcumae 10 g
Cang Zhu	Rhizoma Atractylodis 10 g
Yi Yi Ren	Semen Coicis Lachryma-Jobi 30 g
Chuna Lian Zi	Fructus Meliae Toosendan 10 g
Gan Cao	Radix Glycyrrhizae Uralensis 5 g

The above-mentioned herbs are decocted into herbal juice taken twice daily. After she has improved over the week, she is given patent herbal pills, Chai Hu Shu Gan Pills and Ren Shen Gui Pi pills, until her has recovered.

Insomnia

Sleep is a basic life necessity and could be disturbed in any unfavourable circumstances due to the environmental or thoughts inside one's mind. Sleep quality directly affects health and the development of illness because it is the most important time for the body to repair itself and tidy up the mind, from memory to cognitive capacity. During the COVID-19 pandemic, the normal living environment was a significantly changed for many, from visiting hospitals or being hospitalised to being limited in movement and house-bound, working from home, and being unable to meet friends and family members, including those who needed to care. These are changes in the external world. However, more could happen in the internal world, the mental world, due to the uncertainty, the fear, the confusion due to various information sources, and exhaustion/burnout due to highly demanding workloads. The former, caused by environmental changes or disturbance is called situational insomnia, while the latter is primary insomnia, which means no trigger can be identified. As life goes back to normal, situational insomnia will not be a concern, at least when related to COVID-19. The theme here focuses on primary insomnia.

Sleeping problems are part of the symptom portfolio of anxiety and depression. This has been discussion in the previous two sections in this chapter. However, it can be a prominent problem, not necessarily just one of the symptoms of anxiety and depression.

Sleep is controlled by genes in the combined mechanism of the bio-clock, requires the coordination and communication of different part of the brain (the sleep–wake mechanism), and could be interrupted by many factors. Stress is a major contributor to insomnia.

A human being's day and night cycle is known as Circadian Rhythm and is synchronised by the suprachiasmatic nucleus (SCN) inside the hypothalamus and receives input from the eyes which signal the level of sunlight. Certain genes regulate the production of some proteins that increase overnight and fade during the day. When the eyes sense daylight and send signals through the optic nerve, the SCN then releases those proteins and other chemicals, including cortisol and neurotransmitters of norepinephrine and serotonin. They work together to make and keep the brain alert and awake (NIH, 2021). During the daytime, a different chemical adenosine is constantly released by cells all over the body, accumulating in the bloodstream, which eventually makes every part feel tired. The strongest dip in rhythms of wakefulness happens in the afternoon, namely, the afternoon slump, which leads to a strong desire to have a short sleep. Inside the brain, as the daylight fades in the evening, the hormone melatonin is released helping prepare for sleep (Greene *et al.*, 2017).

In TCM, the sleep awareness circle is the circle mimicking the day and night caused by *Yin* and *Yang* shifting. In the daytime, the *Yang* is in power and warms the body, keeps the mind awake, and deals with all essential responses; at nighttime, the *Yin* steps in to calm down the whole body, rest the *Qi* and *Blood* for restoration, and allow many organs to repair their damage. This circle follows the movement of the Sun. In detail, the *Yang* in the *Heart* rises in the morning, and *Yang Qiao* (yang mobility) opens the eyes to receive messages. In the evening, the *Heart Yang* retreats to the inner part of the *Heart*, resting in *Heart Blood* (part of the *Yin*), and the eyes are closed by the *Yang Qiao* channel to stop disturbance. A peaceful night should be guarded by the liver spirit of *Hun* for any urgent needs, internally and externally. So, the body is not left unprotected.

From this understanding, the *Heart* and *Liver* are the two main organs for facilitating sleep and improving the quality of sleep. The whole mechanism also needs help from other parts of the body, for example, a smooth and quiet digestive system, *Spleen*, and *Stomach*, and a *Kidney* to absorb extra *Yang* accumulated in the daytime.

Because coordination is complicated, a treatment for insomnia in TCM is required.

Diagnosis

Individuals need different amounts of sleep. Some might need more than 8 h per night to feel ready for the next day, while some others might only need 6 h to feel good. It is also differs due to ages — the younger ones need more sleep; in other words, older people need less sleep.

According to DSM-5 (APS, 2016) a complex diagnosis criterion is used for diagnosing insomnia disorder.

Condition A: Must last for 3 months, more than 3 nights a week. The main complaint of poor sleep quantity or quality, with at least one or more of the following three conditions:

- Difficulty initiating sleep.
- Difficulty maintaining sleep, characterised by frequent awakenings or problems returning to sleep after awakenings.
- Early-morning awakening with inability to return to sleep.

Condition B: The insomnia causes distress in daily life and function.
Condition C: The person suffers from insomnia when provided with a good environment and chance to sleep.
Condition D: No other disease or medicine has been established as the cause.

The key point is how a person feels mentally and physically, and if the performance of the next day is maintained at a normal level. If the person feels fresh and ready for a full day of duty, then the sleep quality and amount is right; otherwise, the sleep is poor.

Differentiation syndromes of TCM and herbal treatment

Insomnia should be seen with these patterns.

Liver Qi Stagnation and Liver Fire flare-up

Clinical features and signs: Signs are difficulty falling asleep, headache and dizziness, irritation, easily angered, loss of temper, restlessness, crying, getting triggered by bad news or a stressful thing, aching at coastal areas and upper abdomen, and red tongue with less white or thin yellow coating.

Treatment principle in TCM: Dredge *Stagnated Liver Qi* and clear *Excessive Liver Heat.*

Acupuncture

Main points: Baihui (DU20), Fengchi (GB20).

Assistant points: Hegu (LI4), Taichong (LIV3), Shenmen (HE7), Zuqiaoyin (GB44). If accompanied by Tinnitus, use Yifeng (SJ17), Zhongzhe (SJ3).

Analysis: Baihui is the main point to calm the mind, which can urge the patient to fall asleep. Fengchi dispels stagnated *Liver Qi* and releases *Liver Heat*. Hegu and Taichong are the four gate points and eliminate excessive *Liver Heat* for tranquilising *Liver Qi* to help with sleep. Shenmen clears *Heart Heat*. Zuqiaoyin is the Well-Jing point of the *Gallbladder* meridian and encourages dispelling of *Liver Heat*. All these points can promote sleep by dredging *Liver Qi* and calming *Liver Heat* down.

Treatment: Herbal prescription.

Pinyin: Jia Wei Xiao Yao Decoction variation.

English name for decoction: Rambling Decoction variation.

Role in formula	Name/ Pinyin	Name/Latin	Dose (g)	Function
Chief herb	Chai Hu	Radix Bupleuri	10	Dredges the liver *Qi* and releases stress to promote *Qi* flow in the meridians.
Deputy herb	Dang Gui	Radix Angelicae Sinensis	10	Softens the liver and cultivates the liver *Yin* and blood.
Assistant herb	Chi Shao	Radix Paeoniae Rubrae	10	Activates the blood stasis and softens the liver to help the *Qi* and blood circulation.
	Fu Ling	Sclerotium Poria Cocos	10	Replenishes the spleen and dries the accumulated damp.
	Bai Zhu	Rhizoma Atractylodis Macrocephalae	10	Replenishes the spleen and strengthens the muscles.
	Gan Jiang	Rhizoma Zingiberis Officinalis	10	Warms and agitates the spleen *Qi* and general *Qi*.
	Bo He	Herba Menthae Haplocalycis	5	Leads to ascension of herbs to release the external wind.

(*Continued*)

Role in formula	Name/ Pinyin	Name/Latin	Dose (g)	Function
	Mu Dan Pi	Cortex Moutan Radicis	10	Clears the excessive heat in the middle burns and general heat in the blood.
	Zhi Zi	Fructus Gardeniae Jasminoidis	10	Clears the excessive heat in the liver and heart to create relaxation.
Guiding herb	Gan Cao	Radix Glycyrrhizae Uralensis	5	Harmonises the stomach promoting cohesiveness of all herbs.

Method: The above-mentioned herbal prescription is the main formula, which can be used in combination with decoctions of different variations according to specific individual symptoms, and is then boiled or made into concentrated herbal powders to be consumed with warm water, taken twice daily.

Analysis: Dang Gui and Bai Shao nourish *Liver Yin* and *Blood* to harmonise *Liver Qi* as the main herbs. Chai Hu dredges *Stagnated Liver Qi.* Gan Jiang stimulates *Yang* and *Qi* in the middle burner of the *Liver* and *Spleen*. Bo He evacuates the stagnated Liver *Qi*, unblocking and ascending to the mind and promoting relaxation. Fu Ling and Bai Zhu nourish the *Spleen* and *Stomach Yin* and *Qi* to support and calm *Liver Qi.* Zhi Gan Cao warms the *Stomach* and synthesises all of herbs effectively together. Mu Dan Pi and Zhi Zi dispel excessive *Liver Heat* to calm the mind and promote peace and tranquillity. All herbs can foster immediate relaxation and encourage sleep.

Advice: This is the commonest pattern seen in people experiencing sudden occurrence of insomnia, temporary insomnia, or gentle insomnia. It is also seen with depression or anxiety as a part of a psychiatric disorder, or a part of liver weakness or failure after COVID-19 infection.

Heart Blood and Spleen Qi Deficiency

Clinical features and signs: Signs are difficulty falling asleep, more dreams and easily waking up when asleep, palpitations, forgetfulness, easily sweating, pale face, poor spirit, distension of the upper abdomen, loose bowels, light white tongue with teeth marks and thin white coating, and fine-weak pulse.

Treatment principle in TCM: Reinforce *Spleen Qi*; nourish *Heart Blood*; tranquilise the spirit and calm the mind down.

Acupuncture

Main points: Zhongwan (REN12), Qihai (REN6).

Assistant points: Xinshu (DU15), Pishu (DU20), Shenmen (HE7), Shaohai (HE3). If accompanied by dreams, use Lingdao (HE4), Pohu (BL42). If accompanied by forgetfulness, us Zhishi (BL52), Baihui (DU20).

Analysis: Zhongwan is the front-mu point of the Stomach to reinforce Spleen *Qi* and calm the mind. Qihai strengthens the vitality gate and complements the original *Qi* to promote the main point. Xinshu and Pishu are back-points to reinforce the relevant *Qi* and Blood. Shenmen and Shaohai are the Spring-Shu point and Sea-He point of Heart-meridian and emphasise and promote the Heart to calm the mind and promote sleep.

Treatment: Herbal prescription.

Pinyin: Ren Shen Gui Pi Decoction variation.

English name for decoction: Restore the Spleen Decoction variation with Ginseng.

Role in formula	Name/ Pinyin	Name/Latin	Dose (g)	Function
Chief herb	Ren Shen	Radix Ginseng	10	Replenishes heart *Qi* to complement the heart blood.
	Huang Qi	Radix Astragali Membranacei	10–30	Replenishes the spleen and vitality *Qi*.
Deputy herb	Dang Gui	Radix Angelicae Sinensis	10	Nourishes the blood.
Assistant herb	Bai Zhu	Rhizoma Atractylodis Macrocephalae	10–30	Replenishes spleen and general *Qi*, dries the excessive damp.

(*Continued*)

Role in formula	Name/ Pinyin	Name/Latin	Dose (g)	Function
	Dang Shen	Radix Codonopsis Pilosulae	10	Promotes replenishing of the spleen and vitality *Qi*.
	Fu Shen	Sclerotium Poriae Cocos Paradicis	10	Calms the mind, releases the damp to reinforce the Spleen.
	Long Yan Rou	Arillus Euphoriae Longanae	10	Nourishes the *Yin* and blood to tranquilise the mind and promote good sleep.
	San Zao Ren	Semen Zizyphi Spinosae	10	Nourishes the liver *Yin* and blood to tranquilise the mind.
	Yuan Zhi	Radix Polygalae Tenuifoliae	10	Tranquilises the mind and nourishes the heart.
	Mu Xiang	Radix Aucklandiae Lappae	6–10	Pushes the *Qi* flow in the meridians and supports cohesiveness of tonic herbs.
Guiding herb	Gan Cao	Radix Glycyrrhizae Uralensis	5	Harmonises the stomach and promotes unification of herbs.

Method: The above-mentioned herbal prescription is the main formula used in combination with decoctions of different variation according to specific individual symptoms, and is then boiled or made into concentrated herbal powders to be consumed with warm water, taken twice daily.

Analysis: Ren Shen or Dang Shen is the main herb and reinforces the Heart and *Spleen Q*i. Huang Qi and Bai Zhu strengthen the *Heart* and *Spleen Qi* as well. Dang Gui and Bai Shao nourish the *Heart Blood*. Fu Shen and Yuan Zhi tranquilise *Heart Qi* and calm the mind. Suan Zao Ren tranquilises the *Heart* and *Liver Qi*. Mu Xiang dredges general *Qi Stagnation* and prevents increased herb use, generating further *Qi Stagnation*. Gan Cao stimulates *Heart Qi* and harmonises all herbs. The herbal mixture is a beneficial prescription to encourage good sleep.

Advice: This pattern can be seen in the chronic stage of COVID-19, with patients manifesting additional deficiency symptoms after struggling to heal from the infection. Insomnia can also be accompanied by heart, lung, liver or kidney weakness, or failure, and is commonly involved as part of the multiple organ inflammatory syndrome.

Disharmony in the Stomach

Clinical features and signs: Signs are shallow sleep, easily waking up, distension or soreness in the upper abdomen, indigestion, upset stomach, nausea, belching, reflux with sore discharge, burning in the stomach which disturbs sleep, dizziness, loose bowel or sluggish-loose bowel, red tongue with white or yellow coating, and rolling or wiry pulse.

Treatment principle in TCM: Regulate *Stomach Qi*; Calm the mind.

Acupuncture

Main points: Jiuwei (REN15), Zhongwan (REN12), Baihui (DU20).

Assistant points: Tianshu (ST25), Qihai (REN6), Yinlingquan (SP9), Taibai (SP3); Fenglong (ST40), Lidui (ST45), Yinbai (SP1). If accompanied by nausea, use Neiguan (P5). If accompanied by dizziness, use Yintang (Ext) and Hegu (LI4).

Analysis: "Unsettled stomach can result in disturbed sleep" is a famous proverb of TCM, so Jiuwei (REN15) and Zhongwan (REN12) regulate *Stomach* as the main points, while Baihui (DU20) calms the mind to promote sleep. Tianshu (ST25) dredges *Stagnated Qi* in the middle burner and supports in harmonising the *Stomach.* Qihai (REN6) promotes the *Vitality Qi.* Yinlingquan (SP9) and Taibai (SP3) are the He-sea point and the Spring-Shu point of the *Spleen* meridian and reinforce sleep to promote *Stomach* healing. Lidui is the Well-Jing point of the *Stomach* and Yinbai is the Well-Jing point of the *Spleen*, which will influence which will provide the stronger treatment level to regulate the *Stomach* and *Spleen.* All these points can foster better sleep by harmonising the *Stomach* and spleen to settle sleep.

Treatment: Herbal prescription.

Pinyin: Ban Xia Xie Xin Decoction.

English name for decoction: Pinelliae Decoction to Drain the Epigastrium variation.

Role in formula	Name/ Pinyin	Name/Latin	Dose (g)	Function
Chief herb	Jiang Ban Xia	Rhizoma Pinelliae Ternatae	15–20	Regulates the stomach and calms the mind.
Deputy herb	Huang Qin	Radix Scutellariae Baicalensis	10	Clears the excessive heat in the chest and both upper and middle burners.
Assistant herb	Huang Lian	Rhizoma Coptidis	10	Promotes clearing of excessive heat in the stomach.
	Ren Shen	Radix Ginseng	10	Harmonises and replenishes the vitality *Qi* in the middle burner and in general.
	Gan Jiang	Rhizoma Zingiberis Officinalis	10	Excites and warms the stomach *Qi* to calm the mind.
	Da Zao	Fructus Zizyphi Jujubae	10	Nourishes the stomach *Yin* and warms the stomach *Qi* to harmonise the stomach.
Guiding herb	Zhi Gan Cao	Radix Glycyrrhizae Uralensis	5	Harmonises the stomach promotes cohesiveness of herbs.

Method: The above-mentioned herbal prescription is the main formula used in combination with decoctions of different variations according to specific individual symptoms, and is then boiled or made into concentrated herbal powders to be consumed with warm water, taken twice daily.

Analysis: Jiang Ban Xia is given in a dose of 15–20 g and can regulate the *Stomach* and calm the mind as the main herb. Huang Qin, plus Huang Lian, clears excessive *Heat* from both the *Stomach* and middle burner. Gan Jian is warm in nature and regulates the *Stomach* and harmonises the cold herbs used. Ren Shen strengthens the *Spleen* and general *Qi*, along with Da Zao and Zhi Gan Cao. All the herbs combined promote better sleep by stabilising the *Stomach.*

Advice: This pattern can be seen when insomnia is the causation of stomach or gastrointestinal disorder after COVID-19 infection. Preexisting IBS, Colitis, or other Gastro-intestinal inflammatory disease can be triggered to reoccur during the infection phase of COVID-19, which includes the above-mentioned complication. The sequelae are part of post-COVID-19 syndrome, and are common reasons for insomnia. Therefore, insomnia in this presentation type can be seen in every stage of COVID-19.

Heart and Kidney Yin Deficiency

Clinical features and signs: Signs are difficulty falling asleep and being easily woken up, disturbed sleep early in the morning, warm palms and hot complexion, palpitations, getting easily startled, sweating, dry mouth, dizziness and tinnitus, forgetfulness, nocturnal emission, sore back, red tongue without coating, and fine-rapid pulse.

Treatment principle in TCM: Nourish *Kidney Yin* and clear *Heart Heat*; encourage *Heart* and *Kidney* connection.

Acupuncture

Main points: Baihui (DU20), Sishencong (Ext).

Assistant points: Daling (P7), Shenmen (HE7), Taixi (KI3), Yingu (KI10). If accompanied by dizziness, add Fengchi. If accompanied by tinnitus, add Tinggong. If accompanied by nocturnal emission, add Zhishi.

Analysis: Baihui and Sishencong calm the mind to promote sleep. Daling and Shenman are the Spring-Shu points of the *Pericardium* and *Heart* meridian and nourish *Heart Yin* and clear *Excessive Heat.* Taixi and Yingu are Spring-Shu point and Sea-He point of the *Kidney* meridian and nourish *Kidney Yin.* If *Heart Heat* is eliminated and *Kidney Yin* is building up, the connection of *Heart and Kidney* is preformed, and Yang can easily immerse into *Yin,* so sleep can be accomplished.

Treatment: Herbal prescription.

Pinyin: Huang Lian E Jiao Decoction.

English name for decoction: Coptis and Ass-Hide Gelatin Decoction variation.

Role in formula	Name/ Pinyin	Name/Latin	Dose (g)	Function
Chief herb	Huang Lian	Rhizoma Coptidis	10	Clears excessive heart heat.
Deputy herb	E Jiao	Gelatinum Corii Asini	10	Moistens the kidney *Yin* to hold the heart yang.
Assistant herb	Huang Qin	Radix Scutellariae Baicalensis	10	Promotes and dispels excessive heart heat.
	Bai Shao	Radix Paeoniae Lactiflorae	10	Nourishes the heart, the kidney, and general *Yin.*
Guiding herb	Ji Zi Huang	Egg yolk	10	Nourishes the kidney *Yin* and emboldens herbs to influence the kidney.

Method: The above-mentioned herbal prescription is the main formula used in combination with decoctions of different variations according to specific individual symptoms, and is then boiled or made into concentrated herbal powders to be consumed with warm water, taken twice daily.

Analysis: Huang Lian is the main herb clearing Excessive *Heart Heat.* E Jiao moistens *Kidney Yin.* Huang Qin supports Huang Lian and eliminates excessive *Heat* in the upper burners. Bai Shao nourishes the *Kidney, Heart*, and all the *Yin* and *Blood.* Egg yolk nourishes *Yin* and *Essence;* this combination can affect and clear *Heat*, while moistening *Yin-Blood* to promote good sleep.

Advice: This pattern can be seen in chronic conditions after COVID-19 infection, and is commonly seen in the senior population, such as ladies in the premenopause or post-menopause phase. Some younger people also suffer during extended times of stress giving rise to *Yin Deficiency.*

Case Study

Mrs. S. Lindlen, 73 years old, a retiree, has been suffering from insomnia for more than 10 years. She seldom has enough sleep, including the night before she was infected with COVID-19. Although she has minor coronavirus, lasting only a week, she presents with a cough and sore throat. However, it intensified her sleep disturbance. She now finds it harder to fall asleep, suffering the whole night, with broken sleep. Although her PCR recovered quickly, she feels tired, fatigued, depressed, and lethargic without exerting herself. This is accompanied by confusion in the mind and poor spirit.

Clinical features and signs: Signs are difficulty sleeping and daily broken sleep for a period of 10 years (preexisting disorder), which was worse post-COVID-19. She had a light red tongue with less white coating and wiry-fine pulse.

Diagnosis:

1. Post-COVID-19 syndrome.
2. Refractory insomnia.

Differentiation syndromes of TCM:

1. *Liver Qi Stagnation* with excessive *Heat.*
2. *Heart* and *Kidney Yin* Deficiency with *Empty Heat* flare-up.

Treatment principle in TCM: Eliminate excessive and *Empty Heat* from *Liver* and *Heart*; Nourish *Kidney*, *Heart*, and *Liver Yin* to promote sleep.

Treatment: Herbal prescription and acupuncture.

Acupuncture

Main points: Baihui (DU20), Ershencong (Ext); Hegu (LI4), Taichong (LIV3), Shenmen (HE7), Taixi (KI3), Yingu (KI10), Zhaohai (KI6).

Herbal prescription

Pinyin: Huang Lian E Jiao variated with Sini San.

English name for decoction: Coptis and Ass-Hide Gelatin Decoction variated with Frigid Extremities Powder.

Herbal powders (g):

Huang Lian	Rhizoma Coptidis 10 g
Huang Qin	Radix Scutellariae Baicalensis 10 g
Bai Shao	Radix Paeoniae Lactiflorae 30 g
E Jiao	Gelatinum Corii Asini 10 g
Chai Hu	Radix Bupleuri 10 g
Dang Gui	Radix Angelicae Sinensis 10 g
Chi Shao	Radix Paeoniae Rubrae 10 g
Zhi Qiao F	Ructus Citri Aurantii 10 g

Result: This patient travelled a long distance for treatment and visited 2 weeks later, when she remarked that she feels like a changed person, very relaxed and peaceful, although she still wakes up 2–3 times a night, but feels she has been sleeping better. Having taken herbal powders for 2–3 months, she has had very good sleep.

References

America Psychiatric Society. (2016). Diagnostic and Statistical Manual of Mental Disorders (DSM-5). Available at: https://dsm.psychiatryonline.org/pb-assets/dsm/update/DSM5Update2016.pdf#page=12 (Accessed 2 March 2022).

Dafsari, F. S. and Jessen, F. (2020). Depression — An underrecognized target for prevention of dementia in Alzheimer's disease. *Translational Psychiatry*, 10, 160. https://doi.org/10.1038/s41398-020-0839-1.

Greene, R. W., Bjorness, T. E., and Suzuki, A. (2017). The adenosine-mediated, neuronal-glial, homeostatic sleep response. *Current Opinion in Neurobiology*, 44, 236–242. doi:10.1016/j.conb.2017.05.015.

Hu, G.-T. and Wang, Y. (2021). Advances in treatment of post-traumatic stress disorder with Chinese medicine. *Chinese Journal of Integrative Medicine*, 27, 874–880. https://doi.org/10.1007/s11655-021-2864-1.

Michelen, M., Manoharan, L., Elkheir, N., Cheng, V., Dagens, D., Hastie, C., *et al.* (2020). Characterising long-term covid-19: A rapid living systematic review. *medRxiv* [Preprint]. https://doi.org/10.1101/2020.12.08.20246025.

NICE. (2022). Depression-Diagnosis. National Institute for Health and Care Excellence. Available at: https://cks.nice.org.uk/topics/depression/diagnosis/diagnosis/. (Accessed 2 March 2022).

NIH. (2021). Circadian rhythms. National Institute of General Medical Sciences (NIH). Available at: https://www.nigms.nih.gov/education/fact-sheets/Pages/circadian-rhythms.aspx (Accessed 2 March 2022).

Pereira-Sanchez, V., Adiukwu, F., El Hayek, S., *et al.* (2020). COVID-19 effect on mental health: Patients and workforce. *Lancet Psychiatry*, 7, e29–e30. doi:10.1016/S2215-0366(20)30153-X.

Taquet, M., Geddes, J. R., Husain, M., Luciano, S., and Harrison, P. J. (2021). 6-month neurological and psychiatric outcomes in 236 379 survivors of COVID-19: A retrospective cohort study using electronic health records. *Lancet Psychiatry*. https://doi.org/10.1016/S2215-0366(21)00084-5.

Vadivel, R., Shoib, S., El Halabi, S., El Hayek, S., Essam, L., *et al.* (2021). Mental health in the post-COVID-19 era: Challenges and the way forward. *General Psychiatry*, 34(1), e100424. https://doi.org/10.1136/gpsych-2020-100424.

Whitaker, M., Elliott, J., Chadeau-Hyam, M., Riley, S., Darzi, A., Cooke, G., *et al.* (2021). Persistent symptoms following SARS-CoV-2 infection in a random community sample of 508,707 people. Available at: http://hdl.handle.net/10044/1/89844.

Yang, X.-Y., Yang, N.-B., Huang, F.-F., *et al.* (2021). Effectiveness of acupuncture on anxiety disorder: A systematic review and meta-analysis of randomised controlled trials. *Annals of General Psychiatry*, 20, 9. https://doi.org/10.1186/s12991-021-00327-5.

Chapter 10

Gastrointestinal Disorders

The symptoms of gastrointestinal conditions are part of the digestive disorders. The liver has been excluded from this chapter as it has been discussed in an earlier chapter. Similar to some strands of the influenza virus, the SARS-II virus shows its impairments to the digestive system in COVID-19 as the part of the multi-system damage. The impairment will more or less remain at the post-COVID-19 stage in the form of persistent indigestion, change of bowel movement, diarrhoea, or constipation.

An early systematic review and meta-analysis by Sultan *et al.* (2020) suggested that the prevalence of GI symptoms was broadly presented, with diarrhoea at 7.7%, nausea/vomiting at 7.8%, and abdominal pain at 2.7% among a pooled sample size of 10,890 patients. This report is based on current COVID-19 patients, in other words, acute patients. A related survey by Oshima *et al.* (2021) found functional indigestion at 8.5% and IBS at 16.6% with an overlap of 4% among them in general hospital visitors. Stress during the pandemic was a major contribution to such trends.

According to Yan *et al.* (2021), the digestive tract is rich in the ACE-2 receptor which is the gateway for the SARS-CoV-2 virus to get into cells. The ACE-2 allows the virus to invade the digestive system easily and causing inflammation and related damage. Additionally, this damage could lead to chronic stage.

Some conditions need to be identified from acute kidney injury if nausea is progressive, and some others may be caused by psychological disorders that can significantly disturb the dynamics of the digestive system.

According to the long clinical experience of the authors, digestive tract impairment could also be common to all chronic illness sufferers due to the prolonged use of medicine/drugs, the change in eating habits, and lack of physical exercise. The side effects of many drugs could lead to nausea, diarrhoea, and constipation. The lack of physical exercise and changing to refined foods are two major contributing factors of constipation. A practitioner needs to pay attention to these factors as well.

Irritable Bowel Syndrome (IBS): Constipation and Diarrhoea

Irritable bowel syndrome (IBS) is a clinical condition featuring by a group of symptoms that occur together, including abdominal pain and changes in bowel movements, which may include diarrhoea, constipation, or both. Clinical symptoms could be worse at times and disappear sometimes. The onset of the symptoms is closely related to emotional status, with stress or anxiety being the common triggers of the problem. However, there is no established structural damage in the whole digestive system in the cases of IBS. The condition is therefore to be considered both functional and psychological.

IBS could be further divided into three types: diarrhoea type, constipation type, and mixed type (some days of diarrhoea and constipation on different days).

Diagnosis

Key symptoms:

Symptoms are abdominal pain, abdominal bloating, urgent need to empty the bowels, diarrhoea, or constipation, or alternatively diarrhoea with constipation. Abdominal pain is relieved after a bowel movement.

The Rome IV criteria are the worldwide accepted requirements for the diagnosis of IBS (Lacy & Patel, 2017). The criteria require the following:

Recurrent abdominal pain on average at least 1 day/week in the last 3 months, associated with two or more of the following criteria:

A. Related to defecation.
B. Associated with a change in the frequency of stool.
C. Associated with a change in the form (appearance) of stool.

The above clinical manifestations last 3 months with symptom onset of at least 6 months.

The following medical investigations should be provided to confirm whether any serious damage exists:

- Barium meal X-ray, colorectal transit study, CT or CAT scan, MRI;
- Defecography, lower gastrointestinal series;
- Magnetic resonance cholangiopancreatography (MRCP);
- Oropharyngeal motility (swallowing) study;
- Endoscopic examination.

Syndrome pattern and treatment of TCM

TCM pays attention to irritable bowel syndrome with diarrhoea as the main associated symptom.

We should identify the following:

- Whether the diarrhoea occurred urgently or gradually.
- Whether the diarrhoea belonged to the heat or cold pattern.
- Whether diarrhoea manifested as an excess or deficiency pattern.
- Whether it appeared for a shorter or chronic period.

Common patterns of TCM as IBS of post-COVID-19 syndrome are indicated in the following.

Diarrhoea due to Spleen Deficiency

Clinical features: Features are loose bowels or diarrhoea, interchangeably, which can last for a longer time or be of recurrent appearance, indigestion, distension, feeling worse after eating, increasingly worse after a big or greasy meal, yellow-pale complexion, fatigue, lethargy, a pale tongue with thin white coating, and a weak-fine pulse.

Treatment principle in TCM: Reinforce *Spleen* and build the *Qi* up.

Treatment: Herbal prescription.

Pinyin: Shen Ling Bai Zhu Tang variation.

English name for decoction: Ginseng, Poria, and Atractylodis Macrocephalae Powder variation.

Role in formula	Name/ Pinyin	Name/Latin	Dose (g)	Function
Chief herb	Ren Shen	Radix Ginseng	10	Reinforces the spleen and general qi.
Deputy herb	Bai Zhu	Rhizoma Atractylodis Macrocephalae	10–30	Supports reinforcement of the spleen and general qi and dries the excessive damp.
Assistant herb	Chen Pi	Pericarpium Citri Reticulatae	10	Supports reinforcement of the spleen qi and dredges the stagnated qi in the middle burner.
	Shan Yao	Radix Dioscoreae Oppositae	10	Promotes reinforcement of the spleen qi and dries the damp.
	Fu Ling	Sclerotium Poria Cocos	10	Releases the accumulated dampness.
	Sha Ren	Fructus Amomi	10	Dredges the stagnated stomach and harmonises general qi.
	Yi Yi Ren	Semen Coicis Lachryma-Jobi	10–30	Eliminates the accumulated dampness and promote diuresis.
	Jie Geng	Radix Platycodi Grandiflori	10	Ventilates the stagnated qi in the upper and the middle burners.
	Bai Bian Dou	Semen Dolichoris Lablab	10	Nourishes the spleen yin to ease diarrhoea.
	Lian Zi Rou	Semen Nelumbinis Nuciferae	10	Nourishes the spleen and heart yin to tranquilise the mind.
Guiding herb	Gan Cao	Radix Glycyrrhizae Uralensis	5	Harmonises the stomach and promotes cohesiveness of herbs.

Method: The above-mentioned herbal prescription is the main formula and can be used in combination with a variation of decoctions according to specific individual symptoms where the herbs are boiled and the concentrated herbal powders are taken with warm water twice daily.

Analysis: Ren Shen, Bai Zhu, Fu Ling, and Gan Cao form Si Jun Zi Tang, a famous formula that reinforces *Spleen Qi* and promotes general *Vitality Qi.* Sha Ren and Chen Pi harmonise the *Stomach* and support *Spleen Qi.* Bai Bian Dou and Shan Yao dry *dampness* and promote *Spleen Qi.* Jie Geng dredges the *Stagnated Qi* in the chest. Lian Zi Rou nourishes *Heart Qi* to tranquilise the mind. Yi Yi Ren reinforces *Spleen Qi* and dissipates excessive *dampness* caused by *Spleen Deficiency.*

Advice: This pattern is commonly seen as part of the post-COVID-19 syndrome, one which causes extended suffering as a chronic condition. This pattern can be combined together with the above pattern. If the *Spleen Qi* and general *Vitality Qi* are not sufficient, the patients will easily progress to a chronic state, disturbing their quality of life.

Diarrhoea due to Kidney Deficiency

Clinical features: Features are cramps and urgent diarrhoea early in the morning before dawn, diarrhoea after gurgling, a peaceful feeling after diarrhoea, incomplete control of bowel movements, cold feeling in the body and limbs, weakness and soreness in the back and knees, a pale tongue with white coating, and a deep-fine pulse.

Treatment principle in TCM: Warm and strengthen *Kidney Qi* and *Yang*; relieve diarrhoea with astringent.

Treatment: Herbal prescription.

Pinyin: Si Shen Tang variation.

English name for decoction: Four Miracle Decoction variation.

Role in formula	Name/ Pinyin	Name/Latin	Dose (g)	Function
Chief herb	Bu Gu Zhi	Fructus Psoraleae Corylifoliae	10	Warms and strengthens the yang in the vitality gate to replenish the kidney qi-yang and ease the diarrhoea.
Deputy herb	Wu Zhu Yu	Fructus Evodiae Rutaecarpae	10	Warms and strengthens the middle yang and disburses the internal cold.
Assistant herb	Rou Dou Kou	Semen Myristicae Fragrantis	5–10	Warms and strengthens the spleen and the kidney, constrains the intestines to restrain the diarrhoea.
	Wu Wei Zi	Fructus Schisandrae Chinensis	10	Constrains the intestine and restrains the diarrhoea.
	Gan Jiang	Rhizoma Zingiberis Officinalis	10	Warms and excites vitality qi in the middle and lower burners.
Guiding herb	Rou Gui	Cortex Cinnamomi Cassiae	2–5	Warms the kidney yang and vitality yang.

Method: The above-mentioned herbal prescription is the main formula and can be used in combination with a variation of decoctions according to specific individual symptoms where the herbs are boiled or concentrated herbal powders are taken with warm water twice daily.

Analysis: Bu Gu Zhi warms and strengthens the *Kidney* as the main herb. Wu Zhu Yu warms the middle and lower burners to release excessive retained *Cold*. Rou Dou Kou and Wu Wei Zi constrict the middle *Qi* to support to against diarrhoea. Gan Jiang and Rou Gui warm and excite *Yang Qi* in the *Spleen* and *Kidney*. All herbs in this formula are efficient in any combination to prevent diarrhoea caused by the *Kidney* or both a *Kidney and Spleen Deficiency*.

Advice: This pattern is seen as chronic diarrhoea, accompanying an extended disease history. It always presents as severe diarrhoea during the infection phase of COVID-19 or after. If this diarrhoea cannot be controlled, it can stimulate an inflammatory syndrome in multiple organs and disturb the quality of life of the patients.

Irregular bowel movement due to Liver Qi Stagnation

Clinical features and signs: Signs are distension and soreness at coastal areas, diarrhoea and cramps, belching, eructation, poor appetite, frequent gurgling or wind moving in the abdomen (borborygmus), a light red tongue with less coating, and a wiry pulse. These symptoms are always triggered or aggravated by unstable emotions, restlessness, or nervousness.

Treatment principle in TCM: Regulate *Liver Qi* and reinforce *Spleen.*

Treatment: Herbal prescription and acupuncture.

Pinyin: Tong Xie Yao Fang variation.

English name for decoction: Important Formula for Painful Diarrhoea.

Role in formula	Name/ Pinyin	Name/Latin	Dose (g)	Function
Chief herb	Bai Zhu	Rhizoma Atractylodis Macrocephalae	10–30	Reinforces the spleen and dries the excessive damp.
	Bai Shao	Radix Paeoniae Lactiflorae	10–30	Releases abdominal spasms to ease the pain.
Deputy herb	Chen Pi	Pericarpium Citri Reticulatae	10	Promotes reinforcement of the spleen and excites the stagnated qi.
Assistant herb	Fang Feng	Radix Ledebouriellae Divaricatae	10	Ventilates the internal wind to push the qi to promote blood flow.
	Chai Hu	Radix Bupleuri	10	Dredges the stagnated qi in the middle burner and general body to ease pain.
	Zhi Qiao	Fructus Citri Aurantii	10	Dredges the stagnated qi in the spleen and intestines.
	Xiang Fu	Rhizoma Cyperi Rotundi	10	Dredges the stagnated qi in the middle and lower burners.
	Wu Mei	Fructus Pruni Mume	10	Confines the spleen qi and abdominal qi to ease the diarrhoea.
Guiding herb	He Zi	Fructus Terminaliae Chebulae	5–10	Excites the middle qi and the general qi to stabilise the middle and lower burners.

Method: The above-mentioned herbal prescription is the main formula and can be used in combination with a variation of decoctions according to specific individual symptoms where the herbs are boiled or concentrated herbal powders are taken with warm water twice daily.

Analysis: Bai Shao nourishes *Liver Blood a*nd *Yin* to calm stagnated *Liver Qi* and is the main herb. Bai Zhu reinforces *Spleen Qi* to ease diarrhoea. Chen Pi dredges stagnated *Qi* and excites *Spleen Qi*. Fang Feng increases *Yang Qi* to ease diarrhoea. Chai Hu, Zhi Qiao, and Xiang Fu give emphasis to the dredging of the stagnated *Liver Qi* and general abdominal *Qi*. He Zi confines the intestinal *Qi* to stop diarrhoea. All herbs combined are affective to calm Liver *Qi* and reinforce *Spleen Qi*. This is, therefore, a good formula to ease diarrhoea.

Advice: This pattern can be seen with diarrhoea being easily triggered by stress and unstable emotions as part of post-COVID-19 syndrome. It is commonly seen in people with a combination of both excess and deficiency patterns.

Acupuncture and moxibustion treatment

Moxibustion: Shenque (REN8).

Main points: Jiuwei (REN15), Zhongwan (REN12), Qihai (REN6), Guanyuan (REN4); Tianshu (ST25).

Assistant points: For acute diarrhoea: Shangjuxu (ST37), Xiajuxu (ST39), Yinlingquan (SP9) with increasing warm technology (Shaoshanhuo), Hegu (LI4).

If accompanied by:

- Chronic diarrhoea: Zusanli (ST36), Sanyinjiao (SP6).
- Spleen deficiency: Pishu (BL20), Guanyuanshu (BL26), Gongsun (SP4), Taibai (SP3), Neiting (ST44).
- Liver *Qi* stagnation: Ganshu (BL18), Waiguan (SJ5), Zulinqi (GB41); or Hegu (LI4), Taichong (LIV3).
- Kidney deficiency: Sheshu (BL23), Mingmen (DU4), Taixi (KI3), Zhaohai (KI6), Yingu (KI10).

Analysis: Shenque is warmed by Moxi for excessive *Cold-Damp*, and *Qi* stagnation, but it should be avoided if there is excessive heat accumulated. Jiuwei, Zhongwan and Qihai should be manipulated using special needles technology with the reinforcing *Qi* method, leading the general *Qi* to the Vitality Gate. This is a stronger *Qi* managing treatment to excite the spleen *Qi* and general vitality *Qi*, therefore it can ease diarrhoea which is caused by all patterns in the acute phase. The points on the back, like Pishu, Ganshu, and Shenshu, can build the relevant organic *Qi* up; plus, their *Stream-Ying* point, *Spring-Shu* point, or *Sea-He* point separately should promote and build up the *Qi* in relevant weaker meridians, meaning this acupuncture formula can stop all patterns in a chronic pattern.

Case Study

Ms. Li, a 42-year-old housewife in London, required the support of a TCM consultant for her fever, cough, and breathlessness. The following day, her husband was admitted to an ICU hospital for COVID-19. She had a temperature of 38.3°C, breathlessness, cough, tenderness of chest, nausea, upset stomach, anorexia, nervousness, restlessness, insomnia, and a pale tongue with teeth marks and white greasy coating. After the pandemic, dampness was identified in a cold and damp pattern, and she was giving Huo Xiang Zheng Qi decoction, modified with Wen Dan decoction for treatment. She had a slight loose bowel movement initially, which gradually improved after 2 weeks, and she had a clear and less greasy coating since then. She also had an immune function examination, which demonstrated that she was immunised against COVID-19 with higher IgE. She manifested discomfort in the stomach, which was upset easily, nausea, reflex, and also grief, sorrow, severe anxiety, nervousness, and restless after her husband died in the hospital. She also had a pale tongue with teeth marks and less thin coating.

Diagnosis:

1. Post-COVID-19 syndrome.
2. IBS.

Differentiation syndromes of TCM:

1. Spleen Deficiency and *Liver Qi Stagnation.*
2. Disharmony of the *Stomach.*

Treatment principle in TCM: Strengthening *Spleen* and harmonising the middle burner; dredging *Liver* and promoting *Qi* to mobilise.

Treatment: Herbal prescription and acupuncture.

Pinyin: Bu Zhong Yi Qi Decoction modified with Xiao Yao Wan.

English name for Decoction: Tonify the Middle and Augment the *Qi* Decoction varied with Rambling Powder.

Herbal powders (g):

Huang Qi	Radix Astragali Membranacei 15 g
Dang Shen	Radix Codonopsis Pilosulae 10 g
Bai Zhu	Rhizoma Atractylodis Macrocephalae 10 g
Chen Pi	Pericarpium Citri Reticulatae 10 g
Fu Ling	Sclerotium Poriae Cocos 10 g
Sheng Ma	Rhizoma Cimicifugae 6 g
Chai Hu	Radix Bupleuri 10 g
Xiang Fu	Rhizoma Cyperi Rotundi 10 g
Sha Ren	Fructus Amomi 10 g
Gan Jiang	Rhizoma Zingiberis Officinalis 10 g
Dang Gui	Radix Angelicae Sinensis 10 g
Yuan Hu	Rhizoma Corydalis 10 g
Zhi Gan Cao	Radix Glycyrrhizae Uralensis 5 g

The above herbs are decocted into herbal juice, and taken twice daily.

Result and analysis: This patient had irritable bowel syndrome in the past as a pre-existing disease, so she had *Spleen Deficiency* as part of her basic body constitution. She quickly manifested some symptoms and signs such as a *Cold-Damp* pattern after she was infected with coronavirus. When a relevant herbal prescription was given, her symptoms were controlled in 2 weeks. But she was living with many symptoms and it was hard for her to recover as COVID-19 infected her husband, causing his death. She healed after receiving treatment to strengthen *Qi* and harmonise the *Stomach.*

Constipation

Constipation means difficulty into passing stools, less frequency in passing stools, or in complete passing of stools. It is a common condition affecting a large proportion of the population. However, some suffer chronic functional constipation.

Constipation is not typically a newly added symptom of PCS, but it tends to affect the quality of life (QoL) if present. Newly presenting constipation after COVID-19 might be from prolonged intestine damage due to viral infection, or due to the restricted level of physical movement, dehydration, change of diet, lack of fibre intake, and the side effect of some medicine. It is also important to know that the gut bacteria balance could be altered which could lead to diarrhoea and constipation. Stress and depression are two known factors causing reduced regular physical activities resulting in constipation.

Constipation should be managed not only with acupuncture and herbal medicine but also with a correction to the lifestyle, including an increase of physical activity, regular toilet habits to stimulate the intestinal control mechanism of the bio-clock, increased fibre-rich diet, fixed eating time, and regular habits. In the case of physical restriction due to some other illness, such as being bedridden, a coordinated physical exercise plan should be adjusted to suit the person.

Diagnosis

Clinical features: Features are passing fewer than three stools a week, having lumpy or hard stools, and straining to have a bowel movement. The diagnosis exclusively relies on case history and details of daily life.

Diagnostic criteria for functional constipation (Chronic constipation)

1. Must include two or more of the following:
   a. Straining during more than one-fourth (25%) of defecation.

   b. Lumpy or hard stools (BSFS 12) during more than one-fourth (25%) of defecation.
   c. Sensation of incomplete evacuation during more than one-fourth (25%) of defecation.
   d. Sensation of anorectal obstruction/blockage during more than one-fourth (25%) of defecation.
   e. Manual manoeuvres to facilitate more than one-fourth (25%) of defecation (e.g., digital evacuation, support of the pelvic floor).
   f. Fewer than three spontaneous bowel movements per week.
2. Loose stools are rarely present without the use of laxatives.
3. Insufficient criteria for irritable bowel syndrome (IBS).
4. Criteria fulfilled for the last 3 months with symptom onset at least 6 months prior to diagnosis.

[Rome 5 criteria for functional constipation (Lacy *et al.*, 2016).]

Examinations are conducted to exclude other digestive disorders and possible causes of constipation as a symptom. The same routines listed in IBS should be performed for a final confirmation, plus thyroid function.

Differentiation syndromes of TCM and herbal treatment

Stomach and Liver Qi Stagnation

Clinical features and signs: Signs are sluggish bowel movements with lower frequency, abdominal distension with cramping, lumpy and hard stools, straining to have bowel movement, poor appetite with belching, irritable emotion which always aggravates the constipation, a red tongue with white-thick coating, and a wiry-strong pulse.

Treatment principle in TCM: Dredge stagnated *Liver* and *Stomach Qi*; promote and cleanse accumulated abdominal *Qi*.

Treatment: Herbal prescription.

Pinyin: Da Chai Hu Tang variation.

English name for decoction: Major Bupleurum Decoction variation.

Role in formula	Name/ Pinyin	Name/Latin	Dose (g)	Function
Chief herb	Chai Hu	Radix Bupleuri	10	Dredges the stagnated liver and stomach qi.
Deputy herb	Huang Qin	Radix Scutellariae Baicalensis	10	Clears the excessive heat in the burner.
Assistant herb	Zhi Shi	Fructus Immaturus Citri Aurantii	10	Promotes dredging of the stagnated liver and abdominal qi to purge the bowel movement.
	Da Huang	Radix et Rhizoma Rhei	10	Purges the bowel and eliminates the accumulated stools in the abdomen.
	Ban Xia	Rhizoma Pinelliae Ternatae	10–15	Harmonises the stomach and decreases the turbid qi.
	Bai Shao	Radix Paeoniae Lactiflorae	10–30	Softens the liver yin and blood to ease the pain and stagnation.
Guiding herb	Da Zao	Fructus Zizyphi Jujubae	10	Harmonises the stomach and promotes cohesiveness of herbs.

Method: The above-mentioned herbal prescription is the main formula and can be used in combination with a variation of decoctions according to specific individual symptoms where herbs are boiled or concentrated herbal powders are taken with warm water twice daily.

Analysis: Chai Hu and Huang Qin cleanse stagnated *Liver-Stomach Qi* and relax the mind and emotions. Da Huang as a laxative herb promotes bowel movement. Zhi Shi dredges stagnated abdominal *Qi* to promote bowel movement. Bai Shao nourishes the *Liver* and *Stomach Yin* to moisten the intestine. Ban Xia harmonies the *Stomach* and Da Zhao nourishes the intestines. All herbs in combination are considered a strong formula to promote bowel movement.

Advice: This pattern can be seen patients with acute constipation and a stronger constitution, so they should not suffer this issue for an extended time. Except for organic disease being the diagnosis and cause of constipation, this pattern is commonly seen as being caused by and a side effect of medication, changed lifestyle, less activity, etc.

Stomach Qi accumulation with Spleen Qi-Yin Deficiency

Clinical features and signs: Signs are a bloated stomach and distension around the abdomen, sluggish and lower frequency of bowel movements, indigestion caused easily with poor appetite, tiredness, soreness in the abdomen with a comfort or easing on light touch pressure, soreness or itching around the anus, alight red tongue with white coating and possible teeth marks, and a wiry-fine pulse.

Treatment principle in TCM: Dredge accumulated Stomach and abdominal *Qi*; nourish *Spleen Yin* and reinforce its *Qi*.

Treatment: Herbal prescription and acupuncture.

Pinyin: Da Cheng Qi variated with Zeng Ye Tang.

English name for decoction: Major Order the Qi Decoction variated with Increase the Fluids Decoction.

Role in formula	Name/ Pinyin	Name/Latin	Dose (g)	Function
Chief herb	Da Huang	Radix et Rhizoma Rhei	10	Dredges the stagnated abdominal qi as a laxative.
Deputy herb	Zhi Shi	Fructus Immaturus Citri Aurantii	10	Dredges the stagnated abdominal qi and drives the bowel movement.
Assistant herb	Hou Po	Cortex Magnoliae Officinalis	10	Dredges the stagnated abdominal qi and drives the bowel movement.
	Xuan Shen	Radix Scrophulariae Ningpoensis	10	Nourishes the general yin of the three burners.
	Sheng Di Huang	Radix Rehmanniae Glutinosae	10	Nourishes the kidney yin and original yin to moisten the small and large intestines.

(*Continued*)

Role in formula	Name/ Pinyin	Name/Latin	Dose (g)	Function
	Mai Men Dong	Tuber Ophiopogonis Japonici	10	Nourishes the general yin and fluid in the three burners.
	Bai Shao	Radix Paeoniae Lactiflorae	10–30	Nourishes the liver yin and spleen yin to ease abdominal pain and spasms.
	Yu Zhu	Rhizoma Polygonati Odorati	10	Nourishes the stomach yin.
	Gua Lou Ren	Semen Trichosanthis	10	Nourishes the spleen yin and moistens the intestines to promote bowel movement.
Guiding herb	Huo Ma Ren	Huomaren Semen Cannabis Sativae	10–30	Nourishes the spleen, stomach, and three burners to ease the constipation.

Method: The above-mentioned herbal prescription is the main formula and can be used in combination with a variation of decoctions according to specific individual symptoms where the herbs are boiled or concentrated herbal powders are taken with warm water twice daily.

Analysis: Da Huang dredges stagnated abdominal *Qi* causing a laxative affect and is the main herb. Zhi Shi and Hou Po drive the abdominal *Qi* to support the main herb. Xuan Shen, Mai Dong, and Shen Di Huang nourish the spleen and general *Yin*. Bai Shao and Yu Zhu moisten the intestines. Huo Ma Ren and Gua Lou Ren can also nourish the intestine to promote stool softening for defecation. All herbs combined can dredge accumulated *Qi* and nourish the intestines to ease bowel movement.

Advice: This pattern can be seen as acute constipation or chronic constipation, which is caused by gastrointestinal functional disorder or organic disease. Such constipation is accompanied by deficiency as part of the long post-COVID-19 syndrome.

Lung and Spleen Yin Deficiency

Clinical features and signs: Dry cough and breathlessness still exist, although PCR may indicate a negative result. Other signs are abdominal distension with sluggish bowel movement, dry mouth and dry stools, unsettled or disturbed sleep, a red tongue with less or no coating, and a weaker-fine pulse.

Treatment principle in TCM: Nourish *Lung* and *Spleen Yin*; moisten intestine and promote bowel movement.

Treatment: Herbal prescription.

Pinyin: Ma Zi Ren variated with Run Chang Tang.

English name for decoction: Hemp Seed Pill variated with Moisten the Intestines Decoction.

Role in formula	Name/ Pinyin	Name/Latin	Dose (g)	Function
Chief herb	Huo Ma Ren	Semen Cannabis Sativae	10–30	Moisturises and nourishes the lung and large intestines to promote ease of bowel movement.
Deputy herb	Xin Ren	Semen Pruni Armeniacae	10	Ventilates the lung to promote the lung qi to descend to the large intestine.
Assistant herb	Zhi Shi	Fructus Immaturus Citri Aurantii	10	Regulates the abdominal qi to promote the bowel movement quickly.
	Hou Po	Cortex Magnoliae Officinalis	10	Dredges the stagnated qi from the three burners to promote bowel descending.
	Dang Gui	Radix Angelicae Sinensis	10	Nourishes the yin and blood to ease the pain and spasms.
	Sheng Di Huang	Radix Rehmanniae Glutinosae	10–15	Nourishes the kidney and general yin to drive the bowel movement.
	Tao Ren	Semen Pruni Persicae	10	Moistens the spleen and stomach, activates the blood stasis, drives the bowel movement, and eases the abdominal pain and spasms.
	Bai Shao	Radix Paeoniae Lactiflorae	10–30	Moistens the liver and spleen to promote relaxation and ease the pain and spasms.
Guiding herb	Gan Cao	Radix Glycyrrhizae Uralensis	5	Harmonises the stomach and promotes cohesiveness of herbs.

Method: The above-mentioned herbal prescription is the main formula and can be used in combination with a variation of decoctions according to specific individual symptoms where the herbs are boiled or concentrated herbal powders are taken with warm water twice daily.

Analysis: Huo Ma Ren as the main herb moistens and nourishes the *Lung* and *Large Intestines* to promote ease of bowel movement. Zhi Shi and Hou Po are the main ingredients in the Ze Ye Cheng Qi Tang dredging accumulated abdominal *Qi* and drive bowel movement. Xing Ren and Tao Ren nourish *Lung Yin* and *Spleen-Intestinal Yin*. Dang Gui and Bai Shao nourish *Yin* and *Blood* to soften stools. Gan Cao harmonises all the herbs to promote cohesiveness.

Advice: This pattern is seen as a chronic condition with a prolonged gastrointestinal disorder after being infected with COVID-19, so constipation can be seen as either a functional disorder or an organic disease.

Spleen and Kidney Qi and Yang Deficiency

Clinical features and signs: Signs are sluggish bowel movement, difficulty in defecating accompanied by abdominal bloating, dull aching in the abdomen which is relieved by pressing, a cold-soft abdomen, weakness and breathlessness, feeling worse upon exertion, cold limbs, frequent urination, loss control of bowel movement occasionally, urgent need or increased need to defecate early in the morning, a pale tongue with white coating, and a weaker-fine pulse.

Treatment principle in TCM: Warm *Spleen* and *Kidney Yang* and *Qi*; relax the bowel movement.

Treatment: Herbal prescription and acupuncture.

Pinyin: Ji Chuan Jian variated with Si Shen Wan, Li Zhong Wan, or You Gui Wan.

English name for decoction: Benefit the River Decoction varied with the Four-Miracle Decoction (Pill) and Regulate the Middle Burner Decoction, or Restore the Right Decoction (all the names of formulas).

Role in formula	Name/ Pinyin	Name/Latin	Dose (g)	Function
Chief herb	Rou Cong Rong	Herba Cistanches Deserticolae	10	Replenishes the kidney and moistens the intestines to support bowel movement.
Deputy herb	Dang Gui	Radix Angelicae Sinensis	10	Nourishes the yin and blood to moisten the Intestines.
Assistant herb	Sheng Ma	Rhizoma Cimicifugae	6–10	Raises the yang qi to promote the descent of turbid qi.
	Ze Xie	Rhizoma Alismatis Orientalis	10	Aids in descending of the turbid qi and expels accumulated damp and fluid.
	Zhi Qiao	Zhiqiao Fructus Citri Aurantii	10	Dredges the stagnated qi in the spleen and promotes ease of bowel movement to relieve constipation.
Guiding herb	Chuan Niu Xi	Radix Cyathulae Officinalis	10–15	Aids in descending of the dirty qi and promotes cohesiveness of herbs.

Method: The above-mentioned herbal prescription is the main formula and can be used in combination with a variation of decoctions according to specific individual symptoms where the herbs are boiled or concentrated herbal powders are taken with warm water twice daily.

Analysis: Rou Cong Rong is the main herb warming and strengthening the *Spleen* and *Kidney Yang* to relax bowel movement. Niu Xi also warms *Yang*, relaxes bowel movement, and promotes the descending affect to the lower body. Dang Gui nourishes *Yin* and *Blood* to soften stools. Sheng Ma and Ze Xie are combined to increase the ascension of *Yang Qi* and drive *Turbid Qi*-fluid down. Zhi Qiao promotes general intestinal *Qi* movement. All herbs in combination harmonise to warm *Yang* and strengthen *Qi* promoting soft stools and a relaxed bowel movement.

Advice: This pattern is seen as a chronic condition with prolonged suffering in a patient with deficient. It is mostly caused by organic diseases which are triggered by COVID-19, such as Colonic Diverticulitis and Gastrointestinal bacteria disorders, which form part of the inflammatory cytokine storm response during infectious COVID-19.

Acupuncture treatment

Main points: Zhongwan (REN12), Qihai (REN6) and Tianshu (ST25).

Assistant points:

- Stomach and Liver Qi stagnation: Neiting (ST44), Zusanli (ST36); Xingjian (LIV2), Zhongfeng (LIV4), Jiexi (ST41). Diji (SP8), Shangqiu (SP5), Fujie (SP14).
- Stomach *Qi* accumulation with Spleen Qi-Yin Deficiency: Jiexi (ST41), Hegu (LI4), Yinlingquan (SP9).
- Lung and Spleen Yin Deficiency: Kongzui (LU6), Taiyuan (LU9), Daheng (SP15), Yinlingquan (SP9), Sanyinjiao (SP6).
- Spleen and Kidney Qi and Yang Deficiency: Daheng (SP15), Fujie (SP14). Yinglingquan (SP6), Neiting (ST44), Taixi (KI3), Zhaohai (KI6), Sugu (BL65).

Analysis: Zhongwan, Qihai, and Tianshu are three points surrounding the belly button and dredge accumulated abdominal *Qi* to regulate intestinal *Qi* and are the main points. The assistant points are selected according to points on the *Yang* meridians to treat the symptoms caused by the excess pattern, such as Neiting to treat constipation which is caused by *Stomach Qi Stagnation.* Points on the *Yin* meridians are selected to treat the symptoms caused by the deficiency pattern, such as Yinglingquan and Shangqu, which are selected to treat constipation caused by *Spleen* deficiency. Five shu points in every meridian should be elected as priority.

Case Study

Ms. C. Roberts, 73 years old, a retired university lecturer, suffered from chronic constipation as a pre-existing disease, although her condition was much worse and persisted as part of the post-COVID-19 syndrome after she was infected.

She had been suffering from habitual constipation for two years prior to COVID-19, and colonic diverticulitis was always suspected, but she had never been diagnosed after she accepted TCM treatment. After getting treatment for a half year, she complained of worse constipation with abdominal cramps after she was infected with COVID-19.

Although she had a negative PCR for a while, she still suffered from cough with phlegm, breathlessness in the chest, abdominal distension, constipation, bowel movement only 2–3 times a week, and soreness and discomfort around the anus. She had a light red tongue with many cracks in the middle part with white-greasy coating, and she had a bloated abdomen with softness when palpating. She did not have an X-ray or any other relevant image examination.

Diagnosis:

1. Habitual Constipation as part of the post-COVID-19 syndrome.
2. Incompletely healed and lingering bronchitis.

Differentiation syndromes of TCM:

1. Damp-heat accumulated in the lung and large intestine.
2. Spleen *Qi* and *Yin* deficiency.

Treatment: Herbal prescription and acupuncture.

Acupuncture

Main points: Zhongwan (REN12), Qihai (REN6), Tianshu (ST25); Baihui (DU20), Shanzhong (REN17), Kongzui (LU6), Hegu (LI4); Yinlingquan (SP9), Sanyinjiao (SP6), Taibai (SP3), Neiting (ST44).

Herbal prescription

Pinyin: Ma Zi Ren Wan variated with Er Chen Wan.

English name for decoction: Hemp Seed Pill variated with Decoction of Two Old (Cured) Powders.

Herbal powders (g):

Huo Ma Ren	Semen Cannabis Sativae 30 g
Xuan Shen	Radix Scrophulariae Ningpoensis 20 g
Xing Ren	Semen Pruni Armeniacae 10 g
Bai Shao	Radix Paeoniae Lactiflorae 20 g
Da Huang	Radix et Rhizoma Rhei 10 g
Zhi Shi	Fructus Immaturus Citri Aurantii 10 g
Hou Po	Cortex Magnoliae Officinalis 10 g
Dang Gui	Radix Angelicae Sinensis 10 g
Mai Men Dong	Tuber Ophiopogonis Japonici 10 g
Lai Fu Zi	Semen Raphani Sativi 10 g
Jiang Ban Xia	Rhizoma Pinelliae Ternatae 15 g
Chen Pi	Pericarpium Citri Reticulatae 10 g
Fu Ling	Sclerotium Poriae Cocos 10 g
Bai Zhu	Rhizoma Atractylodis Macrocephalae 10 g
Gan Cao	Radix Glycyrrhizae Uralensis 5 g

The above herbal powder weighs 200 g. She was told to take three teaspoons, of about 7–8 g each time, with warm water, twice daily.

Result: Her chest gradually cleared, her cough and breathlessness also reduced and completely disappeared after a couple of months of regular treatment. She had 1–2 bowel movements daily without cramps, and had much less distension. She was pleased with this result and maintained regular TCM treatment every 2 weeks.

References

Lacy, B. E., Mearin, F., Chang, L., Chey, W. D., Lembo, A. J., *et al.* (2016). Bowel disorders. *Gastroenterology*, 150, 1393–1407. Available at: https://theromefoundation.org/wp-content/uploads/bowel-disorders.pdf. (Accessed 2 March 2022).

Lacy, B. E. and Patel, N. K. (2017). Rome criteria and a diagnostic approach to irritable bowel syndrome. *Journal of Clinical Medicine*, 6(11), 99. https://doi.org/10.3390/jcm6110099.

Oshima, T., Siah, K. T. H., Yoshimoto, T., Miura, K., Tomita, T., *et al.* (2021). Impacts of the COVID-19 pandemic on functional dyspepsia and irritable bowel syndrome: A population-based survey. *Journal of Gastroenterology and Hepatology*, 36(7), 1820–1827. doi:10.1111/jgh.15346.

Sultan, S., Altayar, O., Siddique, S. M., Davitkov, P., Feuerstein, J. D., *et al.* (2020). Rapid review of the gastrointestinal and liver manifestations of COVID-19, meta-analysis of international data, and recommendations for the consultative management of patients with COVID-19. *Gastroenterology*, 159(1), 320–334.e27 doi:10.1053/j.gastro.2020.05.001. Epub 2020 May 11.

Yan, Z., Yang, M., and Lai, C.-L. (2021). Long COVID-19 syndrome: A comprehensive review of its effect on various organ systems and recommendation on rehabilitation plans. *Biomedicines*, 9(8), 966. https://doi.org/10.3390/biomedicines9080966.

Chapter 11

Myalgic Encephalomyelitis (ME) and Fibromyalgia (FM)

Myalgic encephalomyelitis (ME) is also called chronic fatigue syndrome (CFS) depending on the practice environment. ME is preferred among European practitioners, while CFS is more accepted in American and Asian medical circles. It is a set of symptoms of unclear pathology and aetiology, which causes serious problems in maintaining a normal life due to the lack of physical strength and stamina. Many patients are bedridden and rely on help from others (CDC, 2021). The two main symptoms are fatigue and chronic aching. The Institute of Medicine (USA) has proposed a new name of "systemic exertion intolerance disease", in an effort to try to unify ME and CFS.

Fibromyalgia (FM) is a condition characterised by widespread aching/pain or tenderness (sensitive to touch, or feeling pain when touched) in many places of the body without a history of physical injury or other diseases. The two main symptoms are the general aching/tenderness and fatigue (America College of Rheumatology, 2021).

ME/CFS and FM are similar conditions in the clinic, and manifest three key features, *fatigue, pain and mood problem*, so some patients could be diagnosed as both ME and FM. The conditions are also closely linked to depression and sleeping problems (Goldenberg, 2016). It was also suggested that ME/CFS, FM, IBS, depression, anxiety, and insomnia are a cluster of intertwined mind/body conditions. When a patient first reports wide spread pain and is managed by a pain specialist or rheumatologist, the case is more likely to be diagnosed as FM. If the same patient visits a GP for general sickness or fatigue, then ME/CFS would be provided as a diagnosis.

Many clinicians have realised the similarity between PCS and ME/CFS and considered that they are very similar and some patients could eventually be diagnosed as ME/CFS based on the analysis of all symptoms they are suffering. For example, Poenaru *et al.* (2021) quoted fatigue as the most common symptom, followed by dyspnoea, myalgia (general aching), exercise intolerance, sleeping problems, poor concentration, anxiety, etc. Except the dyspnoea, all other symptoms are listed as the symptoms of ME/CFS. With no other clinical findings suggesting physical/structural evidence of damage, they all meet the diagnostic criteria of ME/CFS. The authors strongly agree with what was proposed, and the profile of the symptoms also fits the boot of FM.

In a similar vein, Gonzalez-Hermosillo *et al.* (2021) carried out an assessment on 130 PCS patients and found that 47% of the patients reported fatigue, and on average the patients report nine symptoms at the time of assessment. Eventually, only 13% were convincingly classed as CFS/ME patients if a very strict criterion of "systemic exertion intolerance disease" was applied. There are multiple factors which excluded the patients from being diagnosed as ME/CFS; for example, the duration of suffering fatigue is less than 6 months; the evidence suggests lung impairment still existed. But, when those patients are followed for a longer time, the picture will be much clearer. At the time of the final draft of this chapter, no similar clinic assessment has been reported on co-diagnosis of FM.

In the past, the authors of this chapter have met and treated many ME/CFS and FM patients, and TCM treatments have demonstrated great improvement (Jiang & Franks, 1994). Although the conditions were not known or established before 1985, similar records were available in some TCM documents. Experiences of treating problems after fever diseases (infectious diseases) in the post-infectious stages were discussed in some theses providing precious clues of how the later damage was understood and managed. Because of the invasion of pathogenic factors, the body reacts with a defence response which causes the body to operate on a much higher level of consumption of energy/*Qi* and nutrient/*Yin* and blood. So, *Qi* and *Yin* deficiency was commonly recognised in such situations. And it was also acknowledged that the pathogenic factors might leave some residual parts in the body; meanwhile, some debris is also presented in the body. The pathogenic factors and debris continue to cause body reactions and are commonly classified as dampness remaining/accumulating. If the cause was mainly due to the nature of weak *Qi* and *Yin*, then it was more likely that the patient suffered from ME/CFS, while the presence of dampness can cause broad aching, pointing to FM. However, the two are not separate, and most patients will have both aspects, some showing more weakness while others show more dampness.

Accordingly, the treatment needs to be planned for longer periods as both aspects will need time for the body to readjust and quick solutions might cause more harm than good.

Diagnosis

Diagnostic criteria of ME/CFS (*CDC 2016*)

Diagnosis requires that the patient have the following three symptoms:

A. A substantial reduction or impairment in the ability to engage in pre-illness levels of occupational, educational, social, or personal activities, which persists for more than 6 months and is accompanied by fatigue, which is often profound, with the illness being of new or definite onset (not lifelong), not the result of on-going excessive exertion, and is not substantially alleviated by rest.
B. Post-exertional malaise.*
C. Unrefreshing sleep.*

At least one of the two following manifestations is also required:

A. Cognitive impairment.*
B. Orthostatic intolerance.

Diagnosis of FM and criteria for Diagnosing Fibromyalgia (American College of Rheumatology, 2010):

A. The general aching and pain throughout the body with the level of the severity based on the symptoms for over 6 months.

---

*Frequency and severity of symptoms should be assessed. The diagnosis of ME/CFS (SEID) should be questioned if patients do not have these symptoms at least half of the time with moderate, substantial, or severe intensity.

a. Fatigue.
b. Waking unrefreshed.
c. Cognitive (memory or thought) problems.
Plus, a number of other general physical symptoms.

B. Symptoms lasting at least 3 months at a similar level.
C. No other health problem that would explain the pain and other symptoms.

NICE, the UK equivalent of the CDC, holds similar diagnostic criteria for both ME/CFS and FM. From the diagnostic criteria of both, it is clear that the case has to be newly onset, not from a lingering disease, and the diagnosis is mainly based on case history, with all necessary medical examinations being carried out to exclude any physical damage in any important organ. No biological markers are suggested to be used as a definitive diagnostic tool.

Syndrome Pattern and Herbal Treatment

General muscle aching/Fibromyalgia

We have these diagnoses and treatment principles:

- In diagnosis, the following observation was made: "The more the myalgia, the more the pathogenic dampness".
- In formulating the herbal prescription, the first aim is to resolve dampness and clear pathogenic factors.
- When selecting acupuncture points, expelling pathogenic factors and tonifying the body should be concurrent aims, dealt with according to presentation.
- Use Du Mai and scalp points in addition to other channel points, especially if head symptoms predominate (poor concentration and memory, headache, insomnia, light headedness, mental exhaustion, and depression).

If general aching manifests, the pathogenic factor of dampness should still be existing inside the body, so according to TCM there are excess patterns or mixed excess and deficiency patterns.

The general principle is that the degree of myalgia depends on how much dampness has been accumulated. "The more the pathogenic dampness, the more the myalgia".

Damp-Heat accumulated in the upper burner

Clinical features: Features are sore and dry throat; turbid nasal discharge; tinnitus; headache; pain in the shoulders, neck, and back; light red tongue with scanty yellow-greasy coating; and soggy (Ru) pulse.

Treatment principle in TCM: Clear *Lung Heat* and resolve exterior *Dampness*.

Treatment: Herbal prescription.

Pinyin: Hou Po Xia Ling Tang variation.

English name for decoction: Agastaches, Magnolia Bark, Pinellia, and Poria Decoction.

Role in formula	Name/ Pinyin	Name/Latin	Dose (g)	Function
Chief herb	Huo Xiang	Herba Agastaches seu Pogostemi	10	Dissipates the external damp-wind and ventilates the lung *Qi* and upper burner.
Deputy herb	Hou Po	Cortex Magnoliae Officinalis	10	Dries the external and internal damp and ventilates the upper and middle burners.
Assistant herb	Ban Xia	Rhizoma Pinelliae Ternatae	10	Expels the external and internal damp-phlegm, ventilates the lung, and harmonises the stomach.
	Fu Ling	Sclerotium Poriae Cocos	10	Dissipates the excessive dampness and replenishes the spleen.
	Xing Ren	Semen Pruni Armeniacae	10	Ventilates the lung and dissipates the damp-phlegm to ease cough.
	Yi Yi Ren	Semen Coicis Lachryma-jobi	30	Dissipates the damp-fluid from the three burners.
	Bai Kou Ren	Fructus Amomi Cardamomi	6–10	Dries the dampness in the stomach and harmonises the stomach.
	Zhu Ling	Sclerotium Polypori Umbellati	10	Dissipates the damp-fluid from the three burners and eases the passing of urine.
	Ze Xie	Rhizoma Alismatis	10	Dissipates the damp-fluid from the three burners and eases the passing of urine.
Guiding herb	Dan Dou Chi	Semen Sojae Praeparatum	10	Harmonises the stomach and promotes cohesiveness of the herbs.

Method: The above-mentioned herbal prescription is the main formula and can be used in combination with variations of decoctions made according to specific individual symptoms where the herbs are boiled and concentrated herbal powders are taken with warm water twice daily.

Analysis: Huo Xiang dissipates the external Dampness and is the main herb. Hou Po as the deputy herb promotes drying not only of the external dampness but also of internal dampness. Ban Xia dries the Damp-Phlegm and ventilates the lung, and Fu Ling expels the excessive dampness from the upper and middle burns. Yi Yi Ren, Ze Xie, and Zhu Ling support dissipation of the damp-fluid from the three burners and push the diuresis. Bai Dou Kou harmonises the stomach; Dan Dou Chi also harmonises the stomach and leads all the herbs to the exterior. All the prescriptions should be used for the pathogenic factor dampness-heat invading the exterior or the upper burner.

Advice: This pattern is commonly seen at the early stage of the long COVID-19 syndrome. Although patients feel tiredness, the virus is still reoccurring, which causes general aching.

Damp-Heat accumulated in the middle burner

Clinical features and signs: Signs are poor appetite, fullness and distension in the chest and epigastrium, stuffiness and pain in the hypochondriac region, tiredness and drowsiness, aching muscles, feeling of heaviness in the body and head, loose stools or diarrhoea, sticky taste in the mouth, a muzzy feeling in the brain, red tongue with yellow-greasy coating, thick in the middle portion, and slippery (Hua) and rapid (Shu) pulse.

Treatment principle in TCM: Drain *Dampness* and expel *Heat*; regulate and move the interior *Qi*.

Treatment: Herbal prescription.

Pinyin: Lian Po Yin variation.

English name for decoction: Coptis and Magnolia Bark Drink variation.

Role in formula	Name/ Pinyin	Name/Latin	Dose (g)	Function
Chief herb	Huang Lian	Rhizoma Coptidis	5	Clears the heat and dries the dampness in the middle burner.
Deputy herb	Hou Po	Cortex Magnoliae Officinalis	6	Dissipates the dampness and dredges the stagnated *Qi* from exterior and interior.
Assistant herb	Zhi Zi	Fructus Gardeniae Jasminoidis	6	Clears the excessive damp-heat in the lung and stomach.
	Shi Chang Pu	Rhizoma Acori Graminei	3	Ventilates the lung *Qi* in the upper burner and dries the excessive dampness.
	Ban Xia	Rhizoma Pinelliae Ternatae	6	Dries the dampness and ventilates the lung to ease cough and release phlegm.
	Lu Gen	Rhizoma Phragmitis Communis	12	Eliminates the excessive damp-fluid and promotes diuresis.
	Hua Shi	Talcum	15	Eliminates the excessive damp-fluid and promotes diuresis.
	Mu Xiang	Radix Saussureae seu Vladimirae	5	Excites and dredges the stagnated *Qi* from the middle burner.
Guiding herb	Chai Hu	Radix Bupleuri	6	Dredges the stagnated *Qi* and drives *Qi* flow in the whole body.

Method: The above-mentioned herbal prescription is the main formula and can be used in combination with a variation of decoctions according to specific individual symptoms where the herbs are boiled and concentrated herbal powders are taken with warm water twice daily.

Analysis: Huang Lian clears *Heat* and dries the *Dampness* from the middle burner as the main herb. Hou Po releases the *Stagnated Qi* and *Dampness* also as the main herb. Lu Gen eliminates the *Damp* and clears the *Heat.* Shi Chang Po eliminates the *Dampness* with aromatisation. Ban Xia and Hua Shi expel *Dampness* and harmonise the *Stomach*. Mu Xiang and Chai Hu dredge the *Stagnated Qi* and encourage *Damp* away. This prescription can release the excessive *Dampness* with *Heat* accumulated at the middle burner.

Advice: This pattern can be seen in people who are invaded by pathogenic dampness and affected in the stomach by something like a stomach flu, or in people who have had a weak stomach illness in the past and, therefore, easily accumulate viruses in the stomach as the part of the post-COVID-19 syndrome.

Damp-Heat throughout the three burners

Clinical features and signs: Signs are poor appetite; fullness and distension in the abdomen; loose stools, diarrhoea, or constipation; nausea; aching, heaviness, and stiffness in the limbs and back; weary feeling in the whole body, lack of energy; scanty urine; leucorrhoea; dull blank complexion, dull response; red tongue with yellow-greasy coating; and slippery (Hua) pulse.

Treatment principle in TCM: *Expel Heat* and drain *Dampness*, clear the water passages of the three burners.

Treatment: Herbal prescription.

Pinyin: Chang Pu Yu Jin Tang variation.

English name for decoction: Modified Acorus and Curcuma Decoction variation.

Role in formula	Name/ Pinyin	Name/Latin	Dose (g)	Function
Chief herb	Shi Chang Pu	Rhizoma Acori Graminei	3	Ventilates the lung and dries the damp-phlegm in the upper burner.
Deputy herb	Yu Jin	Tuber Curcumae	6	Dredges the stagnated *Qi* from the upper and middle burners.
Assistant herb	Zhi Zi	Fructus Gardeniae Jasminoidis	6	Clears excessive damp-heat in the upper and middle burners.
	Lian Qiao	Fructus Forsythiae Suspensae	6	Dissipates the external damp-heat-wind.

(*Continued*)

Role in formula	Name/ Pinyin	Name/Latin	Dose (g)	Function
	Hua Shi	Talcum	15	Eliminates the excessive damp and promotes diuresis.
	Zhu Ye	Herba Lophatheri Gracilis	6	Dissipates the heat and dampness from the upper and middle burners.
	Mu Dan Pi	Cortex Moutan Radicis	6	Clears the excessive heat in the upper burner.
	Zhu Ru	Caulis Bambusae in Taeniis	6	Clears the heat and eliminates the damp-phlegm.
	Niu Bang Zi	Fructus Arctii Lappae	6	Dissipates the external and internal damp-wind.
	Che Qian Zi	Semen Plantaginis	9	Eliminates the accumulated dampness and promotes diuresis.
Guiding herb	Huai Shan	Radix Dioscoreae Oppositae	6	Dries the dampness and harmonises the stomach.

Method: The above-mentioned herbal prescription is the main formula and can be used in combination with a variation of decoctions according to specific individual symptoms where the herbs are boiled and the concentrated herbal powders are taken with warm water twice daily.

Analysis: Shi Chang Pu ventilates the *Lung* and dries the *Damp-Phlegm* in the upper burner as the main herb. Yu Jin dredges the *Stagnated Qi* from the upper and middle burners to support the main herb as the deputy herb. Lian Qiao and Niu Bang Zi dissipate the external *Wind-Damp*. Zhi Zu and Mu Dan Pi clear the stagnated *Heat* and accumulated *Dampness*. Zhu Ye, Zhu Ru, and Huai Shang eliminate the *Damp-Phlegm* from the upper and middle burners. Hua Shi and Che Qian Zi release the excessive *Dampness* from the middle and low burners and promote diuresis. All the herbs can eliminate the accumulated *Dampness* from the three burners.

Advice: This pattern can be seen in patients who suffer from severe aching in general with symptoms involving the three burners, always with long

COVID-19 syndrome. The pattern is a combination of excess and deficiency, with predominance of the accumulated pathogenic factor *Damp* and *Heat.*

Predominance of Dampness accumulated in the interior

In this, there is an excess of pathogenic dampness, but no obvious appearance of pathogenic heat. This pattern usually occurs in those who are physically deficient, such as older women.

Clinical features and signs: Signs are soreness and stuffiness in the whole body, vague aches and pains, drowsiness, insomnia, amnesia, blurred vision and dizziness, loose stools, leucorrhoea, a light red tongue with white-greasy coating, and slippery (Hua) pulse.

Treatment principle in TCM: *Drain Dampness* and regulate *Qi.*

Treatment: Herbal prescription.

Pinyin: San Ren Tang variation.

English name for decoction: Three Seed (Nut) Decoction variation.

Role in formula	Name/ Pinyin	Name/Latin	Dose (g)	Function
Chief herb	Xing Ren	Semen Pruni Armeniacae	6	Ventilates the lung and releases the damp.
Deputy herb	Yi Ri Ren	Semen Coicis Lachryma-jobi	15	Eliminates the excessive damp-fluid from the three burners.
	Bai Dou Kou	Fructus Cardamomi Rotundi	3	Dries the dampness, harmonises the stomach, and releases the dampness from the middle burner.
Assistant herb	Hua Shi	Talcum	15	Eliminates the excessive damp-fluid from the three burners.
	Hou Po	Cortex Magnoliae Officinalis	5	Dries the dampness and excites the stagnated *Qi* to ease the general aching.

(*Continued*)

Role in formula	Name/ Pinyin	Name/Latin	Dose (g)	Function
	Tong Cao	Caulis Mutong	5	Eliminates the excessive dampness and promotes the diuresis.
	Ban Xia	Rhizoma Pinelliae Ternatae	6	Dries the damp-phlegm from the lung and the upper burner and harmonises the stomach.
Guiding herb	Zhu Ye	Herba Lophatheri Gracilis	9	Clears the heat and cools the blood.

Method: The nature of the herbs used should not be too cold, but they must be strong enough to remove the dampness. The above-mentioned herbal prescription is the main formula and can be used in combination with a variation of decoctions according to specific individual symptoms where the herbs are boiled and concentrated herbal powders are taken with warm water twice daily.

Analysis: Xing Ren ventilates the *Lung* and releases the *Dampness* as the main herb. Yi Yi Ren eliminates the excessive *Damp-Fluid* from the three burners as the deputy herb. Bai Dou Kou dries the *Dampness,* harmonises the *Stomach,* and releases the *Dampness* from the middle burner as the assistant herb. Hua Shi and Tong Cao release the excessive *Dampness* and promote diuresis. Ban Xia and Hou Po ventilate the *Lung* and harmonise the *Stomach* to support the elimination of excessive *Damp*. Zhu Ye clears the heat to cool the blood. All the herbs are prescribed to eliminate the accumulated *Dampness* in the body.

Advice: This pattern can be seen in the patients who suffer from severe muscular aching, which is worse when *Damp* accumulates without *Heat* as part of with long COVID-19 syndrome. Patients feel tiredness, fatigue, and general aching, with no signs demonstrating a deficiency pattern. This state is commonly seen in young people.

Excessive Cold and Damp

This is excessive pathogenic dampness combined with cold. This pattern is usually seen in patients who have a cold constitution.

Clinical features: Features are blurred vision and dizziness, feeling of bloating and pain in the stomach, chilled and cold limbs, loose stools or diarrhoea, cold sensation in the lower abdomen, soreness and aching in the whole body, lack of energy, tiredness, drowsiness, insomnia, amnesia, a pale tongue with white coating, and slow (Chi) and slippery (Hua) pulse.

Treatment principle in TCM: Warm and dispel *Cold* and *Damp*.

Treatment: Herbal prescription.

Pinyin: Ling Gui Zhu Gan Tang variation.

English name for decoction: Poria, Cinnamon Twig, Atractylodes, and Liquorice Decoction.

Role in formula	Name/ Pinyin	Name/Latin	Dose (g)	Function
Chief herb	Fu Ling	Sclerotium Poriae Cocos	9	Dissipates the excessive damp and replenishes the spleen and middle burner.
Deputy herb	Gui Zhi	Ramulus Cinnamomi Cassiae	6	Warms and excites the *Qi* flowing through the body.
Assistant herb	Bai Zhu	Rhizoma Atractylodis Macrocephalae	6	Dries the excessive damp and replenishes the spleen and the vitality *Qi*.
	Wu Zhu Yu	Fructus Evodiae Rutaecarpae	3	Warms and strengthens the spleen and the kidney *Qi*.
	Dang Shen	Radix Codonopsis Pilosulae	6	Strengthens the spleen *Qi* and vitality *Qi*.
	Gan Jiang	Rhizoma Zingiberis Officinalis	6	Warms and excites the *Qi* from the middle burner and general body.
Guiding herb	Gan Cao	Radix Glycyrrhizae Uralensis	3	Harmonises the stomach and promotes cohesiveness of herbs.

Method: The above-mentioned herbal prescription is the main formula and can be used in combination with a variation of decoctions according to specific individual symptoms where the herbs are boiled and concentrated herbal powders are taken with warm water twice daily.

Analysis: Fu Ling dissipates the excessive *Dampness* and replenishes the *Spleen* and the middle burner as the main herb. Gui Zhi warms and agitates the *Yang Qi* flowing through the body as the deputy herb. Bai Zhu and Dang Shen dry the excessive *Damp* and replenish the *Spleen* and the *Vitality Qi* as the assistant herbs. Wu Zhu Yu and Gan Jiang warm and agitate the *Qi* from the middle burner and general body. Gan Cao harmonises the *Stomach* and leads all herbs to work well together. All the herbs are prescribed together to treat the pattern with an excessive *Damp* and *Cold* accumulation without *Heat.*

Advice: This pattern can be seen in patients who are suffering from severe aching and fatigue, but they feel the cold patterns more, which means they had a stronger constitution in the past, so we need to warm and eliminate the accumulated dampness, so that they will recover quickly.

Excessive Heat in interior

Patients of this type do not have much pathogenic dampness but have excessive pathogenic heat. They are usually habitual smokers or drinkers and are often quick tempered.

Clinical features and signs: Signs are pain and heaviness in the head and body; irritability; insomnia; tinnitus; bitter taste and smell in the mouth; fullness and distension in the chest; constipation; hiccups and sighing; fullness and pain in the hypochondriac region, chest, and back; dry and gritty sensation in the eyes; red tongue with yellow-greasy coating; and wiry (Xian) and rapid (Shu) pulse.

Treatment principle in TCM: Clear *Heat* and dry *Damp*.

Treatment: Herbal prescription and acupuncture.

Pinyin: Long Dan Xie Gan Tang variation.

English name for decoction: Gentiana Longdancao Decoction to Drain the Liver variation.

Role in formula	Name/ Pinyin	Name/Latin	Dose (g)	Function
Chief herb	Long Dan Cao	Radix Gentianae	6	Clears the excessive heat and damp from the middle burner.
Deputy herb	Huang Qin	Radix Scutellariae Baicalensis	6	Clears the excessive heat and dampness from the upper burner.
	Zhi Zi	Fructus Gardeniae Jasminoidis	6	Clears the excessive heat and damp from the upper and middle burners.
Assistant herb	Hua Shi	Talcum	15	Eliminates the excessive damp and promotes diuresis.
	Ze Xie	Rhizoma Alismatis Plantago-aquaticae	6	Eliminates the excessive damp and promotes diuresis.
	Tong Cao	Caulis Mutong	5	Eliminates the excessive damp and promotes diuresis.
	Dang Gui	Radix Angelicae Sinensis	6	Cultivates the liver blood and nourishes the liver *Yin*.
	Shen Di Huang	Radix Rehmanniae Glutinosae	9	Nourishes the liver and kidney *Yin* and general *Yin*.
Guiding herb	Chai Hu	Radix Bupleuri	5	Dredges the stagnated *Qi* and promotes cohesiveness of herbs.

Method: The above-mentioned herbal prescription is the main formula and can be used in combination with a variation of decoctions according to specific individual symptoms where the herbs are boiled and concentrated herbal powders are taken with warm water twice daily.

Analysis: Long Dan Cao clears the excessive *Heat* and *Dampness* from the middle burner and is also the main herb. Huang Qin and Zhi Zi clear the excessive *Heat* and Damp from the upper burner and middle burner as the deputy herbs. Hua Shi, Ze Zie, and Tong Cao eliminate the excessive *Damp* and promote diuresis to drive and eliminate *Dampness.* Dang Gui and Sheng Di Huang cultivate the *Liver Blood* and nourish the *Kidney Yin* and general *Yin* to avoid the cold herbs disturbing the *Liver* and *Stomach.* Chai Hu dredges the *Stagnated Qi* and leads all herbs effectively to the middle burners. This prescription will treat the excessive heat pattern without any deficiency signs.

Advice: This pattern can be seen the patients with a stronger muscular aching and dermatological signs as well as patients with long COVID-19 syndrome. The patients may appear with clinical symptoms for a short time, but more severe signs, so this prescription is given, so that they can quickly recover.

General tiredness/Chronic fatigue syndrome

General exhaustion is the main symptom, along with fatigue, insomnia, amnesia, drowsiness, reduced or even lost capacity to work, easy infection by pathogenic factors, and aching or pains in the muscles.

Qi Deficiency mingled with Dampness

Clinical features: Bloated sensation with pain in the stomach, abdominal distension and gurgling, poor appetite, loose stools, lack of energy, drowsiness, shortness of breath, being too lethargic to speak, pale or puffy complexion, a pale tongue with white coating, and a thready (Xi) and slippery (Hua) pulse.

Treatment principle in TCM: Reinforce *Qi* and dry or drain dampness.

Herbal formula: Xiang Sha Liu Jun Zi Tang variation.

English name for decoction: Six Gentlemen Decoction with Aucklandia and Amomum.

Role in formula	Name/ Pinyin	Name/Latin	Dose (g)	Function
Chief herb	Dang Shen	Radix Codonopsis Pilosulae	10	Replenishes the spleen *Qi* and vitality *Qi* to buildup general *Qi*.
Deputy herb	Bai Zhu	Rhizoma Atractylodis Macrocephalae	12	Replenishes the spleen *Qi* and dries the remained dampness.

(*Continued*)

(*Continued*)

Role in formula	Name/ Pinyin	Name/Latin	Dose (g)	Function
Assistant herb	Chen Pi	Pericarpium Citri Reticulatae	10	Replenishes the spleen *Qi* and agitates the stagnated *Qi* through the body.
	Sha Ren	Fructus seu Semen Amomi	4	Harmonises the stomach and warms and regulates the stagnated *Qi* in the stomach.
	Xiang Fu	Rhizoma Cyperi Rotundi	10	Warms and dredges the general stagnated *Qi*.
	Fu Ling	Sclerotium Poriae Cocos	10	Releases the remaining dampness and supports the building up of the middle *Qi*.
	Ban Xia	Rhizoma Pinelliae Ternatae	10	Dries and releases the dampness and promotes the general *Qi* moving through the body.
Guiding herb	Gan Cao	Radix Glycyrrhizae Uralensis	5	Harmonises the stomach and leads all the herbs to work well together.

If some dampness still remains with minor aching, Che Qian Zi Semen Plantaginis 6 g and Yi Yi Ren Semen Coicis Lachryma-jobi 6 g are given.

Method: The above-mentioned herbal prescription is the main formula where the herbs are mixed as a decoction, which can be varied according to special individual symptoms, and then boiled or made into concentrated herbal powders to be taken with warm water twice daily.

Analysis: Dang Shen is the main herb with Bai Zhu, Fu Ling, and Gan Cao making up the four gentlemen formula, which replenishes the spleen *Qi* and vitality *Qi*. Xiang Fu and Sha Ren warm and agitate the stagnated *Qi*. Ban Xia releases the remained dampness and releases the stagnated *Qi* and phlegm. All the herbs are mixed to replenish the general *Qi* and eliminate stagnation which is caused by accumulated dampness.

Advice: This pattern is commonly seen as part of the long COVID-19 syndrome in gentle and middle stages of the syndrome. Fatigue or tiredness is the main symptom which is part of a deficiency pattern, with minor or no pathogenic factor.

Yin Deficiency mingled with Dampness

Clinical features: Epigastric distress, dry mouth, dull complexion, loss of weight, erratic fever in the afternoon or evening, irritability, insomnia, a deep red tongue with scanty white coating, and a thready (Xi) pulse.

Treatment principle in TCM: Tonify Yin and eliminate dampness.

Herbal formula: Shen Ling Bai Zhu San.

English name for decoction: Ginseng, Poria, and Atractylodis Macrocephalae Powder variation.

Role in formula	Name/ Pinyin	Name/Latin	Dose (g)	Function
Chief herb	Ren Shen	Radix Ginseng	10	Reinforces the spleen and general *Qi*.
Deputy herb	Bai Zhu	Rhizoma Atractylodis Macrocephalae	10–30	Supports reinforcement of the spleen and general *Qi* and dries the excessive dampness.
Assistant herb	Chen Pi	Pericarpium Citri Reticulatae	10	Supports reinforcement of the spleen *Qi* and dredges the stagnated *Qi* in the middle burner.
	Shan Yao	Radix Dioscoreae Oppositae	10	Promotes reinforcement of the spleen *Qi* and dries the dampness.
	Fu Ling	Sclerotium Poria Cocos	10	Releases the accumulated dampness.
	Sha Ren	Fructus Amomi	10	Dredges the stagnated stomach and harmonises general *Qi*.
	Yi Yi Ren	Semen Coicis Lachryma-Jobi	10–30	Eliminates the accumulated dampness and promotes diuresis.
	Je Geng	Radix Platycodi Grandiflori	10	Ventilates the stagnated *Qi* in the upper and the middle burners.
	Lian Zi Rou	Semen Dolichoris Lablab	10	Nourishes the spleen *Yin* to ease diarrhoea.
	Lian Zi Rou	Semen Nelumbinis Nuciferae	10	Nourishes the spleen and heart *Yin* to tranquilise the mind.
Guiding herb	Gan Cao	Radix Glycyrrhizae Uralensis	5	Harmonises the stomach and leads all the herbs to work well together.

If necessary, add Sheng Di Huang Radix Rehmanniae Glutinosae 9 g, Shan Zhu Yu Fructus Corni Officinalis 6 g, Ze Xie Rhizoma Alismatis Plantago-aquaticae 9 g, and Fu Ling Sclerotium Poriae Cocos 9 g.

Method: The above-mentioned herbal prescription is the main formula, which is mixed as a decoction that can be varied according to special individual symptoms, and is boiled or made into concentrated herbal powders to be taken with warm water twice daily.

Analysis: Ren Shen, Bai Zhu, Fu Ling, and Gan Cao form Si Jun Zi Tang — a famous formula to reinforce the spleen *Qi* and promote general vitality *Qi*. Sha Ren and Chen Pi harmonise the stomach and support the spleen *Qi*. Bai Bian Dou and Shan Yao dry dampness and promote the spleen *Qi*. Jie Geng dredges the stagnated *Qi* in the chest and Lian Zi Rou nourishes the heart *Qi* to tranquilise the mind. Yi Yi Ren reinforces the spleen *Qi* and dissipates excessive dampness which is caused by spleen deficiency.

Advice: This pattern is also commonly seen. The patient may suffer from the tiredness for a longer time after he/she heals from COVID-19, the illness is accompanied by some psychiatric disorder, like irritable or insomnia, with chronic fatigue syndrome.

Yang Deficiency mingled with Dampness

Clinical features and signs: Signs are lack of energy, tiredness, the heaviness of the whole body, oedema of the lower legs, thin leucorrhoea, a pale and plump tongue with tooth marks and white coating, and a weak (Xu) and thready (Xi) pulse.

Treatment principle in TCM: Warm the *Yang* and purge water.

Treatment: Herbal prescription and acupuncture.

Pinyin: You Gui Yin variated with Zhen Wu Decoction.

English name for decoction: Restore the Right Kidney Drink varied True Warrior Decoction.

Role in formula	Name/ Pinyin	Name/Latin	Dose (g)	Function
Chief herb	Shu Di Huang	Radix Rhemanniae Glutinosae Praeparata	12	Nourishes the kidney *Yin* as the foundation to promote the kidney yang; complements the kidney essence.
	Rou Gui/ Gui Zhi	Cortex Cinnamomi Cassiae	2–5	Warms and excites the kidney yang.
Deputy herb	Shan Zhu Yu	Fructus Corni Officinalis	6	Supports nourishment of the kidney *Yin* for promoting and building the Kidney yang.
	Sheng Jiang	Rhizoma Zingiberis Officinalis Recens	6	Supports warming and excites the kidney yang.
Assistant herb	Shan Yao	Radix Dioscoreae Oppositae	6	Replenishes the spleen *Qi* and middle burner to release excessive damp.
	Du Zhong	Cortex Eucommiae Ulmoidis	6	Warms and replenishes the kidney yang and strengthens the muscles, tendons, and bones.
	Gou Qi Zi	Cortex Cinnamomi Cassiae	6	Nourishes the kidney and liver *Yin* and blood as the foundation to build the kidney yang.
	Bai Zhu	Rhizoma Atractylodis Macrocephalae	12	Replenishes the spleen and releases excessive damp.
	Bai Shao	Radix Paeoniae Lactiflorae	6	Nourishes both kidney and liver *Yin* and blood.
	Fu Ling	Sclerotium Poria Cocos	6	Releases the excessive damp and replenishes the spleen.
Guiding herb	Zhi Qiao	Cao Radix Glycyrrhizae Uralensis	6	Excites and moves the general *Qi* in the middle and lower burners and prevents tonic herbs from causing stagnation.

Method: The above-mentioned herbal prescription is the main formula and can be used in combination with a variation of decoctions according to specific individual symptoms where the herbs are boiled and concentrated herbal powders are taken with warm water twice daily.

Explanation: Shu Di Huang and Rou Gui, or Gui Zhi, warm and excite *Yang Qi* as the main herb. Bai Zhu reinforces the *Spleen Qi* and dries the retained *Dampness.* Fu Ling and Zhu Ling dredge the fluid passage to disperse the remaining *Dampness.* Shan Zhu Yu and Gou Qi Zi are added to strengthen the *Kidney Qi* and *Yang.* Du Zhong warms and reinforces the *Kidney Qi* and *Yang.* Zhi Gan Cao harmonises all the herbs to warm the *Yang* and reinforces the *Qi* to dispel the retained *Damp.*

Advice: This pattern can be seen in patients with an extended time and severe stage of the post-COVID-19 syndrome of, so *Yang Deficiency* appears with *Cold* symptoms and fluid accumulation.

Acupuncture

Main points: Baihui (DU20), Dazhui (DU14).

Assistant points: Feishu (BL13), Xinshu (BL15), Pishu (BL20), Ganshu (BL18), Shenshu (BL23), Mingmen (DU4).

Analysis: Baihui (DU20) benefits and clears the brain, dispels *Wind,* raises central *Qi,* restores collapsed *Yang,* and calms the spirit. Dazhui (DU14) clears the brain, calms the spirit, clears *Heat* (especially residual heat), dispels *Wind,* and restores collapsed *Yin.* Feishu (BL13) regulates the upper burner, reinforces the *Lung*, dispels *Wind*, transforms *Phlegm,* clears *Heat* and releases the exterior. Xinshu (BL15) regulates the upper burner, reinforces the *Heart,* clears *Heart Heat* and *Fire*, calms the spirit, and strengthens and clears the brain. Pishu (Bl20) reinforces *Spleen Qi* and *Yang*, promotes the *Nutritive* (*Ying*) *Qi* and *Blood*, transforms *Damp-Heat,* and raises the middle *Qi.* Ganshu (BL18) regulates and nourishes the *Liver*, transforms *Damp-Heat*, clears *Heat* (especially the *Liver* and *Gall Bladder*), and disperses *Liver Qi.* Shenshu (BL23) strengthens *Kidney Qi* and *Yang*, regulates the lower burner, reinforces *Yuan Qi* and *Jing*, regulates the water pathways, resolves *Damp*, and strengthens the brain. Mingmen (Du4) strengthens the *Kidneys*, *Yuan Qi*, and *Essence*; regulates the water passages; resolves *Dampness*; calms the spirit; strengthens and clears the brain; and restores collapsed *Yang. In clinical practice*, we will add or reduce points according to symptoms, the areas of pain involved, and the pattern.

Case Studies

Case 1: General muscle aching/Fibromyalgia

Miss. Show, 32 years old, a manager, has suffered from fatigue, headache, and general aching for 3 months. She has severe muscular aching with exertion. Two of her work colleagues from the same office were reported to be infected with COVID-19, although she has not been out since and during the lockdown phase. However, she is always feeling tired, and suffers from headaches, general aching, and discomfort; she has no fever, so she believed that she did not need to go to a GP or the hospital for treatment. Her symptoms were aggravated day by day, until she felt too ill to go shopping and used the aid of a rolling pulley to help her walk. She communicates through the Internet and knows that her friend received some benefits from TCM. She has a pale tongue with less thin white coating.

Diagnosis: Fibromyalgia is caused by an infected or suspected case of COVID-19.

Differentiation syndromes of TCM:

1. Dampness accumulated throughout three burners.
2. Both *Qi* and *Yin* deficiency.

Treatment: Herbal prescription.

Pinyin: Herbal powder prescription: Xiao Chai Hu and San Ren Decoction variation.

English name for decoction: Minor Bupleurum Decoction variated with Three Seed (Nut) Decoction.

Herbal powders (g):

Jiang Ban Xia	Rhizoma Pinelliae Ternatae 15 g
Chai Hu	Radix Bupleur 10 g
Huang Qin	Radix Scutellariae Baicalensis 10 g
Gan Jiang	Rhizoma Zingiberis Officinalis 10 g
Xing Ren	Semen Pruni Armeniacae 10 g
Huo Xiang	Herba Agastachesseu Pogostemi 10 g

Sha Ren	Fructus Amomi 10 g
Bai Dou Kou	Fructus Amomi Cardamomi 10 g
Hua Shi	Talcum 15 g
Tong ao	Medulla Tetrapanacis Papyriferi 10 g
Fu Ling	Sclerotium Poriae Cocos 10 g
Gan Cao	Radix Glycyrrhizae Uralensis 5 g

The above herbal powders are mixed according to the prescription, 6 g per time taken with some warm water, twice daily.

Result and analysis: After she is given the prescribed herbal powders for 2 weeks, she feels much better and gets relief from her headache and general aching; therefore, the prescribed herbs of Xiao Cha Hu and Bu Zhong Yi Qi are given until she feels an increase in energy and better quality of life.

Case 2: Chronic fatigue syndrome/ME

Miss. Boxer, 38 year old, an officer, has suffered from tiredness for over a year after she was infected with COVID-19. She was infected by coronavirus in March 2020 with fever, cough, breathlessness, and was confirmed by a positive PCR. She suffered from the ordinary stage of COVID-19 and was not admitted to the hospital for intensive treatment. She managed by taking some Paracetamol to reduce her temperature and Vitamin C after being told it may be good for her. After 2 weeks, her temperature and cough subsided and the general aching was also gone. However, she remained feeling tired when doing activities, displayed excess sweating, with depression, poor sleep, poor appetite, and lethargy, which prompted her to seek alternative treatment.

Clinical symptoms and signs: Signs were fatigues most of the time since she returned to work, but she still struggled, with the fatigue being worse in late afternoon. She sweat a lot, was breathless, had depression and general heaviness, distension, loose bowel movement, alight red tongue with white coating, and a weak-wiry pulse.

Diagnosis:

1. Post-COVID-19 syndrome.
2. Chronic fatigue syndrome.

Differentiation syndromes of TCM:

1. Spleen *Qi* Deficiency with retained Dampness.
2. Liver *Qi* Stagnation.

Treatment: Herbal prescription and acupuncture.

Acupuncture

Main points: Baihui (DU20), Shenting (DU24).

Assistant points: Jiuwei (REN15), Zhongwan (REN12), Qihai (REN6), Guanyuan (REN4); Yinlingquan (SP9), Sanyinjiao (SP6), Hegu (LI4), Taichong (LIV3).

Herbal prescription

Pinyin: Zhi Bai Di Huang Wan; Qiang Huo Sheng Shi Wan.

Result: She is given regular acupuncture every week with herbal pills to take. She confirms that Astragali (Huang Qi) is very good in building up her energy level. She did see another acupuncturist without herbs before visiting the clinic for 3 months, with minor progress, but she feels she has progressed quickly after acupuncture and herbs. She is maintaining her regular treatment, but she has managed to complete a full day of work with a positive mind and happy emotions.

References

American College of Rheumatology. (2010). 2010 fibromyalgia diagnostic criteria-expert. American College of Rheumatology. Available at: https://www.rheumatology.org/portals/0/files/2010%20fibromyalgia%20diagnostic%20criteria_excerpt.pdf. (Accessed 2 March 2022).

American College of Rheumatology. (2021). Fibromyalgia. American College of Rheumatology. Available at: https://www.rheumatology.org/I-Am-A/Patient-Caregiver/Diseases-Conditions/Fibromyalgia. (Accessed 2 March 2022).

CDC. (2021a). Diagnosis of ME/CFS. Centers for Disease Control and Prevention. Available at: https://www.nap.edu/resource/19012/MECFS cliniciansguide.pdf. (Accessed 2 March 2022).

CDC. (2021b). Myalgic encephalomyelitis/chronic fatigue syndrome. Centers for Disease Control and Prevention. Available at: https://www.cdc.gov/me-cfs/index.html. (Accessed 2 March 2022).

Goldenberg, D. L. (2016). Fibromyalgia, chronic fatigue, and chronic fatigue syndrome. *Practical Pain Management*, 16(10). Available at: https://www.practicalpainmanagement.com/pain/myofascial/fibromyalgia/fibromyalgia-chronic-fatigue-chronic-fatigue-syndrome. (Accessed 2 March 2022).

González-Hermosillo, J. A., Martínez-López, J. P., Carrillo-Lampón, S. A., Ruiz-Ojeda, D., Herrera-Ramírez, S., *et al.* (2021). Post-acute COVID-19 symptoms, a potential link with myalgic encephalomyelitis/chronic fatigue syndrome: A 6-month survey in a Mexican cohort. *Brain Science*, 11(6), 760. doi:10.3390/brainsci11060760.

Jiang, D. and Franks, P. (1994). Analysis of 50 cases of ME treated with Chinese herbs and acupuncture. *Journal of Chinese Medicine (UK)*, 44, 13–20. Available at: http://www.acupunctureinhull.co.uk/study/ANALYSIS%20OF%2050%20ME%20CASES%20TREATED%20BY%20TCM.pdf. (Accessed 2 March 2022).

Poenaru, S., Abdallah, S. J., Corrales-Medina, V., and Cowan, J. (2021). COVID-19 and post-infectious myalgic encephalomyelitis/chronic fatigue syndrome: A narrative review. *Therapeutic Advances in Infectious Disease*, 8, 20499361211009385. doi:10.1177/20499361211009385.

Chapter 12

Loss of Smell, Loss of Taste, and Vision Impairments

Various sensory disorders, like loss of smell and taste, hearing impairment with tinnitus, and vision disorders emerged as a new condition among COVID-19 sufferers, particularly in the post-COVID stage. Among them, the loss of smell and taste is an early symptom of the acute COVID-19 stage. However, many cases have been reported where the recovery of these functions is painfully slow or not progressing at all. Hearing and vision changes, or loss, are dynamic. When fever causes dehydration, the vision changes due to the lens losing water. This could be changed back to normal quickly. It is also worth mentioning that hearing impairment and vision impairment were more commonly seen in the aged population, where the conditions might be part of an accelerated ageing process in the organs and connected to nerves due to the infection.

Loss of Smell and Taste

Observations carried out by Lechien *et al.* (2020) on 417 patients in France revealed how common the loss of smell and loss of taste were in acute infection sufferers. 85% and 88% were found to suffer from the two conditions, respectively. The two symptoms closely overlap, with only 18% of patients reporting loss of taste without nasal complaint. The recovery rate was 44%, with more than half of the patients continuing with the symptoms after the acute infection. Observations in Italy by Vaira *et al.* (2020) reported that on day 10, 40% of the patients had problems of taste and on day 20, this increased to 58%. However, after 60 days of symptom onset, 7.2% of patients still had the loss of the two sensations.

Loss of taste (dysgeusia) and loss of smell (anosmia) were found to be relatively unique to the COVID-19 infection, and they could appear before fever as early symptoms. Braz-Silva *et al.* (2021) reviewed reports and pooled 201 patients; dysgeusia and anosmia were reported in 81% and 75% of Chinese patients, and 64% and 54% of European patients, respectively. It confirmed that the two impairments are very common all over the world. The difference of prevalence might be due to the different variants of the virus.

Fortunato *et al.* (2022) reported results of monitoring those who developed the loss of smell and/or taste in the acute stage in an Italian region. Among the 1,175 COVID-19 cases, 488 cases (41%) experienced such problems. When they were followed up, 178 patients completed the project. Among them, recovery at 90 days was seen in 71% of smell and 74% of taste. This project further confirms the early findings that about 20–25% of the sensory loss will continue into a chronic stage.

From these clinical studies, loss of smell and loss of taste are not only the main symptoms during COVID-19 infection but also presented at a higher percentage in post-COVID-19 syndrome sufferers.

In the clinic, loss of smell and loss of taste always appear together in most patients, but some patients manifest only loss of smell without loss of taste. The sensation of loss is considered to be the result of olfactory nerve damage caused by the SARS-CoV-2 virus directly or indirectly (Othman *et al.*, 2022). The direct damage to the olfactory nerve was due to invasion of the virus into the neuroepithelium/sheath protecting the nerve, while the indirect damage was due to inflammation of tissues from the nose surrounding the olfactory nerve. The recovery of the sensation is easy and quick when it is caused by indirect damage. The direct damage of the nerve might take a very long time to heal or might never happen.

Anosmia and dysgeusia are usually linked, which can have a profound effect on the person's quality of life. Due to not be able to fully taste foods, one may lose interest in eating, so it can also lead to weight loss or malnutrition. It can also lead to depression because it may impair one's ability to smell or taste pleasurable foods.

In TCM, the smell is part of the function of nose which is the beginning part of the airway. Then, the function is supported by the lung system. The taste is the function of the mouth and tongue and is part of the digestive tract; therefore, it is supported by the spleen and stomach system.

When they are both damaged, the invasion of external pathogenic factors (EPFs) is to blame for any acute condition, while the chronic impairments are due to the accumulated poisonous dampness or phlegm in either the lung or spleen in TCM or failure of a weak organ in supporting the functions.

Diagnosis

The clinical symptoms of Anosmia and Dysgeusia could be clearly described by patients. However, the degree of impairment should be tested by specialists whenever possible or one should find a Smell Identification Test kit.

For better measuring of the degree of damage in smelling function, a quantitative University of Pennsylvania Smell Identification Test (UPSIT) is the best currently available tool which is commercially promoted as a Smell Identification Test (Doty *et al.*, 1984). The test could be self-administered and uses micro-encapsulated odorants. By scratching the odour test booklet, odour is released and should be noticed by the patient. Therefore, it is nicknamed "Scratch-sniff" test. The UPSIT is clinically validated and used in research in this area.

A taste test "Sip, spit, and rinse" is a test performed by specialists where chemicals are directly applied to specific areas of the tongue. The sensitivity and damage in various tastes could be measured. A Burghart taste strip is a commercially available test kit that is convenient to use. There is no universal test method recognised worldwide yet.

Specialists in the ENT department will carry out thorough examinations from CT/MRI, nasal scope to functional test of nose and throat, as well as a blood test to exclude other diseases.

Syndrome patterns of TCM and herbal treatment

According to TCM, loss of smell and loss of taste are caused by the upper orifices or sense organs of the upper body when obstructed. The obstruction could be accumulated by the excessive *Dampness* during COVID-19 infection, but most patients can be healed on the abnormal sensation after their coronavirus infection is controlled, but some of them can still have symptoms, like loss of smell and taste, for longer time as part of the post-COVID-19 syndrome. Common patterns of TCM are explained in the following.

Damp-Cold accumulation at the upper burner

Clinical features and signs: Signs are partial or complete loss of smell, blocked nose, and occasional cough with breathlessness. Other signs are loss of taste or strange/abnormal taste, like metallic taste, patients always complain that they cannot smell cooking and cannot taste their food, distension of the *Stomach,* stomach ache, loose bowels, diarrhoea with bloating, A pale tongue with white coating, and a floating-slow pulse. All the symptoms can be aggravated by cold drinks or food and which causes swelling in the stomach.

Treatment principle in TCM: Expel excessive *Dampness* and unblock obstructed orifices.

Treatment: Herbal prescription.

Pinyin: Huo Xiang Zheng Qi Tang variation.

English name for decoction: Agastache Powder to Rectify the *Qi* variation.

Role in formula	Name/ Pinyin	Name/Latin	Dose (g)	Function
Chief herb	Huo Xiang	Herba Agastaches seu Pogostemi	10	Dispels the damp and eliminates the internal cold.
Deputy herb	Hou Po	Cortex Magnoliae Officinalis	10	Dredges the stagnated *Qi* and accumulated dampness.
Assistant herb	Ban Xia	Rhizoma Pinelliae Ternatae	10	Dries the damp, releases the phlegm, and clears the orifices.
	Chen Pi	Pericarpium Citri Reticulatae	10	Dries the damp-phlegm and replenishes the spleen.
	Fu Ling	Sclerotium Poriae Cocos	10	Releases the dampness and replenishes the spleen.
	Bai Zhu	Rhizoma Atractylodis Macrocephalae	10–15	Dries the dampness and replenishes the spleen.
	Da Fu Pi	Pericarpium Arecae Catechu	10	Eliminates the excessive damp and promotes diuresis.
	Bai Zhi	Radix Angelicae Dahuricae	5	Unblocks the accumulated damp-phlegm in the orifices, and leads all herbs to the orifices.

(*Continued*)

Role in formula	Name/ Pinyin	Name/Latin	Dose (g)	Function
	Zi Su	Fructus Perillae Frutescentis	5	Expels the external wind-damp and ventilates the lung.
	Jie Geng	Radix Platycodi Grandiflori	6	Ventilates the lung and eliminates the accumulated damp-phlegm in the lung to unblock the nose.
Guiding herb	Gan Cao	Radix Glycyrrhizae Uralensis	5	Harmonises the stomach and promotes cohesiveness of herbs.

Method: The above-mentioned herbal prescription is the main formula and can be used in combination with a variation of decoctions according to specific individual symptoms where the herbs are boiled and the concentrated herbal powders are taken with warm water twice daily.

Analysis: Huo Xiang dispels *Damp* and eliminates *Cold* as the main herb. Bai Zhu, Ban Xia, Chen Pi, and Fu Ling strengthen the *Spleen* and dry *Damp* as the supporting herbs. Da Fu Pi and Hou Po dredge *Stagnated Qi* and dissolve distension. Zi Su and Bai Zhi relieve external *Cold* and *Cold* at the top of the body. Gan Cao harmonises the *Stomach* and unites all herbs together. Pei Lan, Bo He, and Bai Zhi are added to dredge the blocked orifices. This prescription is the typical formula to eliminate *Dampness* and dredge blocked orifices.

Advice: This pattern can be seen with a loss of smell or taste, or both, for a longer time as a post-COVID-19 syndrome, specifically as a lasting symptom after COVID-19 is controlled, as the orifices are blocked badly without significant *Heat* and *Deficiency*.

Damp-Heat accumulation at the upper burner

Clinical features and signs: Signs are loss of smell and blocked nose with burning sensation, sore throat or dry mouth, occasional cough with phlegm, smoking, general stress, a loss of taste or a nasty taste, headache, light-headedness, loss of taste, waking up during sleep, a red tongue with less yellow or white coating, and a floating-wiry or floating-rapid pulse.

Treatment principle in TCM: Cleanse *Damp-Heat* from upper burner; dredge blocked orifices.

Treatment: Herbal prescription.

Pinyin: Huo Ling Shuang Hua Yin variation.

English name for decoction: Agastaches, Poriae, and Japonicae Decoction variation.

Role in formula	Name/ Pinyin	Name/Latin	Dose (g)	Function
Chief herb	Huo Xiang	Herba Agastaches seu Pogostemi	9	Eliminates the external damp-heat and dredges the blocked orifices.
Deputy herb	Zi Su	Folium Perillae Frutescentis	6	Eliminates the external damp-heat and dredges the blocked orifices.
Assistant herb	Xiang Fu	Herba Elsholtziae seu Moslae	9	Dredges the stagnated *Qi* and promotes general vitality and *Qi* movement.
	Jin Yin Hua	Flos Lonicerae Japonicae	6	Eliminates the external wind-heat to unblock the obstructed orifices.
	Chen Pi	Pericarpium Citri Reticulatae	6	Dries the damp-phlegm to ventilate the lung.
	Huang Jing	Rhizoma Polygonati	6	Nourishes the *Yin* and essence to moisten the orifices.
	Fu Ling	Sclerotium Poriae Cocos	6	Eliminates the damp-phlegm.
	Wu Zhi Mao Yao	Ficus hirta Vahl	6	Clears the toxic heat from the exterior and interior.
	Sheng Jiang	Rhizoma Zingiberis Officinalis Recens	6	Warms and excites the stagnated *Qi* and releases the external wind-damp.
	Cao Guo	Fructus Amomi Tsao-Ko	5	Eliminates the toxic heat and damp.

(*Continued*)

Role in formula	Name/ Pinyin	Name/Latin	Dose (g)	Function
	Jie Geng	Radix Platycodi Grandiflori	5	Ventilates the lung and releases the damp-phlegm.
	Pi Ba Ye	Folium Eriobotryae Japonicae	6	Ventilates the lung and unblocks the obstruction in the respiratory tract.
	Sang Ye	Folium Mori Albae	6	Ventilates the lung and expels the external wind-damp.
	Lai Fu Zi	Semen Raphani Sativi	9	Expels the accumulated damp and purges the intestinal function.
Guiding herb	Mai Ya	Maiya Fructus Hordei Vulgaris Germinantus	9	Harmonises the stomach and collates herbs to work effectively together.
	Da Zao	Fructus Zizyphi Jujubae	6	Harmonises the stomach and promotes cohesiveness of herbs.

Method: The above-mentioned herbal prescription is the main formula and can be used in combination with a variation of decoctions according to specific individual symptoms where the herbs are boiled and concentrated herbal powders are taken with warm water twice daily.

Analysis: Huo Xiang, Zi Su, and Xiang Ru eliminate the external Damp-Heat and dredge the blocked orifices as the main herbs. Jin Yin Hua and Sheng Jiang support dispelling of external Damp-Heat and clear Wind. Fu Ling and Chen Pi agitate and dredge stagnated *Qi* in the upper and middle burners. Wu Zhi Mao Tao and Cao Guo clear excessive heat and blocked orifices. Jie Gen, Pi Ba Ye, and Sang Ye dissipate stagnated lung *Qi* and Lai Fu Zi promotes the large intestine's movement. Da Zao and Mai Ya harmonise the Stomach and promote cohesiveness of herbs to clear orifices that are blocked and promote Upright *Qi* in the upper and middle burners.

Advice: This pattern can be seen when the pandemic dampness still exists as part of the post-COVID-19 syndrome, although patients encounter more stress or stomach problems, so some internal heat is mixed together with dampness. This is the commonest pattern to appear when a patient manifests loss of smell and loss of taste.

Damp accumulated at upper-middle burners with Lung-Spleen Qi Deficiency

Clinical features and signs: Signs are partial loss or reduced smell and taste or loss of smell and taste for an extended time, poor appetite, indigestion, bloated abdomen, loose bowel movement, fatigue and lethargy, general muscle heaviness, breathlessness with minor cough, light red tongue with less white coating, and a weak-fine pulse.

Treatment principle in TCM: Eliminate remaining *Dampness* and clear orifices; reinforce *Lung* and *Spleen Qi.*

Treatment: Herbal prescription.

Pinyin: Shen Ling Bai Zhu Decoction variation.

English name for decoction: Ginseng, Poria, and Atractylodis Macrocephalae Decoction variation.

Role in formula	Name/ Pinyin	Name/Latin	Dose (g)	Function
Chief herb	Ren Shen	Radix Ginseng	10	Reinforces the spleen and general *Qi*.
Deputy herb	Bai Zhu	Rhizoma Atractylodis Macrocephalae	10–30	Supports reinforcement of the spleen and general *Qi* and dries the excessive damp.
Assistant herb	Chen Pi	Pericarpium Citri Reticulatae	10	Supports reinforcement of the spleen *Qi* and dredges the stagnated *Qi* in the middle burner.
	Shan Yao	Radix Dioscoreae Oppositae	10	Promotes reinforcement of the spleen *Qi* and dries the dampness.
	Fu Ling	Sclerotium Poria Cocos	10	Releases the accumulated dampness.
	Sha Ren	Fructus Amomi	10	Dredges the stagnated stomach and harmonises the general *Qi*.

(*Continued*)

Role in formula	Name/ Pinyin	Name/Latin	Dose (g)	Function
	Yi Yi Ren	Semen Coicis Lachryma-Jobi	10–30	Eliminates the accumulated dampness and promotes diuresis.
	Jie Geng	Radix Platycodi Grandiflori	10	Ventilates the stagnated *Qi* in the upper and the middle burners.
	Bai Bian Dou	Semen Dolichoris Lablab	10	Nourishes the spleen *Yin* to ease diarrhoea.
	Lian Zi Rou	Semen Nelumbinis Nuciferae	10	Nourishes the spleen and heart *Yin* to tranquilise the mind.
Guiding herb	Gan Cao	Radix Glycyrrhizae Uralensis	5	Harmonises the stomach and promotes cohesiveness of herbs.

Method: The above-mentioned herbal prescription is the main formula and can be used in combination with a variation of decoctions according to specific individual symptoms where the herbs are boiled and the concentrated herbal powders are taken with warm water twice daily.

Analysis: Ren Shen, Bai Zhu, Fu Ling, and Gan Cao form Si Jun Zi Tang, a famous formula to reinforce *Spleen Qi* and promote general *Vitality Qi.* Sha Ren and Chen Pi harmonise the *Stomach* and support *Spleen Qi.* Bai Bian Dou and Shan Yao dry dampness and promote *Spleen Qi.* Jie Geng dredges the *Stagnated Qi* in the chest. Lian Zi Rou nourishes *Heart Qi* to tranquilise the mind. Yi Yi Ren reinforces *Spleen Qi* and dissipates excessive *Dampness* caused by *Spleen Deficiency.*

Advice: This pattern can be seen in patients exhibiting loss of smell and taste for extended periods of time which may be accompanied by chronic rhinitis or gastroesophageal reflux diseases as a pre-existing disease or complication, which is triggered by corona virus. If he/she has not accepted proper treatment, the loss of smell and loss of taste can easily become a chronic condition as part of the post-COVID-19 syndrome.

Acupuncture

Main points: Yintang (Ext), Lianquan (REN23).

Assistant points:

- If accompanied by loss of smell, use Yingxiang (LI20), Hegu (LI4).
- If accompanied by loss of taste, use Daying (ST5), Qihu (ST13).
- For damp-cold accumulation in the orifices, use Jiuwei (REN15), Zhongwan (REN12), Qihai (REN6), Neiting (ST44).
- For Damp-heat accumulation in the orifices, use Liangmen (ST21), Tianshu (ST25), Shuidao (ST28), Xiangu (ST43).
- For Damp accumulation in the lung and spleen deficiencies, use Kongzui (LU6), Yuji (LU10), Zusanli (ST36), Yinlingquan (SP9), Sanyinjiao (SP6).

Analysis: Yintang with Yingxiang and Hegu can dredge congestion in the nose and promote nasal function. Lianquan with Daying and Qihu can stimulate the *Stomach Qi* to promote blocked taste function. Jiuwei, Zhongwan, and Qihai can drive *Stomach Qi* by removing and eliminating excessive *Damp-Cold.* Liangmen, Tianshu, and Shuidao point along the *Stomach* meridian to encourage its function to eliminate *Damp-Heat.* Kongzui and Yuji agitate *Lung Qi.* Zusanli, Yinlingquan, and Sanyinjiao reinforce *Spleen Qi.* Neiting and Xiangu as the Stream-Ying point or Spring-Shu point of *Stomach* meridian are superior to dispel orifice blockage.

Case Study

Mr. T. Moor, a 58-year-old worker, visits the clinic as his abnormal taste in the mouth and loss of smell have lingered for 2 months. He does not know whether he suffers from COVID-19 or not. He has not had fever, cough, breathlessness, and other clinical symptoms common to COVID-19. He also denies suffering from Gastritis or Sinusitis in the past. He has done a PCR test in the test centre with a negative result that we double-check, confirming the negative result. When asked whether he had this kind of abnormal taste and loss of smell in the past, he recalls that he had similar symptoms in February of the present year, which lasted a couple of weeks, but did not receive treatment for them.

Current symptoms: Symptoms are a nasty taste with distension of the stomach, feeling of indigestion, dry mouth, gradual loss of smell, sluggish bowels with bloated abdomen, disturbed sleep with stress, a red tongue with white coating, and a floating and rolling pulse.

Diagnosis:

1. Post-COVID-19 syndrome.
2. Recurrent sensation disorders — abnormal taste and loss of smell.

Differentiation syndromes of TCM: *Damp-Heat* accumulation in the upper and middle burners.

Treatment: Herbal prescription and acupuncture.

Acupuncture

Main points: Lianquan (REN23), Yintang (Ext); Daying (ST5), Qihu (ST13), Tianshu (ST25), Shuidao (ST28); Baihui (DU20), Yinlingquan (SP9), Sanyinjiao (SP6); Hegu (LI4), Taichong (LIV3).

Herbal prescription

Pinyin: Huo Ling Shuang Hua Yin; Chai Hu Shu Gan Wan.

Result: When he returns to the clinic the following week, he feels 50% relief with regard to the nasty taste and is comfortable in his stomach after his bowel movements. We continue providing the above herbs and acupuncture treatment. All sense disorders are controlled in a month, and he is very pleased with this treatment.

Hearing Loss/Tinnitus

Hearing impairment, deafness, or hearing loss refers to the total or partial inability to hear sound. Symptoms may be mild, moderate, severe, or profound. A patient with a mild hearing impairment may have problems understanding speech, especially if there is a lot of noise in the background. Tinnitus is the patient's experience of ringing or other noises in one or both of ears. This noise does not exist in the environment; in other words, it is not an external sound, so other people cannot hear it. Tinnitus is very often the pre-symptom of deafness and is considered a manifestation of hearing impairment.

Loss of hearing and recurrent or permanent tinnitus can be seen in senior/aged patients after they have suffered from a COVID-19 infection, although it is not common like loss of smell and loss of taste. The development of the hearing impairment is gradual onset after the acute stage. Compared to other topics in previous chapters, this topic is less discussed.

Chirakkal *et al.* (2021) in Qatar reported a case of the damaging impact of the COVID-19 virus on hearing in the inner ear, and this finding has yet to be explored. Hearing loss and Tinnitus area common pathology seen in otolaryngology and there are numerous papers in the literature describing associations with other infections. Jafari *et al.* (2021) reviewed the available reports on Hearing Loss, Tinnitus, and Dizziness in COVID-19. The overall prevalence is hearing loss at 3.1%, tinnitus at 4.5%, and dizziness at 12.2%. The association between hearing loss and tinnitus and COVID-19 is confirmed.

The pathology of hearing impairment in COVID-19 has been speculated upon but not thoroughly investigated. First, inner ear damage is caused by the SARS-CoV-2 virus or autoimmune attack. Second, the ototoxicity side effects due to the use of drugs can cause sensorineural in the sound signal process from the inner ear to the brain. Third, vascular damage (clotting or bleeding) is caused in the brain, which leads to hearing problems in CNS (Fancello *et al.*, 2021).

Diagnosis

Except for a complaint of lower hearing with or without tinnitus, we should confirm the diagnosis of whether an impaired ear has existed and the degree of impairment by doing the following:

i. Inner ears are checked with otoscope.
ii. Special ear examination with ENT specialists.

iii. Audiometer test.
iv. Bone oscillator test.

Syndrome patterns of TCM

Hearing loss and tinnitus always appear together or one after another, and they are considered to be different symptoms of the same illness, so they are discussed together. They are classified as excess pattern and deficiency pattern. The excess pattern mainly reflects the accumulation of pathogenic factors in the *Gallbladder* Channel or *San Jiao* Channel which is distributed around the ear and inside the ear, with the internal links being mostly of the *Liver* and *Gallbladder*. On the contrary, the deficiency pattern is mainly concerned with the *Kidney* which opens into the ear and maintains the hearing. Based on this understanding, acupuncture should be a priority therapeutic choice for the conditions.

Excess pattern

Clinical figures and signs: Signs are sudden lost or lower hearing, distension in the ears, tinnitus-like chirping of cicadas or sound of sea tide, which is not eased if ears are pressed, some appear with a red complexion, dry mouth, annoyance and irritability, cough and breathlessness occasionally with more Phlegm, red tongue with yellow or white coating, and wiry or wiry-rapid pulse.

Treatment principle in TCM: Cleanse *Liver* and *Gallbladder Heat*; eliminate accumulated *Phlegm* and dredge block orifices.

Treatment: Herbal prescription and acupuncture.

Acupuncture

Body acupuncture:
Main points: Yinfeng (SJ17), Tinghui (GB2), Zhongzhu (SJ3), Jiaxi (GB43).

Assistant points: For *Liver* and *Gallbladder* fire flare-up, Taichong (LIV3) and Qiuxu (GB40) are added. For accumulated heat and phlegm, Fenglong (ST40) and Laogong (P2) are added.

Analysis: Yifeng and Zhongzhu are selected from the *San Jiao* meridian. Tinghui and Jiaxi at the Gallbladder meridian are also named as lesser yang meridian of the feet and eliminate the excessive heat and damp-phlegm. They can dredge the yang Qi in the lesser yang meridian and push the yang Qi to the ears as the main points. Taichong clears liver *Qi* and Qiuxu dissipates accumulated damp-heat from the gallbladder. Fenglong eliminates accumulated phlegm and Laogong dredges and agitates the orifices.

Other acupuncture technologies

Hand acupuncture: Ear point (a point at the inner side of the first joint of the thumb). New Hegu (a point at the combined point of the thumb and the forefinger, along the bone) for lower hearing and tinnitus.

Ear acupuncture: Subcortex (Pizhixia), Endocrine (Neifenmi), Liver, Kidney.

Electric acupuncture: Electric current is connected to needles attached to the body or ear acupuncture points, with a stronger stimulation 0.5–1 h, every other day.

Herbal prescription

Pinyin: Long Dan Xie Gan Tang.

English name for decoction: Gentiana Longdancao Decoction to Drain the Liver variation.

Role in formula	Name/ Pinyin	Name/Latin	Dose (g)	Function
Chief herb	Long Dan Cao	Radix Gentianae	6	Clears the excessive heat and dampness from the middle burner.
Deputy herb	Huang Qin	Radix Scutellariae Baicalensis	6	Clears the excessive heat and dampness from the upper burner.
	Zhi Zi	Fructus Gardeniae Jasminoidis	6	Clears the excessive heat and dampness from the upper and middle burners.
Assistant herb	Hua Shi	Talcum	15	Eliminates the excessive damp and promotes diuresis.
	Ze Xie	Rhizoma Alismatis Plantago-aquaticae	6	Eliminates the excessive dampness and promotes diuresis.

(*Continued*)

Role in formula	Name/ Pinyin	Name/Latin	Dose (g)	Function
	Tong Cao	Caulis Mutong	5	Eliminates the excessive damp and promotes diuresis.
	Dang Gui	Radix Angelicae Sinensis	6	Cultivates the liver blood and nourishes the liver *Yin*.
	Shen Di Huang	Radix Rehmanniae Glutinosae	9	Nourishes the liver and kidney *Yin* and general *Yin*.
Guiding herb	Chai Hu	Radix Bupleuri	5	Dredges the stagnated *Qi* and leads herbs to affect the middle burner.

Method: The above-mentioned herbal prescription is the main formula and can be used in combination with a variation of decoctions according to specific individual symptoms where the herbs are boiled and the concentrated herbal powders are taken with warm water twice daily.

Analysis: Long Dan Cao, Huang Qin, and Zhi Zi cleanse the *Liver, Gallbladder*, and all heat from the upper burner. Hua Ṣhi, Ze Xie, and Tong Cao dissipate accumulated *Damp* and *Phlegm*. Dang Gui and Sheng Di soften the *Liver* and *Gallbladder Yin* and *Blood*. Chai Hu leads all the herbs to the *Liver* and *Gallbladder* and dredges accumulated *Qi* through the orifices.

Advice: This pattern can be seen with lost hearing and sudden occurrence of tinnitus with loud noise. If a patient maintains a good constitution without deficiency, the disease cannot last for a long time as part of the post-COVID-19 syndrome.

Deficiency pattern

Clinical features and signs: Signs are gradual diminished hearing or lost hearing, intermittent tinnitus on and off, which is a fine-dull sound aggravated by exertion and eased if ears are pressed, dizziness, sore back, nocturnal emission, more vaginal discharge, light red tongue with white coating, and a weak-fine pulse.

Treatment principle in TCM: Reinforce *Kidney Yin* and *Essence*; fill *Qi* and *Blood* into orifices.

Acupuncture

Main points: Yifeng (SJ17), Tinghui (GB3), Qihai (REN6), Guanyuan (REN4).

Assistant points: Taixi (KI3), Zhaohai (KI6), Yingu (KI10), Zusanli (ST36), Diwuhui (GB42); or Ganshu (BL18), Shenshu (BL23), Mingmen (DU4), Yaoyangguan (DU3).

Analysis: Yifeng and Tinghui are local to ears and the lesser *Yang* meridian in the hand and foot and help to dredge accumulated *Qi* and *Damp-Heat* in the orifices as the main points. Qihai and guanyuan excite the *Vitality Qi* and *Essence* as the main points. Taixi, Zhaohai, and Yingu strengthen the Kidney *Qi* and *Essence*. Zusanli reinforces the *Spleen* to promote the *Post-Heaven Qi.* Diwuhui dredges the *Gallbladder Qi* to support the orifices.

Other acupuncture technologies

Abdomen acupuncture: Jiuwei (REN15), Zhongwan (REN12), Qihai (REN6), Zhongji (REN3) lead *Qi* to the *Vitality Gate.*

Treatment: Herbal prescription.

Pinyin: Yi Qi Cong Ming decoction variation.

English name for decoction: Augment the *Qi* and Increase Acuity Decoction variation.

Role in formula	Name/ Pinyin	Name/Latin	Dose (g)	Function
Chief herb	Huang Qi	Radix Astragali Membranacei	10–15	Builds up vitality *Qi* and general upright *Qi* to excite the self-healing function.
Deputy herb	Ren Shen	Radix Ginseng	6	Replenishes the spleen *Qi*, the kidney *Qi*, and vitality *Qi*.

(*Continued*)

Role in formula	Name/ Pinyin	Name/Latin	Dose (g)	Function
Assistant herb	Bai Shao	Radix Paeoniae Lactiflorae	6	Nourishes the *Yin* and blood to complement the orifices.
	Ge Gen	Radix Puerariae	6	Expels the external and internal damp-wind.
	Huang Bai	Cortex Phellodendri	6	Clears the empty heat and nourishes the kidney to replenish the ears.
	Sheng Ma	Rhizoma Cimicifugae	5	Dredges all stagnated *Qi* and leads to ascension of the herbs affecting the top of the body.
Guiding herb	Man Jing Zi	Fructus Viticis	6	Nourishes the liver and kidney *Yin* and leads to ascension of herbs affecting to the top of the body.
	Gan Cao	Radix Glycyrrhizae Uralensis	5	Harmonises the stomach and promotes cohesiveness of herbs.

Method: The above-mentioned herbal prescription is the main formula and can be used in combination with a variation of decoctions according to specific individual symptoms where the herbs are boiled and the concentrated herbal powders are taken with warm water twice daily.

Analysis: Huang Qi and Ren Shen build up *Vitality Qi* and general *Upright Qi* to agitate the self-healing function as the main herbs. Bai Shao nourishes the *Yin* and softens the *Liver.* Ge Gen, Man Jing Zi, and Sheng Ma lead *Yang Qi* to ascend to the top of body and fill it into the orifices. Hung Bai cleanses the remaining *Heat* and dries the *Damp*. Gan Cao harmonises all herbs to work together. This formula stimulates all the orifices and is a famous formula to treat poor and lost hearing.

Advice: This pattern can be seen in all stages, during, and after a prolonged infection of COVID-19. The herbal prescription can also be used by patients with deficiency and mixed *Essence-Deficiency* as part of post-COVID-19 syndrome, which exhibit loss or poor hearing, or every type of tinnitus.

Case Study

Ms. E. Jorden, 68 years old, a retired teacher, has been suffering from tinnitus for over a year after she was infected with coronavirus. She and her husband were infected with COVID-19, but not a severe infection; they rested, isolated, and self-treated at home after they had a positive PCR, and healed in 2 weeks. However, she still suffered from intermittent tinnitus since then, possibly lower hearing also, which is why she visited the clinic for treatment.

Clinical symptoms: Tinnitus had materialised for her more or less on and off, with loud or soft sounds. She ignored the tinnitus in the daytime due to her busy daily life, but it bothered her a lot during the night, leading to disturbing sleep, waking up a lot during the night, frequent urination, sore back, a light red tongue with less coating, and a wiry-fine pulse.

Diagnosis:

1. Post-syndrome of COVID-19 — Tinnitus.
2. Lower hearing.
3. Back pain.

Treatment: Herbal prescription and acupuncture.

Acupuncture: Baihui (DU20), Yifeng (SJ17), Tinghui (GB3); Jiuwei (REN15), Zhongwan (REN12), Qihai (REN6), Zhongji (REN3); Yingu (KI10), Taixi (KI3), Zhaohai (KI6), Waiguan (SJ5), Zulinqi (GB41).
The above acupuncture is done once every 2 weeks.

Herbal prescription

Pinyin: Zhi Bai Di Huang Wan plus Er Long Zuo Ci Wan.

Result: The patient felt much better after acupuncture. Her tinnitus occasionally disappeared, but recurred after 4–5 days. She felt okay in the daytime, but she still recognised tinnitus during the night; therefore, we agreed to continue the treatment.

Vision Changes

The eyes, nerves relating to vision, and the muscles around the eye socket could all be affected in COVID-19 sufferers. However, Glaucoma, Cataract, and some Retina disorders might be accelerated or triggered if the patients are in the later middle age or early 60–70s. These will lead to vision changes, which are not discussed in this section, for which surgical solution is the best choice. Referring to Ophthalmologist for better diagnosis and treatment is always recommended.

According to Feng *et al.* (2021), among 400 patients of COVID-19, patients with average age of 61 were hospitalised. Ocular signs and symptoms were recognised in 38 (9.5%) patients. The most common ocular problems were conjunctivitis infection, vision changes, and ocular irritation. Among the 38 patients who developed eye and vision problems, 30 (79.0%) developed the problems within 30 days of onset of their COVID-19 symptoms. Analysis showed that age, gender, ocular history, fever, mechanical ventilation, and increasing inflammatory markers were not significantly associated with the presence or development of ocular symptoms. This report echoes some other reports in recognising that conjunctivitis affected 1–3% of people with COVID-19. The infection is not directly caused by the virus as there is not enough evidence on this. Sadhu *et al.* (2020) reported uveitis, a form of eye inflammation affecting the middle layer in the uvea (eye wall), in patients of COVID-19 at a higher than usual rate.

Diagnosis

Conjunctivitis is inflammation produced on the outermost layer of the sclera of the eyes and the inner surface of the eyelids. It makes the eyes appear pink or reddish, and pain, burning, scratchiness, or itchiness may occur. The affected eye may have increased tears or be "stuck shut" in the morning. It can affect one or both eyes. This kind of eye inflammation can be caused by coronavirus or could be a recurrent inflammation as part of the post-COVID-19 syndrome.

Uveitis depends on the type of inflammation. Acute anterior uveitis may occur in one or both eyes and is characterised by eye pain, blurred vision, sensitivity to light, a small pupil, and redness. Intermediate uveitis causes blurred vision and floaters.

Some types of uveitis are caused by allergic reactions, so a special test should be done to identify the cause of this allergic reaction.

MRI, CT scan, and X-ray should be done in some cases to identify whether another disease is the cause.

Differentiation syndromes of TCM and herbal treatment

Inflammatory eye diseases are commonly caused by the *Wind-Heat* accumulated at the upper burner or *Liver Fire* flares with redness in the eyes as the main symptom.

Wind-Heat accumulation at the upper burner

Clinical features and signs: Signs are red eyes suddenly appearing or recurring, with soreness, burning, and itching, much tearing, eyes "stuck shut" in the morning, headache, light-headedness, blurred vision, occasional catarrhal and cough, a light red tongue with less white coating, and a floating-rapid pulse.

Treatment principle in TCM: Cleanse *Wind-Heat* from exterior; ventilate *Lung* and clear eyes.

Treatment: Herbal prescription and acupuncture.

Acupuncture

Main points: Jingming (BL1), Taiyang (Ext), Hegu (LI4), Taichong (LIV3).

Assistant points: Shaoshang (LU11), Shangxing (DU23), Fengchi (GB20), Quchi (LI11).

Analysis: Jingming is the united point for 5 meridians of the *Large Yang* in the hand and feet. *Bright Yang*, *Yin*, and *Yang* heal vessels, so they can quickly cleanse *Wind-Heat* at the exterior as a main point. Taiyang can release external *Wind-Heat* and clear the eyes. Hegu and Taichong as the four gate points eliminate excessive *Heat* and dredge the *Liver Qi* to promote the circulation in the eyes. Shaoshang as the Well-Jing point of the *Lung* meridian dissipates excessive *Wind-Heat* from the exterior. Fengchi can eliminate *Wind* and Quchi can cleanse *Heat*. Shangxing agitates the upper *Yang* to lead the effect of all the needles to the top of the body.

Herbal prescription

Pinyin: Yin Qiao Jie Du Tang variation.

English name for decoction: Honeysuckle and Forsythia Decoction to Overcome Pathogenic Toxicity variation.

Role in formula	Name/ Pinyin	Name/Latin	Dose (g)	Function
Chief herb	Jin Yin Hua	Flos Lonicerae Japonicae	9	Cleanses the external wind and heat to control the virus.
Deputy herb	Lian Qiao	Fructus Forsythiae Suspensae	6	Cleanse the external wind and heat to control the virus.
Assistant herb	Zhu Qe	Herba Lophatheri Gracilis	6	Cleanses the external and internal wind-heat.
	Niu Bang Zi	Fructus Arctii Lappae	6	Expels the external wind-dampness.
	Bo He	Herba Menthae Haplocalycis	5	Cleanses the external wind-heat and unblocks the orifices of the upper head.
	Jing Jie	Herba seu Flos Schizonepetae Tenuifoliae	6	Ventilates the lung and eases the cough.
	Ju Hua	Flos Chrysanthemi Morifolii	9	Expels the external wind-heat, and leads all the herbs towards the head and eyes.
	Lu Gen	Rhizoma Phragmitis Communis	12	Cleanses the internal heat and cools the blood.
Guiding herb	Man Jing Zi	Fructus Viticis	9	Moistens the liver *Yin* and blood to nourish the eyes.
	Gan Cao	Radix Glycyrrhizae Uralensis	5	Harmonises the stomach and promotes cohesiveness of herbs.

Method: The above-mentioned herbal prescription is the main formula and can be used in combination with a variation of decoctions according to specific individual symptoms where the herbs are boiled and the concentrated herbal powders are taken with warm water twice daily.

Analysis: Jin Yin Hua and Lian Qiao cleanse the external Wind and Heat to control the virus as the main herbs. Zhu Ye and Lu Gen support cleansing of the heat and cooling of the blood. Niu Bang Zi dissipates external wind. Bo He and Jing Jie eliminate external wind and dredge accumulated *Qi* in the orifices, or eyes. Man Jing Zi leads all herbs effectively towards the eyes and Gan Cao clears heat and harmonises all of herbs to work cohesively.

Advice: This pattern can be seen in an allergy or viral inflammation occurring in the eyes for a short time, so the acupuncture and herbs should heal them quickly. We can also see that individuals with recurrent eye inflammation have post-COVID-19 syndrome; therefore, acupuncture and herbs can stop the allergic inflammation from getting worse.

Liver Fire flare-up

Clinical features and signs: Signs are redness of the eyes with burning sensation, itching, and tearing; headache; easily getting upset; irritability; loss of temper; bitter taste and dry mouth; constipation; poor sleep during which is it hard to fall asleep or having bad dreams; a red tongue with yellow or dry coating; and a wiry or wiry-heat pulse.

Treatment principle in TCM: Cleanse excessive *Liver Heat;* improve eyesight.

Treatment: Herbal prescription and acupuncture.

Acupuncture

Main points: Baihui (DU20), Shenting (DU24), Tongziliao (GB1), Zanzhu (BL2).

Assistant points: Waiguan (SJ5), Zulinqi (GB42), Jiaxi (GB43), Xingjian (LIV2).

Explanation: Baihui and shenting tranquilise the mind and agitate the general *Yang Qi*. Tongziliao cleanses *Liver Heat* and dredges stagnated *Liver Qi* as the point in the *Gallbladder* meridian near the eyes. Zanzhu as the Stream-Ying point of the *Bladder* meridian dredges the general stagnated *Qi* and improves vision. Waiguan and Zulinqi ventilate the general stagnated *Qi* to calm the mind and bring down the heat. Jiaxi and Xingjian as Stream-Ying points in the *Gallbladder* and *Liver* regulate *Stagnated Qi* in both *Yin* and *Yang* meridians.

Herbal prescription

Pinyin: Jia Wei Xiao Yao Tang variation.

English name for decoction: Rambling Decoction variation.

Role in formula	Name/ Pinyin	Name/Latin	Dose (g)	Function
Chief herb	Chai Hu	Radix Bupleuri	10	Dredges the liver *Qi* and releases the stress to encourage the *Qi* to flow in the meridians.
Deputy herb	Dang Gui	Radix Angelicae Sinensis	10	Softens the liver and cultivates the liver *Yin* and blood to nourish the eyes.
Assistant herb	Chi Shao	Radix Paeoniae Rubrae	10	Activates the blood stasis and softens the liver to help the *Qi* and blood circulation in the eyes.
	Fu Ling	Sclerotium Poria Cocos	10	Replenishes the spleen and dries the accumulated damp.
	Bai Zhu	Rhizoma Atractylodis Macrocephalae	10	Replenishes the spleen and strengthens the muscles.
	Gan Jiang	Rhizoma Zingiberis Officinalis	10	Warms and excites the spleen *Qi* and general *Qi*.
	Bo He	Herba Menthae Haplocalycis	5	Leads all the effective herbs to the top of the body and releases the external wind to unblock *Qi* circulation.
	Mu Dan Pi	Cortex Moutan Radicis	10	Clears the excessive heat in the liver and general heat in the blood to cleanse the heat in the eyes.

(*Continued*)

(*Continued*)

Role in formula	Name/ Pinyin	Name/Latin	Dose (g)	Function
	Zhi Zi	Fructus Gardeniae Jasminoidis	10	Clears the excessive heat in the liver and heart to encourage relaxation and cleanse the heat in the eyes.
	Gan Cao	Radix Glycyrrhizae Uralensis	5	Harmonises the stomach and promotes cohesiveness of the herbs.

If there is severe soreness and redness in the eyes, Man Jing Zi and Bai Zhi should be added. If severe inflammation causes more heat with *Dampness,* Long Dan Cao is added.

Method: The above-mentioned herbal prescription is the main formula and can be used in combination with a variation of decoctions according to specific individual symptoms where the herbs are boiled and the concentrated herbal powders are taken with warm water twice daily.

Analysis: Chai Hu dredges the stagnated *Liver Qi* without using a higher dose. Mu Dan Pi and Zhi Zi cleanse excessive *Liver* and *Blood Heat* as the main herbs. Dang Gui and Bai Shao harmonise the *Liver* and nourish *Liver Blood* and *Yin.* Bai Zhu and Fu Ling reinforce the *Spleen* to stabilise the immune reaction. Sheng Di Huang promotes and nourishes *Liver Yin* and *Blood.* Long Dan Cao promotes and clears excessive Heat-Damp. Mang Jing Zi and Bai Zhi improve the eyesight and lead all herbs to influence the eyes. Gan Cao unifies all herbs, promoting cohesiveness, and harmonises the stomach.

Advice: This pattern can be seen in the acute or chronic stage, with a brief or extended diseased pathology, and is commonly seen in patients with stress. An allergic eye inflammation can be aggravated or triggered by stress or accompanied by negative mood attacks as part of the post-COVID-19 syndrome.

Case Study

Ms. J. Wilson, 64 years old, a retired teacher, was suffering from recurrent conjunctivitis for half a year after she healed from COVID-19. She was infected with COVID-19 at the end of 2020 and manifested fever and cough at the beginning, with red and itchy eyes appearing later. She was given antibiotics and painkillers to control the inflammation and temperature. After a week, her symptoms were controlled well. The higher temperature was not present; however, she suffered from the recurrent red and itching eyes for half a year. An antihistamine was used, but the redness and itching continued for 2 weeks. This is what prompted her to go to the clinic for treatment.

Clinical features and signs: Signs are red and itching eyes with significant tearing, congestion in the eyes and eyelids, itching does not occur all the time, blocked nose with a dull smell, bloated stomach with indigestion, stress, irritability, a red tongue with less white coating, and a wiry-rapid pulse. The PCR is negative.

Diagnosis:

1. Post-COVID-19 syndrome.
2. Recurrent Conjunctivitis.

Differentiation syndromes of TCM:

1. *Liver Qi* stagnation.
2. *Liver Heat* flare-up.

Treatment: Acupuncture only.

Acupuncture:

Main points: Baihui (DU20), Yintang (Ext), Taiyang (Ext); Sangxing (DU24), Fengchi (GB20), Hegu (LI4), Yingxiang (LI20); Ququan (LIV8), Taichong (LIV3).

Result: After she was done acupuncture once a week with a herbal eye drop, she has been recovered completely after 3 weeks.

References

Braz-Silva, P. H., Mamana, A. C., Romano, C. M., Felix, A. C., de Paula, A. V., *et al.* (2021). Performance of at-home self-collected saliva and nasal-oropharyngeal swabs in the surveillance of COVID-19. *Journal of Oral Microbiology*. 13(1), PMC7733974. https://doi.org/10.1080/00016357.2020.1787505.

Chirakkal, P., Al Hail, A., Zada, N., *et al.* (2021). COVID-19 and tinnitus. *Ear, Nose & Throat Journal*, 100(2_suppl), 160S–162S. doi:10.1177/0145561320974849.

Doty, R. L., Shaman, P., Kimmelman, C. P., and Dann, M. S. (1984). University of Pennsylvania smell identification test: A rapid quantitative olfactory function test for the clinic. *Laryngoscope*, 94(2 Pt 1), 176–178. doi:10.1288/00005537-198402000-00004. PMID: 6694486.

Fancello, V., Hatzopoulos, S., Corazzi, V., *et al.* (2021). SARS-CoV-2 (COVID-19) and audio-vestibular disorders. *International Journal of Immunopathology and Pharmacology*. 35, 20587384211027373. Published online 2021 Jun 18. doi: 10.1177/20587384211027373.

Feng, Y., Park, J., Zhou, Y., *et al.* (2021). Ocular manifestations of hospitalized COVID-19 patients in a tertiary care academic medical center in the United States: A cross-sectional study. *Clinical Ophthalmology*, 13(15), 1551–1556. doi:10.2147/OPTH.S301040.

Fortunato, F., Martinelli, D., Iannelli, G., *et al.* (2022). Self-reported olfactory and gustatory dysfunctions in COVID-19 patients: A 1-year follow-up study in Foggia district, Italy. *BMC Infectious Diseases*, 22, 77. https://doi.org/10.1186/s12879-022-07052-8.

Jafari, Z., Kolb, B., and Mohajerani, M. (2021). Hearing loss, tinnitus, and dizziness in COVID-19: A systematic review and meta-analysis. *Canada Journal of Neurological Science*, 12,1–12.doi:10.1017/cjn.2021.63.

Lechien, J., Chiesa-Estomba, C., De Siati, D., *et al.* (2020). Olfactory and gustatory dysfunctions as a clinical presentation of mild-to-moderate forms of the coronavirus disease (COVID-19): A multi center European study. *European Archives of Oto-rhino-laryngology*, 277(8), 2251–2261. doi:10.1007/s00405-020-05965-1.

Othman, B. A., Maulud, S. Q., Jalal, P. J., Abdul Kareem, S. M., Ahmed, J. Q., *et al.* (2022). Olfactory dysfunction as a post-infectious symptom of SARS-CoV-2 infection. *Annals of Medicine and Surgery*, 75, 103352.https://doi.org/10.1016/j.amsu.2022.103352.

Sadhu, S., Agrawal, R., Pyare, R., *et al.* (2020). COVID-19: Limiting the risks for eye care professionals. *Ocular Immunology and Inflammation*, 28(5),714–720. doi:10.1080/09273948.2020.1755442.

Vaira, L. A., Hopkins, C., Petrocelli, M., *et al.* (2020). Smell and taste recovery in coronavirus disease 2019 patients: A 60-day objective and prospective study. *Journal of Laryngology and Otology*, 134(8), 703–709. doi:10.1017/S0022215120001826.

Chapter 13

Reproductive Disorders

It was well known that the reproductive system is vulnerable to viral infection and could be seriously damaged if one is infected. Examples include the damage to testicles in men due to mumps infection. It was observed that male and female reproductive systems could be impaired by infection in the broader context. The impairments could be caused directly by the virus invading into cells in the system or the immune reaction. The COVID-19 virus is infecting people of all age groups, and the damage to the reproductive system was not a concern of acute COVID-19, but is a concern in the long and post-COVID-19 stage.

The existing reproductive conditions might not be the focus of research. However, newly added or diagnosed orchitis and prostatitis were reported in men, related to sperm disorders and hormone disorders. This could eventually result in infertility. Reproductive disorders were less reported in women; however, the authors' observations suggest that there are obvious delays in menstruation cycles in and an increased risk of miscarriage possibly due to the high level of stress or PTSD, which is a known factor for miscarriage. Sexual function is inevitably affected due to the huge influence of the change in personal life, with the lockdown leading to limited social connections, and the stress caused during the infection.

Inflammatory Impairment in Reproductive Organs

It was speculated that due to the existence of the ACE-2 receptor on the membrane of the testicle and prostate gland, the SARS-CoV-2 virus could easily invade into those structures, and it is possible thereafter that the semen could carry the virus. However, He *et al.* (2021) reviewed the available evidence and found that only one report found SARS-CoV-2 in samples. All others did not find the virus in semen. But the infection did lower the sperm count and quality. The findings suggest that most of the damage was caused by non-infectious inflammation resulting from an immune system response to the infection in other systems.

In another review, Sansone *et al.* (2021) investigated the male problem of Ejaculation Disorder (ED) and suggested that ED is possibly much broader than reported and the cause of ED due to COVID-19 could be multifaceted. The endothelial dysfunction, subclinical hypogonadism, could directly lower the function of the male organ. Psychological factors and lower oxygen due to pulmonary impairment and cardiovascular impairment are also strongly linked to the male function. Test results suggested that the testicular function of producing the male hormone and sperm is obviously lower in many cases.

In female cases, it is easy to understand that female hormone production could be suppressed due to acute stress response, the fight or flight response. This could lead to long-term impairments due to the lack of supply of oxygen and nutrition if the blood supply reduction lasted longer.

The whole female system is also rich in blood vessels and could be affected by the whole-body circulatory impairment which was discussed in previous chapters. After the stress stage, the blood vessels could behave differently and blood congestion could happen to those organs.

Diagnosis

Clinical symptoms: For men, symptoms are pain in the scrotum, swelling in the back of the testicle in the coiled tubes (epididymitis), and swelling and pain in one or both testicles (orchitis). A sperm test and ultrasound are commonly used to confirm the diagnosis on inflammation. For women, symptoms are pain around the pelvic region or lower abdomen, discomfort or pain during sexual activity or urination, heavier or painful periods, and more vaginal discharge with white or yellow colour. Internal examination and swabs which are taken from the vagina and the cervix of the uterus are used to confirm the inflammation, after which possibly an internal ultrasound is done.

Syndrome patterns and TCM treatment

Damp-Heat accumulation at the lower burner

Clinical features and signs: Signs for men are pain in the scrotum or testicles; signs for women are pain in the vagina with more discharge of white or yellow colour and burning during urination or increased frequency. Signs for both men and women are lower abdominal pain and aching in the lower back as well, a red tongue with yellow-greasy coating at the base of the tongue, and a rolling-rapid pulse.

Treatment principle in TCM: Dissipate accumulated *Damp* and cleanse excessive *Heat.*

Treatment: Herbal prescription and acupuncture.

Acupuncture

Main points: Qihai (REN6), Zhongji (REN3), Dahe (KI12).

Assistant points: Fuliu (KI7), Rengu (KI2), Jinggu (BL64), Tonggu (BL66).

Analysis: Zhongji accompanied by Dahe as the main point stimulates the conception vessel and *Kidney* to eliminate excessive *Damp* and *Heat.* Qihai supports Zhongji to excite the *Conceptive Vessel* to dredge excess fluid. Fuliu and Rangu as the River-Jing point and Stream-Ying point of the *Kidney* meridian eliminate excessive *Damp* and heat. Jinggu as the original point and Tonggu as the Stream-Ying point of the *Bladder* meridian eliminate the excessive pathogenic *Damp-Heat* with a stronger intensity.

Herbal prescription

Pinyin: Si Miao variated with Long Dan Xie Gan Tang.

English and Latin: Mysterious Four Decoction variated Gentiana Longdancao Decoction to Drain the Liver.

Role in formula	Name/ Pinyin	Name/Latin	Dose (g)	Function
Chief herb	Huang Bai	Cortex Phellodendri	10	Eliminates excessive damp and heat at the lower burner.
Deputy herb	Cang Zhu	Rhizoma Atractylodis	10	Dries the excessive dampness.
Assistant herb	Long Dan Cao	Radix Gentianae	10	Releases the excessive damp-heat from the middle and lower burners.
	Yi Yi Ren	Semen Coicis Lachryma-Jobi	30	Eliminates the damp-fluid and promotes diuresis.
	Hua Shi	Talcum	15	Eliminates the damp-fluid and promotes diuresis.
	Ze Xie	Rhizoma Alismatis Orientalis	10	Eliminates the damp-fluid and promotes diuresis.
	Chai Hu	Radix Bupleuri	10	Dredges the stagnated *Qi* and relaxes *Qi* flow movement.
	Dang Gui	Radix Angelicae Sinensis	10	Softens the liver and nourishes the liver blood.
Guiding herb	Gan Cao	Radix Glycyrrhizae Uralensis	5	Harmonises the stomach and promotes cohesiveness of herbs.
	Chuan Niu Xi	Radix Cyathulae Officinalis	15	Leads all the herbs to descend to the lower burner and activates the blood stasis.

Method: The above-mentioned herbal prescription is the main formula and can be used in combination with a variation of decoctions according to specific individual symptoms where the herbs are boiled and the concentrated herbal powders are taken with warm water twice daily.

Analysis: Huang Bai and Cang Zhu as the main herbs eliminate excessive *Damp* and *Heat* at the lower burner. Chuan Ni Xi leads all of herbal effects to the lower body and activates the *Blood* to ease abdominal pain. Yi Yi Ren dissipates excessive *Damp*. Long Dan Cao is added to support and cleanse *Heat*. Hua Shi and Ze Xie are added to promote *Damp* elimination. Chai Hu dredges and excites *Qi* movement. Dang Gui softens the *Liver* and *Kidney*. Gan Cao harmonises all the herbs and prevents them being too cool in nature to protect the *Stomach*.

Advice: This pattern can commonly be seen in young people who suffer from a systematic inflammation with many organs involved, but they still possess a general good constitution with stronger pathogenic factors, with no deficiency signs during long COVID-19. Therefore, these herbs can take effect quickly.

Empty Heat accumulation over the Liver and Kidney as Yin Deficiency

Clinical features and signs: Signs for men are dull aching at one or both testicles of the scrotums, slower urination, or premature ejaculation; signs for women are, frequent urination, more vaginal discharge, tinnitus, hot flashes, and waking up during the night or early morning. Signs for both men and women are recurring inflammation of reproductive organs, a dull aching at the lower abdomen, and lower back, a red tongue without coating, and a wiry-fine pulse.

Treatment principle in TCM: Nourish *Liver* and *Kidney Yin*; cleanse *Empty Heat* from lower burner.

Treatment: Herbal prescription and acupuncture.

Acupuncture

Main points: Baihui (DU20), Guangyuan (REN4), Qixue (KI13).

Assistant points: Yanyangguan (DU3), Liver (BL18), Kidney (BL23), Yingu (KI10); Taixi (KI3), Zhaohai (KI6), Houxi (SJ3), Shenmai (BL62).

Analysis: Baihui accompanied by Yaoyangguan excites the general *Yang Qi* to eliminate *Damp-Heat*. Guanyuan accompanied by Qixue promotes *Qi* flow in the conception vessel and excites *Vitality Qi*. Taixi as the original Yuan point accompanied by Zhaohai strengthens the *Kidney*. Houxi and shenmai as 8 cross points dissipate empty *Damp-Heat*. All points can be efficient in eliminating *Damp-Heat* and reinforcing the *Kidney* and *Liver* to treat chronic and recurrent inflammation.

Herbal prescription

Pinyin: Zhi Bai Di Huang Tang variation.

English name for decoction: Anemarrhena, Phellodendron, and Rehmannia Decoction variation.

Role in formula	Name/ Pinyin	Name/Latin	Dose (g)	Function
Chief herb	Sheng Di Huang	Radix Rehmanniae Glutinosae	10–30	Nourishes the kidney *Yin* and clears the empty heat.
	Huang Bai	Cortex Phellodendri	10	Releases the empty heat and dries the dampness.
Deputy herb	Mu Dan Pi	Cortex Moutan Radicis	10	Clears the heat in the blood, kidney, and lower burner.
	Zhi Mu	Radix Anemarrhenae Asphodeloidis	10	Emphasises to nourish the kidney *Yin* and clears the empty heat.
Assistant herb	Zhan Zhu Yu	Fructus Corni Officinalis	10	Nourishes the kidney *Yin* and essence.
	Shan Yao	Radix Dioscoreae Oppositae	10	Replenishes the spleen *Qi* and dries the dampness.
	Fu Ling	Sclerotium Poria Cocos	10	Dries the dampness and replenishes the spleen.
	Ze Xie	Rhizoma Alismatis Orientalis	10	Dredges the stagnated *Qi* and accumulated dampness.
	Tu Fu Ling	Rhizoma Smilacis Glabrae	15–30	Dries the dampness and releases excessive discharge from the vagina.
	Ku Shen	Radix Sophorae Flavescentis	10	Dries the damp-heat and eases the itchiness outside the vagina.

Method: The above-mentioned herbal prescription is the main formula and can be used in combination with a variation of decoctions according to specific individual symptoms where the herbs are boiled and the concentrated herbal powders are taken with warm water twice daily.

Analysis: Huang Bai and Zhi Mu dry *Damp*, cleanse *Heat*, and nourish *Yin* as the main herbs. Sheng Di Huang nourishes the *Kidney Yin and* stabilises the immune system with a bigger dose. Shan Zhu Yu and Shan Yao reinforce the *Kidney* and *Spleen* to promote *Damp* diuresis. Mu Dan Pi cleanses heat. Ze Xie and Fu Ling dissipate *Damp*. Tu Fu Ling and Ku Shen are added into the formula to promote dry *Damp* and cleanse *Heat* to stop the inflammation from occurring at the lower burner.

Advice: This pattern is commonly seen in chronic or recurrent inflammation of reproductive organs in both men and women with long COVID-19. This pattern is a mixture of excess and deficiency in which there is a robust pathogenic factor, but deficiency of general constitution.

Case Study

Mr. W. He, 28 years old, Ph.D. student, requests help for his fever and dull aching of the lower abdominal and groin, present for a week. He has a fever of 37.4, a dull pain of the low abdomen, distension, and pain at the groin and testicles. He says he has been worried since some classmates suffered from COVID-19. He is confused whether these symptoms can indicate infection or not, and whether he needs treatment.

After further enquiry, he confirms he feels some abdominal discomfort while he is running, and soreness and pain when the left of his scrotum is pressed. He has a red tongue with white greasy coating, thick at the base. Due to worry regarding COVID-19, he has not gone to a hospital for a PCR test.

Diagnosis:

1. Suspected COVID-19.
2. Seminal vasculitis.

Differentiation syndromes of TCM: *Heat* and *Dampness* accumulated within and spread throughout the three burners.

Treatment: Herbal prescription.

Pinyin: Hou Po Xia Ling Tang variated with Si Miao Decoction.

English name for decoction: Agastaches, Magnolia Bark, Pinellia, and Poria Decoction variated with Si Miao Mysterious Four Decoction.

Herbal powders (g):

Huang Lian	Rhizoma Coptidis 10 g
Hou Po	Cortex Magnoliae Officinalis 10 g
Huang Bai	Cortex Phellodendri 10 g
Cang Zhu	Rhizoma Atractylodis 10 g
Chuan Niu Xi	Radix Cyathulae Officinalis 15 g
Yi Yi Ren	Semen Coicis Lachryma-Jobi 30 g
Ze Xie	Rhizoma Alismatis Orientalis 10 g
Chi Shao	Radix Paeoniae Rubrae 10 g
Dan Shen	Radix Salviae Miltiorrhizae 10 g
Jiang Ban Xia	Rhizoma Pinelliae Ternatae 15 g
Fu Ling	Sclerotium Poriae Cocos 10 g
Gan Cao	Radix Glycyrrhizae Uralensis 5 g

The above herbs are made into a herbal juice and taken twice daily, for a week.

Result and analysis:
After he takes the herbal decoction for a week, pain at the abdomen, groin, and scrotum is less, the temperature has gone down to normal, and the greasy coating on his tongue is less as well. He is told to consume Si Miao Pills and Chai Hu Shu Gan Pills until all his symptoms are completely controlled.

According to reports in China, many young men who are infected with COVID-19 have complications relating to inflammation of the reproductive organs, leaving them with post-COVID-19 syndrome after they have healed from the infection in the lungs. The inflammation of the reproductive organs can gradually heal, but leaves some adhesion and scars in the testicle(s) or prostate(s), which may disturb stored sperm. This causes issues with producing sperm, causing malformation and low sperm count, contributing to the potential for infertility. If this presentation occurs, this will influence the later life of this young man. Therefore, adding Dan Shen and Chi Shao to the main prescription is important, and so is using Si Miao with Chai Hu Shu Gan pills for preventing adhesion and inflammation in the reproductive organs after eliminating coronavirus in the whole body in addition to the main prescription.

Irregular Menstruation

Irregular menstruation means some abnormal menstrual circles, of shorter or longer duration than the normal cycles, heavier or lighter in menstrual volume, unusual clotting of period blood, or worsened premenstrual syndromes (PMS). Most cases of menstruation cycle changes take place immediately after the infection. Some found that their menstruation stops and starts long after the infection is cleared. The irregularity is a long trend in the post-COVID-19 stage. For almost all who had premenstrual tension/stress (PMT/PMS), their condition is worsened due to the emotional upheaval.

Regulating of menstruation is a very complex mechanism. The cyclical alteration of oestrogen and progesterone in a month to feature a blood stream at the end and the follicle development in the ovary is matched with the growth of the endometrial layer in the uterus. The hormonal and structural changes are all driven by the gonadotropin (GnRH) produced in the hypothalamus via the FSH and LH then produced in the pituitary. The hypothalamic–pituitary–ovarian feedback mechanism regulates the female monthly functional cycle. The regulating mechanism could be easily disturbed by stress response, intensive brain activities, and changes in the ovaries. All those could happen during an infection of COVID-19.

According to the authors' observation, the most common change is delayed menstruation, which is commonly defined as expected menses delay of more than 7 days. This is in line with a report from Li *et al.* (2021) with 237 subjects, 28% of whom experienced menstruation cycle prolongation and 25% of whom experienced reduced volume of discharge. Furthermore, the changes were not considered to be linked to any other organ damage, which is a hint that most of the changes might be due to the emotional and stress response.

Diagnosis

The patients complain of changed menstrual cycles, shorter or longer, changed menstrual volume, heavier or lesser, menstrual nature, more clots or not, or abnormal symptoms around menstruation, PMS or pain.

Whether there is a gynaecological disease, or hormonal disorder, this should be identified by general hormonal tests, such as FSH, LH, E2, Progesterone, and TSH. If necessary, vaginal ultrasound and X-ray should be done.

Differentiation syndromes of TCM and herbal treatment

Qi Deficiency of Spleen and Kidney, accumulation of Fluid and Stasis of Blood

Clinical features and sign: Signs are shorter or longer menstrual cycle, less blood during menstruation without pain, fatigue, lethargy, poor concentration, loose bowel movement, pale tongue with teeth marks and white-slippery coating, and a rolling-fine pulse.

Treatment principle in TCM: Reinforce *Spleen Qi* and eliminate excessive *Dampness*; activate *Blood* to release *Stasis.*

Treatment: Herbal prescription and acupuncture.

Pinyin: Jin Kui/Gui Shen Qi Tang variation.

English name for decoction: *Kidney Qi* Decoction from the Golden Cabinet variation.

Role in formula	Name/ Pinyin	Name/Latin	Dose (g)	Function
Chief herb	Shu Di Huang	Radix Rhemanniae Glutinosae Praeparata	10–30	Nourishes the kidney *Yin* and complements the kidney essence.
Deputy herb	Shan Zhu Yu	Fructus Corni Officinalis	10	Promotes nourishment of the kidney *Yin* and holds the kidney essence.
Assistant herb	Shan Yao	Radix Dioscoreae Oppositae	10	Replenishes the spleen and dries the damp.
	Fu Ling	Sclerotium Poria Cocos	10	Releases excessive dampness and replenishes the spleen to support Shanyao.
	Mu Dan pi	Cortex Moutan Radicis	10	Eliminates the liver fire and general fire in the lower burner.

(*Continued*)

Role in formula	Name/ Pinyin	Name/Latin	Dose (g)	Function
	Ze Xie	Rhizoma Alismatis Orientalis	10	Eliminates the kidney fire and general fire in the lower burner.
	Xiang Fu	Rhizoma Cyperi Rotundi	10	Warms the kidney yang which is a replacement for Fu Zi in the original formula.
	Du Zhong	Cortex Eucommiae	10	Promotes replenishment of the kidney yang and dries the accumulated damp.
	Tu Si Zi	Semen Cuseutae	10–30	Promotes replenishment of the kidney yang to prepare for conceiving.
	Cang Zhu	Rhizoma Atractylodis	10	Dries the damp and reinforces the spleen.
	Ban Xia	Rhizoma Pinelliae	10	Dries the damp and reinforces the spleen.
Guiding herb	Gui Zhi	Ramulus Cinnamomi Cassiae	6–10	Warms the kidney yang and agitates the general yang *Qi* in the lower burner.

Method: The above-mentioned herbal prescription is the main formula and can be used in combination with a variation of decoctions according to specific individual symptoms where the herbs are boiled and the concentrated herbal powders are taken with warm water twice daily.

Analysis: Sheng Di Huang and Shan Zhu Yu as the main herbs strengthen *Kidney Qi.* Shanyao reinforces *Spleen Qi.* Du Zhong and Tu Si Zi support the main herbs and reinforce the *Kidney* and promote ovary function. Mu Dan Pi cleanses the empty *Heat* and *Blood* to reduce heavier periods. Ze Xie and Fu Ling eliminate accumulated *Dampness*. Xiang Fu dredges *Stagnated Qi.* Cang Zhu and Ban Xia dry *Dampness* and support *Kidney* and *Spleen* function.

Advice: This pattern is the commonest one and manifests as irregular menstruation with long COVID-19. Patients possess some *Qi* deficiency in general, but more so in the kidney and spleen.

Kidney Yang Deficiency and accumulation of Fluid and Phlegm

Clinical features and signs: Signs are a prolonged menstrual cycle, possible amenorrhea, cold limbs, aversion to cold, darkened complexion, acne on the face, chest, and back, sometimes obesity, swelling of lower legs, excess hair, heavy feeling in general, A pale tongue with white-slippery coating, and a deep-rolling pulse.

Treatment principle in TCM: Strengthen *Kidney Yang*; release excessive *Fluid* and *Phlegm.*

Treatment: Herbal prescription.

Pinyin: Er Xian variated with Gui Zhi Fu Ling Tang.

English name for decoction: Two Immortals Decoction variated with Cinnamon and Poria Decoction.

Role in formula	Name/ Pinyin	Name/Latin	Dose (g)	Function
Chief herb	Xian Mao	Rhizoma Curculiginis	10	Warms and strengthens the kidney yang to agitate yang qi movement in the uterus.
	Yin Yang Huo	Herba Epimedii	10–30	Warms the kidney yang to promote ovulation.
Deputy herb	Gou Qi Zi	Fructus Lycii	10	Nourishes the kidney *Yin* and reinforces the kidney *Qi.*
Assistant herb	Ba Ji Tian	Radix Morindae Officinalis	10	Warms and strengthens the kidney yang and *Qi.*
	Ai Ye	Folium Artemisiae Argyi	10	Warms the kidney and the whole of the lower burner.
	Ban Xia	Rhizoma Pinelliae	10	Dries the damp-phlegm and reinforces the spleen.

(*Continued*)

Role in formula	Name/ Pinyin	Name/Latin	Dose (g)	Function
	Tao Ren	Semen Persicae	10	Activates the blood stasis to rebuild the menstrual cycle.
	Hong Hua	Flos Carthami	10	Activates the blood stasis to unblock the fallopian obstruction and ease menstrual pain.
	Chuan Xiong	Rhizoma Chuanxiong	10	Activates the blood stasis to ease menstrual pain and softens the lining of the uterus.
	Fu Ling	Poria	10	Dries the dampness and reinforces the spleen.
Guiding herb	Gui Zhi	Ramulus Cinnamomi	5–10	Warms and agitates the general yang qi in the lower burner.

Method: The above-mentioned herbal prescription is the main formula and can be used in combination with a variation of decoctions according to specific individual symptoms where the herbs are boiled and the concentrated herbal powders are taken with warm water twice daily.

Analysis: Xian Mao and Yin Yang Hua warm and strengthen *Kidney Yang* to agitate *Yang Qi* movement in the uterus. Gou Qi Zi, Ba Ji Tian, and Ai Ye support the main herbs to warm and promote *Kidney Qi* to recover ovary function. Tao Ren, Hong Hua, and Chuan Xiong activate Blood circulation to release Blood stasis. Gui Zhi agitates general *Yang Qi* to release stasis. Fu Ling reinforces the *Spleen* and releases *Dampness* to clear blocked meridians.

Advice: This pattern can be seen in patients with elongated or severely irregular menstruation. Some females can manifest amenorrhea after being infected with COVID-19. If a patient does not recover quickly, she can develop polycystic ovary syndromes as a real disease with hormonal disorder.

Liver Qi Stagnation and Blood Stasis

Clinical features and signs: Signs are shorter or prolonged menstrual cycles, in some cases amenorrhea, heavier or lighter blood during periods, stress, irritability, agitation, depression, restlessness, weeping, swollen breasts with PMS and dysmenorrhea, headache, acne on cheeks, infertility, a light red tongue with thin white coating, and a wiry or wiry-fine pulse.

Treatment principle in TCM: Dredge *Stagnated Liver Qi*; activate *Blood* circulation to release *Blood Stasis*.

Treatment: Herbal prescription and acupuncture.

Pinyin: Chai Hu Ji variations.

English name for decoction: Bupleuri Decoctions.

Role in formula	Name/Pinyin	Name/Latin	Dose (g)	Function
Chief herb	Chai Hu	Radix Bupleuri	10	Dredges the liver *Qi* and releases the stagnated *Qi* in general.
Deputy herb	Bai Shao	Radix Paeoniae Alba	10	Softens the liver blood and nourishes the liver *Yin*.
Assistant herb	Dang Gui	Radix Angelicae Sinensis	10	Cultivates the blood and nourishes the liver *Yin*.
	Zhi Qiao	Fructus Aurantii	10	Unblocks the stagnated *Qi* and purges the large intestines to promote elimination.
	Chi Shao	Radix Paeoniae Rubra	10	Activates the blood stasis and regulates the menstrual cycles.
	Sheng Di Huang	Radix Rehmanniae	10–30	Nourishes the kidney *Yin* and essence to prepare the body for ovulation.
	Chuan Xiong	Rhizoma Chuanxiong	10	Activates the blood stasis to ease menstrual pain and softens the lining of the uterus.
	Mu Dan Pi	Cortex Moutan	10	Cleanses the heat in the blood and nourishes the liver *Yin*.
Guiding herb	Yi Mu Cao	Herba Leonuri	10	Activates the blood circulation and regulates menstruation.

Method: The above-mentioned herbal prescription is the main formula and can be used in combination with a variation of decoctions according to specific individual symptoms where the herbs are boiled and the concentrated herbal powders are taken with warm water twice daily.

Analysis: Chai Hu as the main herb in the prescription dredges the *Liver* and *Stagnated Qi* in general. Bai Shao, Chi Shao, and Dang Gui soften the *Liver* and nourish *Liver Yin* and *Blood.* Sheng Di Huang reinforces the *Kidney* to nourish *Kidney Yin* and *Essence*. Zhi Qiao promotes the main herbs to dredge *Stagnated Qi.* Chuan Xiong and Yi Mu Cao release Blood Stasis to regulate menstruation. Mu Dan Pi clears *Stagnated Heat.* This formula can regulate menstruation, specifically when triggered by stress or mood swings.

Advice: This pattern can be seen in patients who manifest irregular menstruation with stress and irritability, among many emotional symptoms; therefore, some empty heat may exist within. It can occur in a shorter or longer diseased periods as long COVID-19.

Acupuncture treatment

Main points: Baihui (DU20), Moxibustion at Shenque (REN8); Zhongji (REN3), or Guanyuan (REN4), Qihai (REN6); Guilai (ST28) or Zigong (Ext).

Associated points:

- Strengthen the *Spleen* and remove the excessive fluid: Xuehai (SP10), Yinlingquan (SP9), Sanyinjiao (SP6), Taibai (SP3).
- Replenish the *Kidneys* and Warm *Yang*: Yingu (KI10), Zusanli (ST36), Fuliu (KI7), Zhaohai (KI6), Taixi (KI3).
- Remove the *Liver Qi* and dissolve the *Blood Stasis*: Waiguan (SJ5), Zulinqi (GB41); Hegu (LI4), Taichong (LIV3).

Analysis: Baihui agitates general qi in all the *Yang* meridians. Moxibustion at Shenque warms and supports the *Vitality Gate* to excite the original *Qi.* Zhongji and Qihai promote the original *Qi* in the *Conception Vessel* and stimulate the uterus. Guilai or Zigong promotes *Spleen Qi* and stimulates the ovaries to regulate menstruation. Xuehai and Taibai encourage *Spleen*

Qi. Yingu and Taixi reinforce *Kidney Qi.* Waiguan and Zulinqi dredge stagnated *Liver Qi.* Hegu and Taichong cleanse *Liver Heat.* All the assistant points can accompany the main points to regulate the menstrual cycles.

Case Study

Ms. Y. Yu, 29 years old, master's degree student who has come to UK half a year ago.

She has had amenorrhea for 2 months after healing from COVID-19. Her PCR gave a negative result. She has a fever of 38.6°C, cough, and breathlessness. She has controlled the COVID-19 infection well by taking a herbal prescription, but her menstrual cycle has not arrived since she was infected with COVID-19. She had a regular menstrual cycle before she was infected with the virus. Then, she came to the UK for stressful studies and research. She feels her symptoms are worse after the virus; therefore, she contacted the clinic for further treatment.

Clinical symptoms: Her symptoms are no menstrual cycles for 2 months, stress, annoyance, irritability, restlessness, disturbed sleep, distended abdomen and breasts, red tongue with less white coating, and a wiry pulse.

Diagnosis:

1. Post-COVID-19 syndrome.
2. Irregular menstrual cycles, suspected Polycystic Ovary (PCO).

Treatment: Herbal prescription and acupuncture.

Acupuncture

Main points: Moxibustion at Shenque (REN8), Guanyuan (REN4), Qihai (REN6), Guilai (ST28), Baihui (DU20), Shenting (DU24). Waiguan (SJ5), Zulinqi (GB41), Yanglingquan (GB34), Hegu (LI4), Taichong (LIV3).

Analysis: Shenque warms the *Yang* and stops a collapse from taking place. Guanyuan is the meeting point of the *Conception Vessel,* benefiting the uterus and *Kidney*. Qihai is the sea of *Blood* and regulates *Qi* and *Blood* and fortifies *Yang*. Guilai regulates the lower jiao, dispelling stagnation and benefits the uterus. Baihui is the *Sea* of *Marrow*, pacifies the *Wind* and calms the mind. Shenting calms the spirit. Waiguan is the Luo-connecting point and linking point to the *Yang* vessel, expels *Wind*, and releases the exterior. Zulinqiis is the shu-stream and disburses *Liver Qi*. Yanglingquan is the He-sea earth point of the *Gallbladder*, clears *Damp Heat*, and spreads *Liver Qi*. Hegu and Taichong are the famous "four gates" and promote the free flow of *Qi* to promote good circulation and reduce stress.

Herbal prescription

Pinyin: Chai Hu Shu Gan variation.

English name for decoction: Bupleurum Decoction to Spread to the *Liver*.

Herbal powders (g):

Chai Hu	Radix Bupleuri 10 g
Xiang Fu	Rhizoma Cyperi Rotundi 10 g
Zhi Shi	Fructus Immaturus Citri Aurantii 10 g
Chi Shao	Radix Paeoniae Rubrae 10 g
Shu Di Huang	Radix Rhemanniae Glutinosae Praeparata 30 g
Dang Gui	Radix Angelicae Sinensis 10 g
Chuan Xiong	Radix Ligustici Wallichii 10 g
Tao Ren	Semen Pruni Persicae 10 g
Hong Hua	Flos Carthami Tinctorii 10 g
Gui Zhi	Ramulus Cinnamomi Cassiae 10 g
Da Huang	Radix et Rhizoma Rhei 10 g
Zhi Gan Cao	Radix Glycyrrhizae Uralensis 5 g

Advice: The above-mentioned herbal powders were given in a 6 g dose to be taken with warm water twice daily. Her menstrual circles restart with normal blood for 5 days. Chai Hu Shu Gan and Ren Shen Gui Pi are then given to her for 2 months, after which regular menstruation returns.

Prevention of Miscarriage Among Post-COVID-19 Women

Miscarriage refers to spontaneous abortion and, in most clinical discussions, is loss of a foetus before 20 weeks of pregnancy with no clear cause. There is another category of miscarriage, septic miscarriage, which is considered to be caused by infection in the uterus or another reproductive organ. Both are closely related to the pandemic sufferers. The clinical symptoms indicating miscarriage are lower abdominal pain, vaginal bleeding, and vaginal fluid discharge. Pain may also be present in the lower back.

A pregnant woman has a higher-than-normal risk of blood clotting, and this was well recognised. When infected with the COVID-19, another potentially increased risk of maternal venous thromboembolism is added. This can cause a very threatening change to the foetus and can lead to abnormal changes. Another potential factor is anxiety and stress when COVID-19 leads to isolation and a hospital stay. The authors observed that stress and anxiety were common among all pregnant women during clinic visits.

According to Antonakou (2020), early studies summarised and indicated that there is not enough evidence to conclude that COVID-19 increased the risk of miscarriage, possibly due to the policies in place to reduce infection. The topic was followed later by Wang *et al.* (2021), and similarly no conclusion was reached on how much risk is increased to miscarriage resulting from COVID-19. But Hakari K (2021) reported that there is an increased risk of miscarriage and preterm delivery with their clinical comparison study. The authors' opinion is that the risk of spontaneous miscarriage is high for about 15% of pregnancies, and a small increase will not change the statistical profile. Quenby (2021) report only after the world moves into the post-COVID-19 era will a large sample reveal the real picture. However, miscarriage is extremely frustrating to any individual, and the event commonly leads to anxiety disorders like PTSD and depression, and an increased risk of developing cardiovascular diseases in the long run (Antonakou, 2020).

The authors have accumulated a rich experience in treating spontaneous miscarriage and have observed great outcomes in the last 20 years of practice in the UK. Many cases were associated with infection and trauma, and the whole system of TCM approaches that the authors used demonstrated very good success. So, when the pandemic continued, many pregnant women approached the authors and received good results.

Diagnosis

Clinical symptoms:
Symptoms include heavy spotting, vaginal bleeding, discharge of tissue or fluid from the vagina, severe abdominal pain or cramping, and mild to severe back pain, all of which are clinical signs of miscarriage. In general, miscarriage can appear before 20 weeks.

Hormonal tests and ultrasound are necessary to confirm whether the miscarriage has occurred or make a prediction on its occurrence.

If a women has a previous record of miscarriage or is in the high-risk category of miscarriage, such as older than 35 years, a BMI that is too high or too low, smoking and alcoholism, and contact with chemicals, and COVID-19 has then been confirmed, it is always advisable to take preventive measures for a safe pregnancy, even when one does not display any symptom of miscarriage.

Some tests might shed light on the risk of miscarriage, which are mainly the tests for infection and genetic abnormality. When these tests indicate a higher risk of miscarriage, preventive measures should be taken, because the combined risk of COVID-19 and those risks might be very real.

TCM management for promoting a normal pregnancy with herbal medicine

Clinical signs' appearance during the earlier pregnancy

Clinical features and signs: Signs are abdominal cramps, pain, back pain, heavy spotting, vaginal bleeding, light red tongue with less white coating, and a wiry-fine pulse.

Treatment principle in TCM: Strengthen *Spleen* and *Kidney Qi*; prevention of miscarriage.

Treatment: Herbal prescription.

Pinyin: Bao Tai Tang.

English name for decoction: Protecting Foetus Decoction.

Role in formula	Name/ Pinyin	Name/Latin	Dose (g)	Function
Chief herb	Huang Qi	Radix Astragali Membranacei	20–30	Replenishes the spleen, kidney *Qi*, and the vitality *Qi* to strengthen foetal growth.
Deputy herb	Dang Shen	Radix Codonopsis Pilosulae	10–15	Replenishes the spleen and general *Qi*.
Assistant herb	Bai Zhu	Rhizoma Atractylodis Macrocephalae	10–15	Replenishes the spleen and the vitality *Qi* to support foetal growth.
	Shan Yao	Radix Dioscoreae Oppositae	10–15	Dries the dampness and replenishes the spleen *Qi*.
	Shu Di Huang	Radix Rhemanniae Glutinosae Praeparata	10–15	Nourishes the kidney *Yin* and the essence to feed foetal growth.
	Du Zhong	Cortex Eucommiae Ulmoidis	10–15	Strengthens the kidney yang qi to prevent miscarriage.
	Sang Ji Sheng	Ramulus Loranthi	10–15	Strengthens the kidney yang qi to prevent miscarriage.
	Sha Ren	Fructus Amomi	10	Cultivates the embryo to promote and relax the stomach.
Guiding herb	Da Zao	Fructus Zizyphi Jujubae	4–6	Harmonises the stomach and leads to cohesiveness of herbs.

If accompanied by *Yin* deficiency, add: E Jiao (Gelatinum Corii Asini) 10 g, Huang Jing (Aurum Metalicum) 10 g.

If accompanied by *Kidney* and *Spleen* severe deficiencies, add: Tu Si Zi (Semen Cuscutae Chinensis) 10 g, Fu Pen Zi (Fructus Rubi Chingii) 10 g, Rou Dou Kou (Semen Myristicae Fragrantis) 10 g, Yi Zhi Ren (Fructus Alpiniae Oxyphyllae) 10 g.

If it is colder in the uterus, add: Yin Yang Huo (Herba Epimedii) 10 g, Bu Gu Zhi (Fructus Psoraleae Corylifoliae)10 g, Rou Gui (Cortex Cinnamomi Cassiae) 5–10 g.

If there is too much bleeding, add: Di Yu Tan (Radix Sanguisorbae Officinalis) 10 g, Huang Qin Tan (Radix Scutellariae Baicalensis

(Carbonis)) 10 g, Xian He Cao (Herba Agrimoniae Pilosae) 10 g, Ai Ye (Folium Artemisiae Argyi) 10 g.

Method: The above-mentioned herbal prescription is the main formula and can be used in combination with a variation of decoctions according to specific individual symptoms where the herbs are boiled and the concentrated herbal powders are taken with warm water twice daily.

Analysis: Huang Qi as the main herb replenishes the *Spleen,* the *Kidney,* and *Vitality Qi* to feed the growing embryo. Dang Shen, Bai Zhu, and Shan Yao promote replenishment of the *Spleen Qi* and dry the *Dampness*. Shu Di Huang nourishes the *Kidney Yin* and *Essence* to cultivate the embryo. Du Zhong and Sang Ji Sheng strengthen the *Kidney Yang*. Sha Ren harmonises the *Stomach* to ease the nausea and other reactions of pregnancy. Da Zao harmonises the *Stomach* and promotes cohesiveness of all herbs.

Advice: Due to coronavirus disturbing multiple organs, an embryo may be affected, so this formula is always given to a lady in early pregnancy when she is suffering from abdominal cramps with minor vaginal bleeding and if a lady displays signs of miscarriage at the early stage of the pregnancy after she has been infected with coronavirus or has had contact with someone who may be infected with coronavirus.

Patients who experienced more than one miscarriage in the past

Clinical features and signs: When a woman conceives, at the earlier stage of pregnancy, she has mild symptoms or no symptoms; however, she worries that miscarriage may occur again during the COVID-19 pandemic phase.

Treatment principle in TCM: Reinforce *Spleen Qi* and *Nourish Liver Blood*; support pregnancy and prevent miscarriage.

Treatment: Herbal prescription.

Pinyin: Fang Tai Tang.

English name for decoction: Preventing Miscarriage Decoction.

Role in formula	Name/ Pinyin	Name/Latin	Dose (g)	Function
Chief herb	Huang Qi	Radix Astragali Membranacei	15	Replenishes the spleen and the vitality *Qi* to nourish the foetus.
Deputy herb	Dang Shen	Radix Codonopsis Pilosulae	15	Replenishes the spleen and the vitality *Qi* to nourish the foetus.
Assistant herb	Bai Zhu	Rhizoma Atractylodis Macrocephalae	15	Replenishes the spleen and the vitality *Qi* to nourish the foetus.
	Dang Gui	Radix Angelicae Sinensis	10	Nourishes the *Yin* and blood to soften the lining of the uterus.
	Bai Shao	Radix Paeoniae Lactiflorae	10	Nourishes the *Yin* and blood to soften the lining of the uterus.
	Tu Si Zi	Semen Cuscutae Chinensis	10	Strengthens the kidney to promote the kidney essence.
	Chuan Bei Mu	Bulbus Fritillariae Cirrhosae	10	Dries the dampness and calms the mind down.
	Chuan Xiong	Radix Ligustici Wallichii	10	Cultivates the blood and activates the blood stasis to release any stasis that may cause a miscarriage.
	Gan Jiang	Radix Glycyrrhizae Uralensis	3	Warms and agitates the spleen *Qi* and yang, and harmonises the stomach.
	Ai Ye	Folium Artemisiae Argyi	3	Warms and strengthens the kidney and whole basin to comfort the local environment for pregnancy.
	Qiang Huo	Rhizoma et Radix Notopterygii	3	Warms the yang qi and dries the damp.
	Jing Jie	Herba seu Flos Schizonepetae Tenuifoliae	3	Warms the yang qi and unblocks the stagnation.
	Zhi Qiao	Fructus Citri Aurantii	3	Dredges the stagnated *Qi* and purges the bowel movement.
Guiding herb	Hou Po	Cortex Magnoliae Officinalis	3	Warms and agitates the general stagnated *Qi* and promotes cohesiveness of tonic herbs.

Method: The above-mentioned herbal prescription is the main formula and can be used in combination with a variation of decoctions according to specific individual symptoms where herbs are boiled and the concentrated herbal powders are taken with warm water twice daily.

Analysis: Huang Qi as the main herb replenishes the *Spleen* and the *Vitality Qi to* feed the embryo. Dang Shen and Bai Zhu support it to replenish the *Spleen* and *Vitality Qi.* Dang Gui and Bai Shao nourish the *Kidney* and the *Liver Yin*, plus Chuan Xiong activates the *Blood Stasis* to soften the lining of the uterus. Tu Si Zi and Ai Ye strengthen the *Kidney* by warming it to prevent miscarriage. Gan Jiang and Qiang Huo warm and agitate the stagnated *Qi*. Zhi Qiao and Hou Po dredge the *Stagnated Qi* and unblock all the *Stasis* that may cause a miscarriage. Jing Jie agitates the *Qi* flowing through the body. This formula uses stronger herbs to activate the *Blood Stasis* and release the stasis that may cause a miscarriage.

Advice: Some ladies may show minor symptoms and signs of miscarriage; however, there may be no symptoms and signs at all, but one is worried that it may occur after one is infected with coronavirus or has close contact with infected people, or even if there is a miscarriage history. This formula can help prevent miscarriage.

Case Study

Mrs. X. Li, a 38-year-old officer in a London company, seeks support from a TCM consultant with an urgent enquiry. Due to being diagnosed with infertility issues 5 years ago, she has not been able to conceive after marriage. She has gone through a 2-year treatment for her infertility with Chinese herbal medicine. In the first lockdown phase, she was worried about her husband who became infected with coronavirus in a gentle stage. She found out she is pregnant and is told that this foetus may not be strong enough to mature. She starts vaginal bleeding with minor abdominal pain for 2 days in 2 months of pregnancy. Due to such difficulty in conceiving, she is reluctant to terminate her pregnancy and she enquires whether TCM can help her continue with the pregnancy and protect her baby.

Clinical features and signs: Although COVID-19 restrictions state that physical contact with her is not possible, we have technology and therefore are able to see that she has a red tongue with less white coating and we are not sure if she is infected with coronavirus. She has manifested a series of typical signs of miscarriage since she conceived and might have been infected with COVID-19 by her husband, so she and her foetus are in a dangerous state. If she decides to keep her pregnancy, we can help treat her, prevent miscarriage, and protect her foetus.

Diagnosis:

1. Close contact with COVID-19.
2. The early stage of miscarriage.

Differentiation syndromes of TCM:

1. *Spleen* and *Kidney Qi* and *Yin Deficiency.*
2. *Liver Qi Stagnation.*

Treatment: Herbal prescription.

A week's supply of a herbal prescription for protecting her foetus is sent to her.

Herbal powders (g):

Huang Qi	Radix Astragali Membranacei 20 g
Dang Shen	Radix Codonopsis Pilosulae 10 g
Bai Zhu	Rhizoma Atractylodis Macrocephalae 10 g
Shan Yao	Radix Dioscoreae Oppositae 10 g
Shu Di Huang	Radix Rhemanniae Glutinosae Praeparata 15 g
Du Zhong	Cortex Eucommiae Ulmoidis 10 g
Sang Ji Sheng	Ramulus Loranthi 10 g
Sha Ren	Fructus Amomi 10 g
Da Zao	Fructus Zizyphi Jujubae 4 g

Result: After she takes the herbal prescription, the vaginal bleeding and abdominal pain gradually decrease, but she still suffers from more nausea and dizziness as pregnancy reactions. Ganjiang Shenqu and Shanzha are added into the secondary prescription, completely stopping her abdomen cramps and vaginal bleeding in 2 weeks. An ultrasound is done for her at

12 weeks which confirms a normal pregnancy with a healthy baby of a suitable size for her pregnancy month.

Intrauterine Growth Restriction (IUGR)/Foetal Growth Restriction

The condition of intrauterine growth restriction (IUGR) is also called foetal growth restriction (FGR), and refers to a situation where an unborn baby is growing slower which makes the baby smaller than it should be inside the mother's womb. This can only be diagnosed by a routine check-up with special equipment.

Diagnosis

IUGR can have serious consequences such as premature birth, underdevelopment of the baby, weak immune function in childhood, and stillbirth, which is the worst-case scenario. So, it should be treated immediately after been diagnosed. The cause of it could be simply that the mother's body is not in a favourable condition to support the pregnancy, mentally and physically, including malnutrition. There could also be a problem of genetic disorders. However, there are many cases in which no cause could be identified.

TCM management for supporting foetal growth

Clinical features and signs: The patients are checked using an ultrasound showing the foetus size being smaller compared to its clinical size relevant to the month of development, although the foetus is alive.

Differentiation syndromes of TCM: *Spleen* and *Kidney Qi* and *Essence Deficiency*.

Treatment principle in TCM: Reinforce *Spleen* and strengthen *Kidney Qi* and *Essence*; promote foetal growth.

Treatment: Herbal prescription and acupuncture.

Pinyin: Shou Tai Wan.

English name for decoction: Promoting Embryo Decoction.

Role in formula	Name/Pinyin	Name/Latin	Dose (g)	Function
Chief herb	Tu Si Zi	Semen Cuscutae Chinensis	5	Warms and replenishes the kidney to feed the foetus.
Deputy herb	E Jiao (Dissolved)	Gelatinum Corii Asini	5	Nourishes the kidney *Yin* and the essence to cultivate the foetus.
Assistant herb	Shu Di Huang	Radix Rhemanniae Glutinosae Praeparata	15	Nourishes the kidney *Yin* and essence.
	Dang Shen	Radix Codonopsis Pilosulae	12	Replenishes the spleen *Qi* to feed the foetus.
	Huang Qi	Radix Astragali Membranacei	12	Replenishes the spleen *Qi* and general vitality *Qi*.
	Sang Ji Sheng	Ramulus Loranthi	12	Strengthens the kidney yang and *Qi*.
	Bai Zhu	Rhizoma Atractylodis Macrocephalae	10	Reinforces the spleen and general vitality *Qi*.
	Dang Gui	Radix Angelicae Sinensis	10	Nourishes the *Yin* and blood to feed the foetus.
	Xu Duan	Radix Dipsaci Asperi	10	Strengthens the kidney yang and *Qi*.
Guiding herb	Sha Ren	Fructus Amomi	3	Agitates the yang qi and harmonises the stomach promoting cohesiveness of herbs.

Method: The above-mentioned herbal prescription is the main formula and can be used in combination with a variation of decoctions according to specific individual symptoms where the herbs are boiled and the concentrated herbal powders are taken with warm water twice daily.

Analysis: Tu Si Zi replenishes the *Kidney Qi* and *Vitality Qi* to feed the foetus as the main herb. E Jiao and Shu Di Huang nourish the *Kidney Yin* and *Essence* to cultivate the foetal growth. Dang Shen, Huang Qi, and Bai Zhu reinforce the *Spleen.* Sang Ji Sheng and Xu Duan strengthen the *Kidney Qi* and *Essence.* Dang Gui nourishes the *Blood* and *Yin.* Sha Ren agitates all the herbs, harmonises the *Stomach,* and promotes cohesiveness of the herbs.

Advice: Due to a coronavirus infection, or some other reason, the foetus may be disturbed and might grow slower. This is demonstrated in an ultrasound, identifying smaller foetal growth than the clinical age growth should be. Therefore, this prescription is given to promote foetal growth and prevent foetal death during early pregnancy.

Acupuncture and moxibustion

Moxibustion: Shenque (REN8).

Main points: Baihui (DU20), Shenting (DU24), Qihai (REN6), Zhongji (REN3), Zigong (Ext).

The points on the lower abdomen should be used before 12 weeks of pregnancy, and are forbidden after 12 weeks of pregnancy.

Assistant points: Yinlingquan (SP9), Sanyinjiao (SP6), Zusanli (ST36); Yingu (KI10), Zhaohai (KI6), Taixi (KI3), Rangu (KI2); Waiguan (SJ5), Zulinqi (GB41), Neiguan (P6), Neiting (ST44).

Analysis: Yinlingquan is a He-sea point of the *Spleen* and benefits the *Lower Jiao*. Sanyinjiao harmonises the *Lower Jiao*, promotes the *Blood* and *Liver,* and tonifies the *Kidney.* Zusanli is the earth point and tonifies and nourishes the *Blood* and *Yin*, fortifying the *Spleen* and raising the *Yang*. Yingu activates the *Kidney* and is used for uterine urgency. Zhaohai will regulate the general *Yin* vessel and calm the spirit. Taixi is the supreme stream of the *Kidney* and will tonify *Yang*. Rangu will help regulate and promote the *Lower Jiao.* Waiguan, a Luo-connecting point and a *Yang*-linking vessel point, will support in reducing *Kidney Deficiency.* Zulinqi will support the spread of *Liver Qi* in the body. Neiguan will calm the mind and alleviate nausea. Neiting calms the spirit and prevents cold.

References

Antonakou, A. (2020). The latest update on the effects of COVID-19 infection in pregnancy. *European Journal of Midwifery*, 4, 12. https://doi.org/10.18332/ejm/120973.

Hazari, K. S., Abdeldayem, R., Paulose, L., *et al.* (2021). Covid-19 infection in pregnant women in Dubai: A case-control study. *BMC Pregnancy Childbirth*, 28;21(1):658. doi: 10.1186/s12884-021-04130-8.

He, Y., Wang, J., Ren, J., *et al.* (2021). Effect of COVID-19 on male reproductive system — A systematic review. *Frontier of Endocrinology (Lausanne)*, 27(12), 677701. doi:10.3389/fendo.2021.677701.

Li, K., Chen, G., Hou, H., Liao, Q., Chen, J., *et al.* (2021). Analysis of sex hormones and menstruation in COVID-19 women of child-bearing age. *Reproductive BioMedicine Online*, 42(1), 260–267. doi:10.1016/j.rbmo.2020.09.020.

Quenby, S., Gallos, I. D., Dhillon-Smith, R. K., Podesek, M., Stephenson, M. D., *et al.* (2021). Miscarriage matters: The epidemiological, physical, psychological, and economic costs of early pregnancy loss. *The Lancet*, 397(10285), 1658–1667. https://doi.org/10.1016/S0140-6736(21)00682-6. S Lancet 2021 May 1;397(10285):1658–1667. doi: 10.1016/S0140-6736(21)00682-6.

Sansone, A., Mollaioli, D., Ciocca, G., *et al.* (2021). Addressing male sexual and reproductive health in the wake of COVID-19 outbreak. *Journal of Endocrinological Investigation*, 44(2), 223–231. doi:10.1007/s40618-020-01350-1.

Wang, C. L., Liu, Y. Y., Wu, C. H., Wang, C. Y., Wang, C. H., and Long, C. Y. (2021). Impact of COVID-19 on pregnancy. *International Journal of Medical Sciences*, 18(3), 763–767. https://doi.org/10.7150/ijms.49923.

Chapter 14

Skin/Dermatological Disorders

In the long historic records of TCM relating to pandemic illness, skin impairments were recorded as a valuable sign of some patterns in TCM diagnosis; for example, red patches on the skin were sign of pathology developing to cause damage to the blood system, indicating an unfavourable prognosis of multiple organ system damage that was difficult to treat or manage. This opinion was described in Warm Disease documents (Wen Bing Xue). However, it was not clear how long the skin conditions would remain after the feverish period of illness, although it was clear that the skin damage left over by smallpox was permanent but not bothersome as there was no itchiness or disturbance in daily life.

The skin conditions that developed after infection were mainly psoriasis and blistering. The experience might have been similar to COVID-19 as many of the infections were viral from a modern perspective.

In an early global study by Zoe COVID Study app (2020), skin conditions were considered to be very common affecting about 8.8% of patients of COVID-19, significantly higher than people without COVID-19 at 5.4%. And more interestingly, 17% of all COVID-19 patients who experienced skin problems found the skin problem to be the first symptom. The same research report classified all COVID-19-related skin conditions into three main categories: hive-type rashes (similar to urticarial), erythematous-papular/vesicular rashes, and chilblains (COVID finger and toes). They all last well into the chronic stage.

Virus Rashes

Skin rashes, hives, and erythematous plaque (red patched) were commonly reported in the early stage of the pandemic and some suggest that skin rashes should be considered for early diagnosis purposes. Gisondi *et al.* summarised early findings and proposed that all skin impairments in COVID-19 patients could be classified into four groups: exanthema (blister like), vascular (chilblain-like, purpuric/petechial and livedoid lesions), urticarial, and acro-papular eruption (rashes). For existing skin conditions like psoriasis or atopic dermatitis, it is unclear where the skin conditions could lead to more COVID-19 or less, and it also remains unknown if such conditions could be triggered by COVID-19.

The cause of such skin impairments was mainly the immune system response, particularly the master cells (Gokahle, 2020; Sanghvi, 2020). Investigation also suggested that many such cases are actually not related to the SARS-CoV-2 virus, but to the hygienic products which cause contact dermatitis. These skin impairments from COVID-19 infection were not due to viral presence in the skin, but caused by immune system overreaction and therefore will last longer than the infection itself (Silva Andrade *et al.*, 2021). Gül's (2020) review suggested that there are three pathways for skin conditions that developed in COVID-19 sufferers, the viral infection itself, the use of personal hygienic products which is well above the ordinary level, and the side effects of medicines used for the treatment. It was also worthy of mention that even in people showing no COVID-19 symptoms, skin conditions are still common.

TCM treatment of skin conditions caused by viral infection, contact dermatitis, and allergic dermatitis has been popular in the past 20 years with acupuncture, oral herbal medicine, and atopic herbal remedies. Acupuncture has proven to be helpful.

Diagnosis

Rashes related to COVID-19 are in the following three forms:

- Hive-type rash (urticaria): Sudden appearance of raised bumps of pale colour on the skin which can disappear quite quickly over hours and can be very itchy.

- Small itchy skin raised bumps scattered over an area. It was described as Prickly Heat, similar to chickenpox rash but not with water bubbles on top.
- COVID fingers and toes (chilblains): Reddish and purplish bumps on the fingers or toes, which may be sore but not usually itchy.

The most of the skin conditions that occur during COVID-19 infection can be relieved without treatment when acute COVID-19 is cleared. However, some do remain long after other symptoms vanish.

No biomarkers are used in clinical diagnosis for those skin impairments. Diagnosis is mainly based on the case history, the experience of the dermatologist, and his/her observation of the skin lesion.

Differentiation syndromes of TCM and herbal treatment

Wind-Heat is explored at the exterior

Clinical features and signs: Some rashes gradually or suddenly appeared on the upper part of the body, chest, the upper back, and arms with or without itchy, red, or pink rashes in a small purpura. Other signs are a sore throat, minor fever, cough, a light red tongue with less white coating, and a floating-rapid pulse.

Treating principle in TCM: Release *External Wind* and *Heat*; eliminate rashes and ease itching.

Treatment: Herbal prescription.

Pinyin: Xiao Feng San variation.

English name for decoction: Eliminate Wind Decoction.

Role in formula	Name/ Pinyin	Name/Latin	Dose (g)	Function
Chief herb	Fang Feng	Radix Ledebouriellae Divaricatae	6	Dissipates the external wind and eases the itching.
Deputy herb	Jing Jie	Herba seu Flos Schizonepetae Tenuifoliae	6	Dissipates the external wind and eases the itching.

(*Continued*)

(*Continued*)

Role in formula	Name/ Pinyin	Name/Latin	Dose (g)	Function
Assistant herb	Sheng Di Huang	Radix Rehmanniae Glutinosae	12	Nourishes the kidney yin and stabilises the immune system.
	Dang Gui	Radix Angelicae Sinensis	6	Nourishes the blood and general yin to moisten the skin.
	Niu Bang Zi	Fructus Arctii Lappae	6	Supports dissipation of the external wind-damp.
	Chai Tui	Periostracum Cicadae	3	Leads all the herbs to the exterior and dissipates the external wind.
	Shi Gao	Gypsum Fibrosum	12	Cleanses the internal heat and cools the blood.
	Huo Xiang	Herba Agastaches seu Pogostemi	6	Dissipates the external wind-damp from the upper and middle burners.
	Chen Pi	Pericarpium Citri Reticulatae	6	Harmonises the stomach and dries the dampness.
	Jie Geng	Radix Platycodi Grandiflori	6	Dredges the stagnated qi in the chest and lung to ventilate the external qi.
Guiding herb	Gan Cao	Radix Glycyrrhizae Uralensis	5	Harmonises the stomach and promotes cohesiveness of the herbs.

Method: The above-mentioned herbal prescription is the main formula and can be used in combination with a variation of decoctions according to specific individual symptoms where the herbs are boiled and the concentrated herbal powders are taken with warm water twice daily.

Analysis: Jing Jie and Fang Feng dissipate external Wind and ease itching as the main herbs. Qiang Huo and Chan Tui support the main herbs to cleanse internal and *External Wind* in the *Blood* and joints. Huo Xiang eliminates external *Wind* and *Damp* and harmonises the Stomach. Shi Gao cleanses the *Blood Heat*. Jie Gen regulates *Lung Qi* and dissipates internal and *External Wind* to eliminate rashes. Sheng Di Huang and Dang Gui nourish *Yin* and *Blood* to moisturise the skin. Gan Cao harmonises all herbs and promotes cohesiveness.

Advice: This pattern can be seen in the patients who manifest rashes throughout the body in a brief time. The rashes can recur as part of the post-COVID-19 syndrome and they may not be very itchy, but they can easily reoccur if the situation is not controlled well.

Internal Liver Wind-Heat flare-up

Clinical features and signs: Dizziness, anxiety, easily angered, red face, Bitter taste in the mouth, Tinnitus, insomnia, disturbed dreams, red tongue, yellow complexion, wiry pulse.

Treatment: Herbal prescription and acupuncture.

Pinyin: Dao Chi San variation.

English name for decoction: Guide Out the Red Decoction variation.

Role in formula	Name/ Pinyin	Name/Latin	Dose (g)	Function
Chief herb	Sheng Di Huang	Radix Rehmanniae Glutinosae	30	Cleanses the heat and nourishes the yin which can stabilise the immune reaction.
Deputy herb	Dan Zhu Ye	Herba Lophatheri Gracilis	10	Promotes cleansing of the blood heat and dissipates the external wind-damp.
Assistant herb	Chi Shao	Radix Paeoniae Rubrae	10	Cools the blood and activates the blood stasis.
	Fang Feng	Radix Ledebouriellae Divaricatae	10	Dissipates the external wind to release the dermatological rashes and eases the itching.
	Jing Jie	Herba seu Flos Schizonepetae Tenuifoliae	6	Dissipates the external wind to release the dermatological rashes and eases the itching.
	Wei Ling Xian	Radix Clematidis	10	Promotes dissipation of the external wind to ease the itching and release the rashes.
	Mu Dan Pi	Cortex Moutan Radicis	10	Cleanses the blood heat and eliminates the rashes.
	Lu Gen	Rhizoma Phragmitis Communis	10	Emphasises cleansing of the blood heat.
	Zi Cao	Radix Arnebiae seu Lithospermi	10	Cools the blood and cleanses the excessive heat.
Guiding herb	Gan Cao	Radix Glycyrrhizae Uralensis	5	Harmonises the stomach and promotes cohesiveness of the herbs.

If accompanied by a red tongue, Shi Gao is added; if itching is more, Bai Xian Pi is added.

Method: The above-mentioned herbal prescription is the main formula and can be used in combination with a variation of decoctions according to specific individual symptoms where the herbs are boiled and the concentrated herbal powders are taken with warm water twice daily.

Analysis: Sheng Di Huang cleanses *Heat* and nourishes *Yin* which can stabilise the immune reaction as the main herb. Chi Shao, Mu Dan Pi, and Zi Cao cleanse *Heat* in the *Blood.* Fang Feng and Jing Jie eliminate External *Wind* to ease Itching. Lu Gen emphasises to *Cool Blood.* Wei Ling Xian dissipates Internal *Wind.* Gan Cao harmonises all herbs and comforts the *Stomach.* All herbs work cohesively to *Cool* the *Blood* and cleanse *Wind-Heat,* so they can ease rashes in the whole body.

Advice: This pattern can be seen as recurrent rashes which may be triggered by stress or other internal reasons as a common pattern in the post-COVID-19 syndrome. In general, if rashes appear, on and off, in patients when they are infected with coronavirus, they have an impaired immune system, and therefore, recurrent dermatological reactions occur. Sheng Di Huang is the main herb that can effetely stabilise an impaired immune system.

Acupuncture

As part of the post-COVID-19 syndrome, these recurrent rashes can be treated by acupuncture to regulate and recovery the immune system.

Main points: Fengchi (GB20), Quchi (LI11), Hegu (LI4); Xuehai (SP10), Yinlingquan (SP9), Sanyinjiao (SP6), Taichong (LIV3).

If accompanied by heat, Dazhui (DU14) is added. When itching is present, Yanglingquan (GB34) and Zulinqi (GB41) are added. When rashes are triggered by stress, Waiguan (SJ5) and Baihui (DU20) are added.

Analysis: Fengchi eliminates external and internal *Wind* as the main point. Quchi and Hegu cleanse internal *Blood Heat.* Xuehai, Yinlingquan, and

Sanyinjiao cool *Blood* to dissipate rashes. Taichong with Hegu cleanses *Heat*.

Atopic TCM herbs (external herbs)

Chinese herbs are used for skin rashes and eczema as a routine practice. There are two common types of external herb usage: washing liquid using Chinese herbs and creams.

Most recommended herbal washing liquids are based on the principle of cooling down *Heat*, clearing *Dampness*, and moistening (protecting) the skin. The formula prescribed by the author is as follows:

- Huang Bai (Cortex Phellodendri) 20 g
- Ku Shen (Radix Sophorae Flavescentis) 20 g
- Cang Zhu (Rhizoma Atractylodis) 10 g
- Xing Ren (Semen Pruni Armeniacae) 10 g
- Huo Ma Ren (Semen Cannabis Sativae) 10 g
- Bai Xian Pi (Cortex Dictamni Dasycarpi Radicis) 10 g
- Ma Chi Xian (Herba Portulacae Oleraceae) 10 g

Method:
The above-mentioned herbal powders should be placed into a source pan with 1000 ml of water, brought to a boil, and then simmered for 30 min. The decoction/liquid is gathered into 300 ml × 2. When the liquid is warm, soak a few face tissues in the liquid, apply the tissue on the skin rashes, and keep on the skin for 30 min.

Afterwards, immediately apply E45 cream on the affected skin.

The author's preferred skin cream is the Three Yellow Cream (San Huang Gao):

Ingredients:

- Huang Lian (Rhizoma Coptidis) 30 g
- Huang Qin (Radix Scutellariae Baicalensis) 30 g
- Huang Bai (Cortex Phellodendri) 30 g

Method: The raw herbs are placed in a frying pan to which 300 ml sesame oil is added. Heat it to the point where the steam from the herbs has stopped and the temperature of the oil reaches about 180°C. Remove from the heat and let it cool down naturally. The oil is then filtered and blended into base cream of 200 ml.

The cream is kept in small jar in the fridge and applied to the affected skin when there is itching or after washing the affected skin.

Case Study

Ms. S. Terries, a 56-year-old solicitor, was infected with COVID-19 and healed from it. She experienced rashes on the upper chest, upper back, and shoulders, which had not disappeared 3 months later. She was taking herbs for healing from the COVID-19 infection for a week, after which her PCR rapidly became negative and fever and cough had gone completely. Due to a busy and stressful workload, she always felt irritable, restless, and suffered from anxiety attacks and depression; the rashes on her upper body never disappeared.

Clinical symptoms: Symptoms are many pink rashes and small papules spreading on her upper chest, back, and shoulders which are not raised on the skin, accompanied by some itchiness, stress, nervousness, irritability, some anxiety and depression occasionally, a red tongue with less white coating, and a wiry-rapid pulse.

Diagnosis:

1. Post-COVID-19 syndrome.
2. Persistent papular signs, like urticarial rashes.
3. Anxiety and depression.

Differentiation syndromes of TCM:

1. Mixed external and *Internal Wind* and *Heat* accumulated in the *Blood*.
2. *Liver Qi Stagnation* and internal heat flare-up.

Treatment: Herbal prescription and acupuncture.

Acupuncture

Main points: Baihui (DU20), Shenting (DU24), Touwei (ST8), Fengchi (GB20); Quchi (LI11), Hegu (LI4), Yanglingquan (GB34), Taichong (LIV3).

Herbal prescription

Pinyin: Dao Chi San variated with Chai Hu Shu Gan Decoction.

Herbal powders (g):

Shen Di Huang	Radix Rehmanniae Glutinosae 30 g
Mu Dan Pi	Cortex Moutan Radicis 10 g
Chuan Lian Zi	Fructus Meliae Toosendan 10 g
Huang Qin	Radix Scutellariae Baicalensis 10 g
Fang Feng	Radix Ledebouriellae Divaricatae 10 g
Jing Jie	Herba seu Flos Schizonepetae Tenuifoliae 6 g (Later)
Dang Gui	Radix Angelicae Sinensis 10 g
Chi Shao	Radix Paeoniae Rubrae 10 g
Zhi Shi	Fructus Immaturus Citri Aurantii 10 g
Tu Fu Ling	Rhizoma Smilacis Glabrae 30 g
Bai Xian Pi	Cortex Dictamni Dasycarpi Radicis 10 g
Gan Cao	Radix Glycyrrhizae Uralensis 5 g

The above-mentioned herbs are boiled into herbal juice to be consumed twice daily, for 2 weeks.

Result: The patient's rashes gradually decreased. At the beginning of the treatment, she felt itchy, then her rashes turned into a lighter colour, and finally faded away. The prescription was changed to Jia Wei Xiao Yao wan and Qiang Huo Sheng Shi Wan which continue to regulate her psychiatric disorder.

Virus Blistering

A blister, or vesicle, is a raised portion of skin filled with fluid (water bubble). Many viral infections, including COVID-19, can cause blisters in the mouth and on the lips. However, blisters can also appear on the toes, heels, or fingers with red-purple, tender, or itchy bumps, commonly called COVID toes. Most of the blisters will dry up in a couple of days, with no skin lesions. However, some do return and last months, thereby becoming chronic.

Diagnosis

Clinical symptoms: Patients manifest local itching, sores, and even burning pain, or are asymptomatic.

Dermatological signs: Some blisters have swelling and discharge, and itching or pain may occur on one or several toes or fingers. Some develop painful raised bumps or areas of rough skin. Initially, they may be red in colour and might gradually turn purple. A tissue biopsy may need to be done for confirmation of the diagnosis.

Differentiation syndromes of TCM and herbal treatment

In general, blisters are the main signs, and TCM believes pathogenic damp-heat or damp accumulation to be the cause; therefore, the three burners should be identified in the Damp Syndrome as the differentiation syndrome of TCM. We should differentiate which burner should be treated according to where the blister is occurring.

Damp-Heat accumulation at upper and middle burners

Clinical features and signs: Ulcerations and blisters occur in the mouth, with pain in the palate, tongue, and lips. Blisters can also occur at corners of the mouth, with other signs being headache, sore throat, thirst and dry mouth, aversion to drinking, distension of the stomach, constipation or loose greasy stools, a red tongue with greasy-yellow coating, and a floating-rolling pulse.

Treatment principle in TCM: Dissipate the *Damp* and cleanse the *Heat*; dredge and calm the *Stomach.*

Treatment: Herbal prescription.

Pinyin: Huang Lian Shang Qing Wan Decoction.

English name for decoction: Coptis Decoction to Clear the Upper Burner variation.

Role in formula	Name/ Pinyin	Name/Latin	Dose (g)	Function
Chief herb	Huang Lian	Rhizoma Coptidis	10	Cleanses the excessive heat from the three burners and dries excessive damp.
Deputy herb	Huang Qin	Radix Scutellariae Baicalensis	10	Cleanses the excessive heat from the three burners and dries excessive damp.
	Huang Bai	Cortex Phellodendri	10	Cleanses the excessive heat from the three burners and dries excessive damp.
Assistant herb	Shi Gao	Gypsum Fibrosum	30	Eliminates the excessive heat in the upper and middle burners.
	Da Huang	Radix et Rhizoma Rhei	10	Emphasises dissipation of the excessive heat in the intestines and purges the bowel movement.
	Lian Qiao	Fructus Forsythiae Suspensae	10	Dissipates the external wind-heat to ease the rashes and blisters.
	Ju Hua	Flos Chrysanthemi Morifolii	10	Dissipates the external wind-heat to ease the rashes and blisters.
	Jing Jie Sui	Herba seu Flos Schizonepetae Tenuifoliae	6	Dissipates the external wind to stop the itching.
	Bai Zhi	Radix Angelicae Dahuricae	6	Dissipates the external wind and leads all the herbs to work on the exterior.
	Man Jing Zi	Fructus Viticis	10	Dissipates the wind and the damp at the top of the body.
	Chuan Xiong	Radix Ligustici Wallichii	10	Activates the blood stasis to release the pain.
	Fang Feng	Radix Ledebouriellae Divaricatae	10	Dissipates the external wind to ease itching.
	Bo He	Herba Menthae Haplocalycis	5	Dissipates the external wind and opens the orifices.
	Jie Geng	Radix Platycodi Grandiflori	10	Dissipates the external wind to ease itching.
Guiding herb	Gan Cao	Radix Glycyrrhizae Uralensis	5	Harmonises the stomach and promotes cohesiveness of herbs.

Method: The above-mentioned herbal prescription is the main formula and can be used in combination with a variation of decoctions according to specific individual symptoms where the herbs are boiled and the concentrated herbal powders are taken with warm water twice daily.

Explanation: Huang Lian, Qin, and Bai as the main herbs cleanse the excessive *Heat* from the three burners and dry excessive *Damp.* Shi Gao and Da Huang promote the main herbs to cleanse *Heat.* Lian Qiao and Ju Hua release external *Heat.* Fang Feng, Bo He, and Man Jing Zi eliminate the *Wind-Heat* from the upper burner and dredge the orifices. Jie Geng dredges the *Stagnated Qi* at the upper burner. *Gan Cao* harmonises all herbs and protects the *Stomach* from the *Cold* nature of the herbs.

Advice: This pattern can be seen in patients who suffer from recurring blisters as a dermatological disorder for a brief time and possess a stronger constitution.

Damp-Heat accumulation at lower burner

Clinical features and signs: Blisters appear along coastal areas, out of the vagina or the top of the penis, and also on the toes with red-purple rashes or bumps, herpes, itching or sores, or pain; the discharge from the blisters is clear or turbid. The patient is in a bad mood, is easily upset, has a red tongue with greasy-yellow coating, and a wiry-rapid pulse.

Treatment principle in TCM: eliminate excessive dampness and cleanse excessive heat; dredge liver and regulate stomach.

Treatment: Herbal prescription.

Pin Yin: Si Miao variated with Long Dan Xie Gan Tang.

English name for decoction: Mysterious Four Decoction variated Gentiana Longdancao Decoction to Drain the Liver.

Role in formula	Name/ Pinyin	Name/Latin	Dose (g)	Function
Chief herb	Huang Bai	Cortex Phellodendri	10	Eliminates excessive damp and heat at the lower burner.
Deputy herb	Cang Zhu	Rhizoma Atractylodis	10	Dries the excessive dampness.
Assistant herb	Long Dan Cao	Radix Gentianae	10	Releases the excessive damp-heat from the middle and lower burners.
	Yi Yi Ren	Semen Coicis Lachryma-Jobi	30	Eliminates the damp-fluid and promotes diuresis.
	Hua Shi	Talcum	15	Eliminates the damp-fluid and promotes diuresis.
	Ze Xie	Rhizoma Alismatis Orientalis	10	Eliminates the damp-fluid and promotes diuresis.
	Chai Hu	Radix Bupleuri	10	Dredges the stagnated qi and relaxes the qi flowing through the body.
	Dang Gui	Radix Angelicae Sinensis	10	Softens the liver and nourishes the liver blood.
Guiding herb	Gan Cao	Radix Glycyrrhizae Uralensis	5	Harmonises the stomach and promotes cohesiveness of herbs.
	Chuan Niu Xi	Radix Cyathulae Officinalis	15	Leads all herbs down to the lower burner and activates the blood stasis.

Method: The above-mentioned herbal prescription is the main formula and can be used in combination with a variation of decoctions according to specific individual symptoms where the herbs are boiled and the concentrated herbal powders are taken with warm water twice daily.

External herbal prescription:

- Qing Dai (Indigo Pulverata Levis) 10 g
- Bing Pian (Borneolum) 10 g
- Ming Fan (Alumen) 10 g

Method: The above-mentioned herbal powders are mixed with warm water and applied on the location of the blisters to dry the blister quickly and ease the pain.

Analysis: Huang Bai and Cang Zhu as the main herbs eliminate excessive *Damp* and *Heat* at the lower burner. Chuan Niu Xi leads all the herbal to affect the lower body and activates blood to ease abdominal pain. Yi Yi Ren dissipates excessive *Damp.* Long Dan Cao is added to support and cleanse *Heat.* Hua Shi and Ze Xie are added to promote *Damp* elimination. Chai Hu dredges and agitates *Qi* movement. Dangui softens the *Liver* and *Kidney.* Gan Cao harmonises all the herbs and prevents the cool nature of the herbs from harming the *Stomach.*

Advice: This pattern can be seen the most in dermatological disorders when blisters manifest as the main signs, such as various kinds of herpes simplex and herpes zoster. When these blisters occur in relation to coronavirus, they are affected as damp-heat as per TCM, so external and internal herbal treatment should be supplied.

Excessive Damp accumulation with Spleen Deficiency

Clinical features and signs: Signs are blisters occurring at the truck, limbs, toes, or fingers. Signs in women are increased discharge from the vagina; signs in men are blisters on the top of penis in men and abdominal distension. Other general signs are loose bowel with greasy stools, lethargy, tiredness, heaviness in general, a light red or pale and plump tongue with teeth marks and white-greasy coating, and a rolling-weak pulse.

Treatment principle in TCM: Dissipate excessive Damp; reinforce Spleen.

Treatment: Herbal prescription.

Pinyin: Chu Shi Wei Ling Tang variated with Wu Ling San.

English name for decoction: Eliminate *Dampness* Decoction by combining Calm the *Stomach* Powder variated with Five Ingredient Powder with Poria.

Role in formula	Name/ Pinyin	Name/Latin	Dose (g)	Function
Chief herb	Cang Zhu	Rhizoma Atractylodis	10	Dries the dampness and dredges the accumulated qi in the middle burner.
Deputy herb	Hou Po	Cortex Magnoliae Officinalis	10	Dries the dampness and dredges the accumulated qi in the middle burner.
Assistant herb	Chen Pi	Pericarpium Citri Reticulatae	10	Dries the dampness and replenishes the spleen.
	Bai Zhu	Rhizoma Atractylodis Macrocephalae	10–30	Dries the dampness and replenishes the spleen.
	Ze Xie	Rhizoma Alismatis Orientalis	10	Eliminates the excessive dampness and promotes diuresis.
	Fu Ling	Sclerotium Poriae Cocos	10	Eliminates the excessive dampness and replenishes the spleen.
	Zhu Ling	Sclerotium Polypori Umbellati	10	Eliminates the excessive dampness and promotes diuresis.
	Rou Gui	Cortex Cinnamomi Cassiae	2–5	Agitates the yang qi and dredges the stagnated qi.
	Hua Shi	Talcum	10–15	Dissipates the excessive dampness.
Guiding herb	Gan Cao	Radix Glycyrrhizae Uralensis	5	Harmonises the stomach and promotes cohesiveness of herbs.

Method: The above-mentioned herbal prescription is the main formula and can be used in combination with a variation of decoctions according to specific individual symptoms where the herbs are boiled the concentrated herbal powders are taken with warm water twice daily.

Analysis: Cang Zhu, Hou Po, and Chen Pi as the Ping Wei San formula dry Damp and dredge accumulated Qi in the middle burner. Bai Zhu, Ze Xie, Hua Shi, Fu Ling, and Zhu Ling as the Wu Ling San formula dry and dredge accumulated qi in the lower burner. Rou Gui excites Yang Qi and dredges general stagnated Qi. Gan Cao harmonises all the herbs and calms down the Stomach. All these herbs work together to potently eliminate accumulated Dampness.

Advice: This pattern can be commonly seen in patients with an extended time of disease, whose blisters are triggered or recur as a chronic state of the post-COVID-19 syndrome. The patient suffers from *Dampness* with *Spleen Deficiency*, with minimal *Heat* presenting.

Acupuncture

Body acupuncture:
Main points: Qihai (REN6), Guanyuan (REN4), Guilai (ST28).

Assistant points:

- For damp-heat: Quchi (LI11), Hegu (LI4), Xuehai (SP10), Sanyinjiao (SP6).
- For damp with spleen deficiency: Taodao (DU13), Feishu (BL13), Geshu (BL17), Pishu (BL20), Taibai (SP3), Shenmen (HE7).

Auricular acupuncture: Lung, Shenmen, Shenshangxian (adrenal point).

Analysis: Qihai and Guanyuan as the main points in the conception vessel nourish yin and agitate general vitality qi. Guilai accompanied by Quchi and Sanyinjiao eliminated dampness. Hegu cleanses heat. Taodao cleanses the external wind-heat to eliminate external pathogenic factors. Feishu and Pishu dredge the water passage to dissipate dampness. Geshu releases accumulated qi and damp. Shenmen is the main point to clear skin blisters.

Case Study

Ms. S. Scrostocial, a 59-year-old retired actress, had recurrent herpes of the vagina for over a half a year after healing from a COVID-19 infection. She was infected with coronavirus while travelling in Europe. Her infection was not severe, with only mild fever of 37.6°C accompanied by tiredness and cough. After 1 week of illness, she healed, although she felt discomfort outside her vagina, with increased discharge, herpes/blisters, mild lower abdominal aching which was worse at times and less sometimes. She sought TCM treatment because the outer side of her vagina was not completely clear.

Clinical symptoms and signs: Herpes occurred severely for 2 weeks with itching, sores, no increased vaginal discharge, a dull sensation of smell and taste, loose bowels 2–3 times daily, poor appetite, tiredness, dry mouth in the night, and a red tongue with greasy-white coating.

Diagnosis:

1. Post-COVID-19 syndrome.
2. Herpes simplex.

Differentiation syndromes of TCM:

1. *Damp-Heat* accumulation at middle and *Lower Burner*.
2. *Spleen* and *Kidney Deficiency*.

Treatment: Herbal prescription and acupuncture.

Acupuncture

Main points: Qihai (REN6), Guanyuan (REN4), Guilai (ST28); Xuehai (SP10), Yinlingquan (SP9), Sanyinjiao (SP6); Taixi (KI), Zhaohai (KI6), Waiguan (SJ5), Zulinqi (GB41).

Herbal prescription

Pinyin: Herbal pills: Long Dan Xie Gan Wan; Shen Ling Bai Zhu Wan.

Herbal washing liquid made with six herbs is given for daily washing of the outside of the vagina.

Result: The blisters outside the vagina are completely controlled for the patient in a month. She continued taking these herbs for another 3 months to prevent blister recurrence.

References

Gisondi, P., Plaseribo, S., Bordin, C., *et al.* (2020). Cutaneous manifestations of SARS-CoV-2 infection: A clinical update. *The Journal of Association Physicians India*, 34(11), 2499–2504. https://doi.org/10.1111/jdv.16774.

Gokhale, Y., Patankar, A., Holla, U., Shilke, M., Kalekar, L., *et al.* (2020). Dermatomyositis during COVID-19 pandemic (a case series): Is there a cause effect relationship? *Journal of Association of Physicians India*, 68(11), 20–24.

Gül, Ü. (2020). COVID-19 and dermatology. *Turkish Journal of Medical Science*, 50(8), 1751–1759. https://doi.org/10.3906/sag-2005-182.

Sanghvi, A. R. (2020). COVID-19: An overview for dermatologists. *International Journal of Dermatology*, 59, 1437–1449. https://doi.org/10.1111/ijd.15257.

Silva Andrade, B., Siqueira, S., de Assis Soares, W. R., de Souza Rangel, F., Santos, N. O., *et al.* (2021). Long-COVID and post-COVID health complications: An up-to-date review on clinical conditions and their possible molecular mechanisms. *Viruses*, 13(4), 700. https://doi.org/10.3390/v13040700.

Zoe-COVID-Study. (2020). Skin rash should be considered as a fourth key sign of COVID-19. Zoe-COVID Study. Available at: https://covid.joinzoe.com/post/skin-rash-covid#:~:text=Researchers%20discovered%20that%208.8%25%20of,with%20a%20negative%20test%20result. (Accessed 5 March 2022).

Appendices

Appendix 1. Instructions on Preparing and Administrating Chinese Herbal Prescriptions

Given to patients to make the decoction and drink the herbal tea.

Tonifying herbal prescription — Instructions for cooking the herbs and administration

- This cooking method is commonly used for herbs to tonify the *Qi*, blood, *Yin*, and yang.
- All herbs are dispensed in packages containing all prescribed ingredients. The practitioner should include only the appropriate amount of each herb to suit the patient's prescription.
- One package is prescribed for the use of 1/2/3 days of administration of oral intake.
- Please empty the herbal package into a deep saucepan. Wash with water and drain the water away. Then, add 0.5/0.75/1 l of water, soaking the contents for 30/60/120 min.
- For the best clinical effect, 3/6/9 slices of ginger and 3 white stems of spring onions should be chopped and added to the saucepan before the boiling.
- Then, place the saucepan on the medium flame and heat it to boiling point. Then, simmer for 45/60/120 min. In between, stir the contents of the saucepan to make sure the herbs do not stick at the bottom.
- Then, turn the fire off, leaving the pan to cool down naturally till it is warm.

- Using a kitchen filter, drain the cooked herbal liquid (decoction now) into a mug.
- The remaining herbs should be cooked again with 0.5/1 l of water, repeating the same procedure to get the second mug of herbal decoction.
- Then, one can throw the cooked herbs into a green garden waste bin (as they are plants).
- Mix the first mug and second mug, then separate into 2/4/6 equal portions.
- Consume one portion at the nearest time (mostly in the evening) and drink it warm.
- The remaining portions are kept in a glass bottle in the fridge. Take the 2nd/3rd/4th/5th/6th dosage out of the fridge, heat it till lukewarm, and then drink it, at the set times of taking the herbs.
- The herbal tea (herbal decoction or herbal drink) should be orally ingested 2/3 times a day.
- When the herbal decoction is finished, open another package and repeat the same cooking procedure, and drink herbal tea of the same amount at the same time.

Reducing herbal prescription — Instructions for cooking the herbs and administration

- This method is applied for the herbs that clear heat/dampness or damp-heat/phlegm/wind/cold.
- All herbs are dispensed in packages containing all prescribed ingredients.
- One package is prescribed for the use of 1 day's dosage of oral intake.
- Please empty the herbal package into a deep saucepan. Wash the contents with water and drain the water away. Then, add 0.75/1 l of water, soaking the contents for 30 min.
- For the best clinical effect, three slices of ginger and two white stems of spring onions should be chopped and added into the saucepan before boiling.
- Then, place the saucepan on a medium flame and heat it to boiling point. Then, simmer for 30 min. In between, stir the contents to make sure the herbs do not stick at the bottom.
- Then turn the fire off, leaving the pan to cool down naturally till warm.
- Using a kitchen filter, drain the cooked herbal liquid (decoction now) into 1 mug.

- Then, throw the cooked herbs into a green garden waste bin (as they are plants).
- Mix the first mug and second mug, then separate into two equal portions.
- Take one portion at the nearest time (mostly in the evening) and drink it warm.
- The rest is kept in a glass bottle in the fridge. Take the 2nd dosage out of the fridge, heat it till lukewarm, and then drink it at the set time of the dosage.
- When the herbal decoction is finished, open another package, repeat the same cooking procedure, and drink herbal tea of the same amount at the same time.

Regulating herbal prescription

- The regulating/balancing herbs are mostly for moving *Qi* and blood and are mixed herbs of warm/cool nature. So, the instructions might be the same as that given above.
- When soaking, traditionally, rice wine/vinegar is added for promotion of *Qi* and blood flow. In current practice, red wine or white wine can be used for the same purpose.
- Many of the herbs contain volatile oils which will dissipate into the air when heated. To preserve them, please use a lid to cover the saucepan and limit the cooking time accordingly.

Appendix 2. Concentrated Herbal Powder Guidelines for Practitioners

Concentrated powders have become popular in modern times among both patients and practitioners, due to their stable quality, convenience in carrying, and avoiding the lengthy time and effort required for cooking. Clinical research has supported the use of such powders.

The powders are the products of individually processed raw herbs. Water boiling, oily distiller, and/or other extracting methods are used to get the active ingredients out of the raw herbs into blended crystals and dry oil. Then they are grinded into fine powder mixture. By using the modern extracting methods, the active ingredients of the herbs which bear the functional effects of the herbs are taken out from the raw plants. The fibres and plant structures are not considered to be the active ingredients and therefore are not needed. Processed in abovementioned methods, the concentrated powders hold the original therapeutic effects of the raw herbs, but are reduced to 10–30% of the weight of raw herbs. For example, 100 g of raw Ginseng is reduced to 30 g concentrated powder, but the 30 g of Ginseng concentrate powder will deliver the same treatment potency that 100 g of raw ginseng can achieve.

Before ordering the concentrated powder, please ask the suppliers to clarify the concentration ratio.

When prescribing herbal powder, please divide the normal dosage according to the ratio, and then calculate the dosage of the powder.

An alternative way of prescribing the herbal powder is to prescribe the dosage for 1 week or 1 month.

When prescribing concentrated herbal powder for 1 week, if all the herbal ingredients added up to 60 g a day and the concentration ratio of powder to raw herbs is 1:5, then 12 g of powder is equivalent to the 60 g of raw herbs. The patient is told to take 6 g in the morning and 6 g in the evening for the 12 g of herbal powder if twice a day is the ideal way of separating the herbs into separate dosages.

On a weekly prescription, 12 * 7 = 72 g. This could be dispensed to the patient in a plastic bottle or a resealable plastic bag.

A common method to measure the weight of herbal powders is that 1 flat full teaspoon of powder equals 2 g. Then, 6 g measures to 3 teaspoons.

Appendix 3. The Instructions for Patients Taking Concentrated Powders

72 g/actual dispensed herbal powder amount of herbal powder is prescribed to … for a week's dosage.

You are advised to take the powder twice a day. 6 g (3 tea spoons) in the morning and 6 g in the evening.

The powder is mixed into ¼ mug of warm water. After blending well, drink the whole mixture.

Please reseal the bag/tighten up the cap of the bottle, and keep it in cool dry place, away from children. The fridge is the best place to store it.

Appendix 4. Understanding the Patient Reaction to Herbs and Managing the Bad Response

Generally, Chinese herbs are very safe, particularly in European countries, thanks to the strict regulations restricting most potentially toxic herbs. Liver and kidney impairments were reported many years ago, but they have not been a concern in the last 10 years. However, some minor side effects are still possible in some patients.

Stomach irritation/heart burn/nausea. This is mainly a direct physical and chemical irritation in the stomach. When this happens, suggest the patients take the herbs half an hour to one hour after food. Most of them will find that the reaction is no longer a concern.

Constipation, dry mouth. When the body's dynamic balance is changed, and body fluid is redistributed, some parts of the body could become dehydrated/dry. Increased water intake would be suggested.

Hot sensation, palpitation. Many herbs are hot natured and can increase the heat in the body. So, this might be the expected effect if the patient is suffering from cold syndrome. If the patient is very weak, palpitation suggests that the dosage is a bit too strong. Then, reducing the dosage is recommended.

Light-headed sensation. When stress and pressure are well managed, the blood pressure might reduce. This is mostly the expected effect. However, even for patients of hypertension, the lowering of blood pressure is more likely to cause a weak or light-headed sensation. The body needs a few days to adjust to this newly achieved level of blood pressure.

Skin rashes and breathlessness. These are most likely due to allergy to some ingredients in the herbal medicine. Whole plants are collected of some herbs, and therefore, some herbal seeds might be presented in the mixture, although the seed is not mentioned. If this happen, stop the herbs immediately.

Appendix 5. Concerns About Potential Interactions Between Prescribed Medications/Drugs and Herbal Medicine

Many patients and practitioners worry about the potential interaction between drugs and herbs, and therefore are reluctant to take TCM herbs or Chinese herbal medicine (CHM). Medical professionals are also aware of such concerns. When a patient asks their doctors, most of them advice to "not use herbs when taking medication".

The issue is to avoid any interaction between drugs and biomedicine, and not that there is anything wrong with herbs. Actually, according to a survey by Charlesworth *et al.* (2015), the average use of prescription drugs among patients over 65 was 4 in the USA, up from 2 in 2000, and they are for different treatment purposes. This trend is continuing and according to AgedUK (Petchey & Gentry, 2019), in their report "More harm than Good", more than 2 million patients over 65 were prescribed more than seven drugs to be used at the same time, and if we take the number of patients taking five drugs, the number is 4 million patients. This is a world-wide trend due to the multiple illnesses and the medical model of reductionism which break down all illnesses into different categories and every medical practitioner only looks at her/his own speciality, and prescribes drug for that condition only. The phenomenon is called polypharmacy and has long been a source of concern among patients' groups. The main concern is the overload of drugs that might cause heavy damage to important organs such as the liver and kidney, unexpected/unknown side effects due to the combination of so many drugs, and the burden of taking so many drugs in a strict timetable (Petchey & Gentry, 2019).

The above mentioned polypharmacy is a problem in biomedicine itself, and no research has been done on the combination of any three drugs in clinical practice yet, and it is impossible to do that simply because the possible combinations in reality are too numerous and it is impossible to investigate those combinations of solutions. In this way, it is not possible to then investigate the possible interactions in detail. All available knowledge is from clinical case reports of potential interactions of herb and drug combinations.

Generally speaking, there are three points to note on this issue: First, some herbs might reduce the effect of prescribed drugs by increasing the rate of detoxification in the liver. Second, some herbs could increase the clinical effect of some drugs; for example, when some herbs are used together with blood thinning drugs, the total effect could be more than expected and bleeding could happen. Third, most herbs become inactive because of the chemical reaction between them and other drugs.

From clinical observations, we do not ask the patients to change their medication/drug regime, and when taking CHM remedy, we suggest that the patients take the herbs well after the medicine, for example, 1 h after their medicine. This makes sure some important drugs will not be affected and will minimise the possibility of chemical interaction between them. The prescription of CHM is also closely monitored on weekly returning visits. So, if there is any side effect, even from the CHM, it could be reduced or better managed.

In the management of PCS, CHM is considered to be an essential part, so practitioners should fully explain the safety of herbs when they are prescribed, if the patients are already on medicines due to existing diseases.

It is also important to inform the patients that our herbal prescription is dynamic and adjusted weekly or every 2 weeks. That is totally different from the prescribed drugs which could be used for the rest of one's life. Therefore, the accumulated side effect or interaction is minimum.

Appendix 6. The Acupuncture Treatment Aftercare Information

When patients with PCS receive acupuncture treatment, the common advice of aftercare still applies. However, due to the clinical characteristics of the broad profile of patients, the following information should be given to the patients:

a. Patients might experience more exhaustion after acupuncture treatment. This is because they are in deficiency, and the needling has moved *Qi* and blood around. However, most patients would report that the exhaustion is followed by good recovery. It is not suggested to change the treatment plan.
b. Patients are advised to not drive immediately after acupuncture. A 10-min break is suggested. The reason is that brain fog or cognitive impairment might already happen to patients. With acupuncture and a long break, some patients might not feel alert enough to concentrate on the task or have problems of orientation.
c. Patients should not expose themselves to coldness/cold environment/cold water directly immediately afterwards. The immune function/resistance to infection is lowered among PCS patients. When relaxed after acupuncture, the defence system is not tuned to a high level, and exposure to coldness could easily invite pathogenic factors to cause new trouble.
d. Do not drink alcohol at all, or reduce the amount of alcohol intake by half. The reason is that acupuncture changes personal experience

based on alcohol intake. It has been observed that when alcohol was taken in the evening of acupuncture treatment, the patients found that their reaction to alcohol is different, and they might be unaware of being over their usual limit, leading to an overdose of it.

e. Do not leave the window open when sleeping even if this was part of their usual sleep environment. The reason is that acupuncture can make the patient very relaxed and not react to the coldness after mid-night. When not protected, the coldness could take hold and lead to stiff neck or similar problem, or blocked nose and headache the next day. In Chinese medicine, the usual level of external pathogenic factor cannot cause trouble when our defensive *Qi* is on guard; however, it could find a chance to invade the body when a relaxed body is not protected.
f. Patients are advised not to bathe after acupuncture on the same day. There are two reasons. One is that the puncture hole is dry when coming home, but not sealed with a mini scar yet. This could open it and lead to an increased chance of skin irritation and possible infection. The second is that most patients will feel very relaxed, and a double relaxation could lead to over-dispatch of *Qi* and the patient might feel very exhausted the next day.
g. A light meal is more suitable in the evening. The reason is that the *Qi* and blood need time to continue reacting to the acupuncture treatment. This might continue for 24 h or longer even if the patient is not feeling any particular change. It takes place inside. If a heavy meal is ingested, the *Qi* and blood are forced into the digestive system, which might not favour the treatment.

References

Charlesworth, C. J., Smit, E., Lee, D. S., Alramadhan, F., and Odden, M. C. (2015). Polypharmacy among adults aged 65 years and older in the United States: 1988–2010. *The Journals of Gerontology. Series A, Biological Sciences and Medical Sciences*, 70(8), 989–995. https://doi.org/10.1093/gerona/glv013.

Petchey, L. and Gentry, T. (2019). More harm than good — Why more isn't always better with older people's medicines. AgeUK. Available at: https://www.ageuk.org.uk/globalassets/age-uk/documents/reports-and-publications/reports-and-briefings/health--wellbeing/medication/age-uk_more_harm_than_good.pdf. (Accessed 8 March 2022).

Index

M

Q

CPSIA information can be obtained
at www.ICGtesting.com
Printed in the USA
JSHW010020040723
43825JS00001B/99

9 781800 613485